GASTRIC CANCER: DIAGNOSIS, EARLY PREVENTION, AND TREATMENT

CANCER ETIOLOGY, DIAGNOSIS AND TREATMENTS

CANCER ETIOLOGY, DIAGNOSIS AND TREATMENTS

GASTRIC CANCER: DIAGNOSIS, EARLY PREVENTION, AND TREATMENT

VICTOR D. PASECHNIKOV
EDITOR

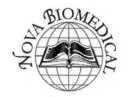

Nova Science Publishers, Inc.
New York

For permission to use material from this book please contact us:
Telephone 631-231-7269; Fax 631-231-8175
Web Site: http://www.novapublishers.com

NOTICE TO THE READER

The Publisher has taken reasonable care in the preparation of this book, but makes no expressed or implied warranty of any kind and assumes no responsibility for any errors or omissions. No liability is assumed for incidental or consequential damages in connection with or arising out of information contained in this book. The Publisher shall not be liable for any special, consequential, or exemplary damages resulting, in whole or in part, from the readers' use of, or reliance upon, this material. Any parts of this book based on government reports are so indicated and copyright is claimed for those parts to the extent applicable to compilations of such works.

Independent verification should be sought for any data, advice or recommendations contained in this book. In addition, no responsibility is assumed by the publisher for any injury and/or damage to persons or property arising from any methods, products, instructions, ideas or otherwise contained in this publication.

This publication is designed to provide accurate and authoritative information with regard to the subject matter covered herein. It is sold with the clear understanding that the Publisher is not engaged in rendering legal or any other professional services. If legal or any other expert assistance is required, the services of a competent person should be sought. FROM A DECLARATION OF PARTICIPANTS JOINTLY ADOPTED BY A COMMITTEE OF THE AMERICAN BAR ASSOCIATION AND A COMMITTEE OF PUBLISHERS.

Additional color graphics may be available in the e-book version of this book.

LIBRARY OF CONGRESS CATALOGING-IN-PUBLICATION DATA

Gastric cancer : diagnosis, early prevention, and treatment / [edited by]
Victor D. Pasechnikov.
  p. ; cm.
 Includes bibliographical references and index.
 ISBN 978-1-61668-313-9 (hardcover)
 1. Stomach--Cancer. I. Pasechnikov, Victor D.
 [DNLM: 1. Stomach Neoplasms--diagnosis. 2. Stomach Neoplasms--surgery.
 3. Early Diagnosis. 4. Gastroscopy--methods. WI 320 G2557 2010]
 RC280.S8.G3765 2010
 616.99'433--dc22
                              2010013748

Published by Nova Science Publishers, Inc. ✦ New York

CONTENTS

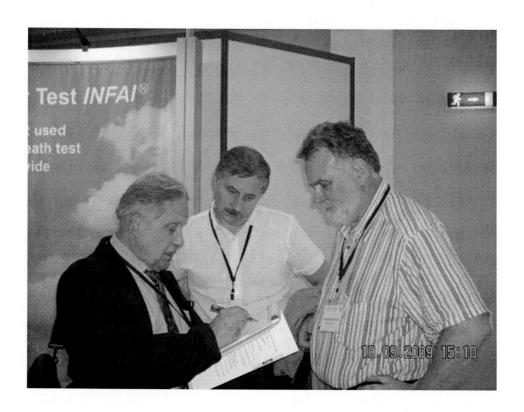

PREFACE

Gastric cancer is a disease often incurable at its first detection, because the diagnosis is made at the advanced stage of tumor. The explanation of such a late diagnosis is that the majority of so-called gastric precancerous conditions, mainly, chronic atrophic gastritis, are asymptomatic. When symptoms are present, they may not be specific enough to diagnose certain disease. In general, there is a common syndrome called dyspepsia. Many strategies have been proposed for the management of out-patients with dyspeptic symptoms, considering H.pylori status and the patient's characteristics (e.g. age, alarm symptoms, assumption of gastric injuring drugs). Some recommendations on this topic were made during a Consensus Conference of gastroenterologists, held in Maastricht in 2000. In spite of the apparent usefulness of this chart, it is not always appropriate in every patient.

To date, we have an excellent example of secondary preventative measures, such as mass screening programs (including radio-graphic and endoscopic examination) for those above 40 years old, which have been extensively implemented in Japan to reduce gastric cancer mortality. Almost half of the gastric cancer patients in Japan are now diagnosed as early gastric cancer and many of them can be treated with minimally invasive measures such as endoscopic mucosal resection. Even when they require operation and/or chemotherapy their survival rates are much better than those of Western countries. However, for more effective disease prevention, primary prevention by interfering with the mechanisms of gastric carcinogenesis is necessary. Eradication of H.pylori seems to be the true primary preventative measure. Epidemiological evidence indicates that the proportion of all gastric cancers attributable to H.pylori infection and hence potentially preventable upon elimination of this risk factor is somewhere in the range of 60-90%. This portends significant benefit in terms of morbidity and mortality, not least in populations with high prevalence of H.pylori infection coupled with high incidence of gastric cancer. While there is some discordance regarding who should undergo a search and treat strategy with the current available therapy, there is broad agreement that cure of the infection reduces the risk for gastric cancer development.

Earlier the only means of diagnosing atrophic gastritis has been gastroscopy and the histological examination of endoscopic biopsy specimens. Until now, diagnosing the diseases of the stomach mucosa has only been possible through H.pylori tests and trial medication (the "test-and-treat" strategy) and limited endoscopic resources. However, the diagnosis of H.pylori infection and its treatment alone (i.e., the "test-and-treat" strategy) is not a safe and ethical treatment without the diagnosis of dyspepsia, atrophic gastritis, and related risks (e.g., metaplasia, intraepithelial neoplasia, gastric cancer). This serious medical problem should be solved by elaborating the reliable diagnostic and screening tests for gastric precancerous conditions and early gastric cancer.

The subject of the present book is early diagnosis of the morphological changes in gastric mucosa that are believed to be precursors of gastric cancer development, and also, the use of modern imaging techniques for revealing and treatment of early gastric cancer. Besides, the book includes some ideas about staging the gastric precancerous lesions with estimating risk of gastric cancer development.

The purpose of this book is to review the modern data on gastric cancer prevention by means of screening gastric precancerous conditions and changes, and also, estimating the risk of gastric cancer development in individual patient with subsequent proper management for reducing the possibility of neoplastic progression.

The book is divided into eight chapters.

Chapter I – "Gastric Cancer Epidemiology" – describes gastric cancer epidemiology: its world-wide prevalence, incidence and mortality rates; the role of environmental, age-, sex-, socioeconomics- adjusted factors; individual risk of cancer.

Chapter II – "Gastric Cancer Etiology and Pathogenesis" – is dedicated to gastric cancer etiology and includes the data on recent advances in molecular carcinogenesis in gastric carcinoma. It describes genetic predisposition to gastric cancer; familial gastric cancer; the role of H.pylori infection; the data concerning Epstein–Barr virus – associated gastric carcinoma. Also, the Chapter contains the data about the pathogenetic role of chronic inflammation and of the precancerous changes of stomach mucosa – atrophy, metaplasia, dysplasia (intraepithelial neoplsia) – in the gastric carcinoma development. There are also modern data concerning recent advances in molecular carcinogenesis in gastric carcinoma and precancerous conditions.

Chapter III – "Pathology of Gastric Cancer, Precancerous Conditions and Precancerous Mucosal Lesions" – includes information about morphology of gastric cancer, precancerous conditions and precancerous mucosal lesions. It provides basic information on the natural history of both precancerous and cancerous lesions, and their clinical context, and on the diagnostic issues and prognostic implications providing the biological rationale for their follow-up and treatment.

Chapter IV – "Strategies for Screening and Early Detection of Gastric Cancer" – includes the description of known screening methods: their sensitivity, specificity, predictive value, cost-effectiveness, acceptability to patients and health-care providers.

Chapter V – "Primary and Secondary Prevention of Gastric Cancer and Early Gastric Cancer Recurrence After Endoscopic RemovaL" – elucidates the modern sight on the problem of the prevention of gastric cancer develoment and evasion of early gastric cancer recurrence after endoscopic removal. It includes data on international consensuses concerning H.pylori eradication therapy, and additional methods of the prevention of the precancerous changes of stomach mucosa (antisecretory and antioxidant therapy, dietary improvement, etc.).

Chapter VI – "Endoscopic Diagnosis of Early Gastric Cancer and Gastric Precancerous Lesions" – contains data about imaging techniques in diagnosis of gastric cancer, and ideas about gastric cancer staging based on imaging techniques data. The Chapter describes the current data on routine and novel technologies in gastric cancer imaging.

Chapter VII – "Endoscopic Treatment For Early Gastric Cancer" – describes the methods of endoscopic treatment for early gastric cancer, with the special emphasis on the methods of endoscopic resection: strip biopsy, endoscopic mucosal resection (EMR), and endoscopic submucosal dissection (ESD).

Chapter VIII – "Surgical Treatment Of Early Gastric Cancer" – contains review on surgical approaches for gastric cancer, short- and long-term results after surgery for EGC; assessment of quality of life according to type of reconstruction after gastrectomy; describes minimally invasive approach to EGC treatment.

The authors hope that the book will be useful for scientists and practical gastroenterologists, endoscopists, pathologists, general practitioners, etc., in areas of gastric cancer screening and prevention, estimating the risk of gastric cancer development, and treatment of early gastric cancer.

In: Gastric Cancer: Diagnosis, Early Prevention, and Treatment   ISBN 978-1-61668-313-9
Editor: V. D. Pasechnikov, pp. 1-42   © 2010 Nova Science Publishers, Inc.

Chapter I

GASTRIC CANCER EPIDEMIOLOGY: THE GLOBAL BURDEN OF THE DISEASE

M. Leja

University of Latvia, Latvia, Riga, Latvia

ABSTRACT

Gastric cancer is still remaining a significant health issue globally, and during the coming decades it is still going to remain such. The incidence and mortality of this cancer have declined significantly in age-standardized rates. Still due to the aging population, in absolute figures the number of new cases *per anum* is still growing.

This chapter is addressing the descriptive epidemiology issues of gastric cancer worldwide as well as the trends for incidence and mortality. Intestinal and diffuse type cancers as well as cancers located distally and those at esophago-gastric junction are discussed. The factors responsible for gastric cancer are analyzed; the role of *H.pylori*, pre-malignant lesions, lifestyle, socio-economic and occupational factors is discussed.

INTRODUCTION

Even though globally the gastric cancer incidence is declining and in many Western countries the disease is not considered among the major health issues any more, globally the cancer of the stomach is still continuing to be an important healthcare problem. Gastric cancer is remaining the second leading cause of mortality worldwide within the group of malignant diseases after the lung cancer, and is accounting for almost 10% of cancer related deaths or 866 000 annual deaths in absolute figures as for 2007. Among men gastric cancer is the second (after lung cancer), but among women – the third leading (after breast and lung) cause of cancer-related deaths [1].

Today gastric cancer is the fourth leading cancer type in incidence (after the lung, breast and colorectal cancers), accounting for 8.6% of all the cancers. Close to a million new gastric cancer cases are diagnosed annually (934 000 cases as reported by the International Agency for the Research on Cancer (IARC) in 2002) [2,3].

Substantial differences are observed between developed and developing countries - altogether 65-70% of the cancer cases are arising in less developed countries [2,3].

CLASSIFICATIONS AND SUBTYPES

Considering the linkage between the subtypes of the cancer and the trends in epidemiology, we will initially briefly look into the classifications used for subtyping tumors of the stomach.

The major part of gastric cancers is adenocarcinomas (90-95%), remaining being lymphomas, carcinoids and leiomiosarcomas. Further on we are going to concentrate exclusively on the adenocarcinomas of the stomach.

The *WHO classification* distinguishes tubular, papillary, mucinous adenocarcinomas, and signet-ring cell carcinoma [4]. Grading into well-differentiated, moderately-differentiated and poorly differentiated adenocarcinoma applies primarily to tubular carcinomas; other types of carcinoma are not graded [4].

Traditionally used *Lauren classification* proposed back in 1965 [5] distinguishing intestinal (glandular epithelium composed of absorptive cells and goblet cells) and diffuse type (poorly differentiated small cells in a dissociated noncohesive growth pattern) gastric adenocarcinomas. Tumors containing approximately equal quantities of intestinal and diffuse components are classified as mixed carcinomas, but those that are too undifferentiated to fit into either category are considered indeterminate. Lauren classification is still in use either for clinical or epidemiological purposes due to differences in patient populations, results of the management and outcome; additionally to morphological also biological differences between these cancer types are considered responsible for the above [6].

Intestinal type cancers are differentiated or moderately differentiated, sometimes with poorly differentiated tumor at the advancing margin, while diffuse type cancers consist of poorly cohesive cells diffusely infiltrating the gastric wall with little or no gland formation; diffuse type tumors resemble signet-ring cell cancers in the WHO classification [4].

The recent validation study for a epidemiological gastric and esophageal cancer (EPIC) [7] has confirmed that the original Lauren's classification is still useful for the reflection of close association between the epidemiology and histopathology.

T.Hattori [8] has been adding "gastric type" cancers to the initial sub-types of the Lauren classification; these cancers are originating primarily from gastric mucin-producing cells and only in more advanced stages; they can be secondarily converting to mixed gastric and intestinal differentiated or purely intestinal differentiated carcinomas [9]. Since the proportion of primary gastric-type carcinomas among early gastric cancers is reported to be 40-50%, the importance of the original Lauren's classification may be challenged [10].

There are *rare variants* of carcinomas not included to either the WHO or Lauren's classifications. These are adenosquamous carcinoma, squamous cell carcinoma and undifferentiated carcinoma [4]. Also endocrine tumors, including carcinoid and small cell carcinoma as well as mesenchymal tumors (mostly gastrointestinal stromal tumors - GIST or smooth muscle type tumors) and metastasis from tumors outside the stomach could be found in this organ.

The *Carneiro classification* [11] distinguishing glandular, isolated-cell type, mixed and solid type adenocarcinomas of the stomach is much less frequently used. The EPIC/EUR-GAST validation study reported good correlation between the cancer histotypes this and the original Lauren's classifications, in particular between intestinal and glandular as well as diffuse and isolated type carcinomas [7].

The first *Japanese classification* dates back to year 1963, and until so far there are at least 13 editions of the classification have been issued by the Japanese Research Society for Gastric Cancer (JRSGC) [12]. This classification is more detailed and incorporating clinical and surgical as well as pathological and final findings. This should be mentioned that category 4 and 5 epithelial neoplasia according to the Vienna classification [13] are classified adenocarcinomas according to the Japanese classification.

Early gastric cancer is a carcinoma limited to the mucosa or mucosa and submucosa of the stomach, regardless of the nodal status [4].

According to the localization the tumors are subtyped into the carcinoma of esophagogastric junction, proximal and distal stomach. The WHO classification [4] defines that an adenocarcinoma crossing esophagogastric junction regardless of where the bulk of the tumor lies is classified as adenocarcinoma of esophagogastric junction, while adenocarcinoma located entirely above the junction is considered esophageal adenocarcinoma, but the one entirely below the junction – adenocarcinoma of gastric origin. This should be mentioned than until so far the terms of "cardia" and "non-cardia" adenocarcinomas have been widely used (correspondingly being reflected in this chapter), although these terms may be misleading and their use is discouraged by the WHO classification.

There are previous classifications defining adenocarcinoma of cardia somewhat different, e.g. as a lesion with its center located within 1 cm proximal and 2 cm distal of esophagogastric junction [14]. Therefore different definitions and interpretations may result in diverse statistics and interpretations.

THE GLOBAL INCIDENCE OF THE DISEASE

Significant geographical differences are observed in gastric cancer incidence and mortality worldwide (See table 1), the high-incidence areas (ASR in male > 20 per 100 000 world standardized population) being Eastern Asia (China, Japan, Korea), Eastern Europe (Belarus, the Baltic States, Ukraine, Russia) and parts of Central and South America (including Chile, Ecuador, Costa Rica). Low gastric cancer incidence areas (ASR in male < 10 per 100 000 world standardized population) are Southern and Eastern Asia (Bangladesh, Indonesia, Thailand), North and East Africa, North America and Oceania. Moreover there might be substantial incidence and mortality differences within one geographical area, e.g. within Asia, Eastern Europe, and Africa [2].

Globally the standardized incidence (ASR world population) is 22 per 100 000 in males and 10.3 in females [2]. The cancer incidence figures in general are not substantially differing between more and less developed areas (in males: 22.3 in more developed areas vs. 21.5 in less developed; in female: 10.0 vs. 10.4 correspondingly) due to the geographical differences; yet the corresponding mortality is worse in less developed countries (See table 1). With the exception of North America the mortality versus incidence ratio is not below 70% in the less developed areas reaching and exceeding 80% (the data from Japan are included to the Asian data-set, country specific data are not considered in the table below).

Since the incidence is higher in males, few further comparisons between geographical areas will be conducted in males.

Chart 1 is demonstrating the highest gastric cancer incidence areas globally (ASR 100 000 world male population) with the incidence above 35 per 100 000 world standard population.

Considering the above mentioned differences several areas deserve interest to look into the epidemiology of the cancer in more detail.

Table 1. Gastric cancer regional incidence, mortality (ASR per 100 000 world population) and the mortality / incidence ratio (source: *GLOBOCAN 2002*)

	Incidence		Mortality		Mort./inc. ratio	
	MALE (ASR)	FEMALE (ASR)	MALE (ASR)	FEMALE (ASR)	MALE (%)	FEMALE (%)
World	**22.0**	**10.3**	**16.3**	**7.9**	**74.1%**	**76.7%**
More developed	**22.3**	**10.0**	**14.5**	**6.9**	**65.0%**	**69.0%**
Less developed	**21.5**	**10.4**	**17.0**	**8.3**	**79.1%**	**79.8%**
Western Europe	12.8	6.6	8.9	5.0	69.5%	75.8%
Northern Europe	12.4	5.9	9.2	4.6	74.2%	78.0%
Eastern Europe	29.6	12.8	25.2	10.8	85.1%	84.4%
Southern Europe	18.0	8.7	12.9	6.3	71.7%	72.4%
North America	7.4	3.4	4.2	2.2	56.8%	64.7%
Central America	15.2	10.8	11.7	8.3	77.0%	76.9%
South America	24.2	12.2	18.1	9.3	74.8%	76.2%
Eastern Asia	46.1	20.6	32.5	14.8	70.5%	71.8%
South-Eastern Asia	8.5	4.5	7.4	3.9	87.1%	86.7%
Western Asia	11.6	6.4	9.8	5.4	84.5%	84.4%
Middle Africa	13.4	12.6	12.6	12.0	94.0%	95.2%
Southern Africa	8.2	3.7	7.2	3.2	87.8%	86.5%
Western Africa	3.4	3.6	3.2	3.4	94.1%	94.4%

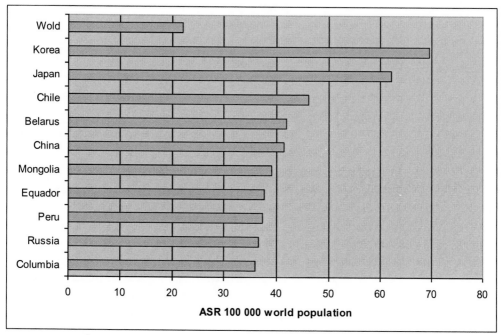

Source: GLOBOCAN 2002.

Chart 1. Gastric cancer incidence in males of high-incidence countries globally (ASR world standard).

Europe and Adherent Areas

There are substantial geographical variations in gastric cancer incidence and mortality figures found throughout Europe. Chart 2 is reflecting the incidence in male in different areas of Europe. The East European area has hot the highest incidence rate, and countries outside the European Union (EU), including Russia, Ukraine and Belarus are devoting to these numbers. In Southern Europe Macedonia, Portugal, Croatia is leading in the standardized incidence figures. This incidence is substantially lower in most of West and North European countries. Although the three Baltic countries (Estonia, Latvia, and Lithuania) with relatively high gastric cancer incidence are included to the group of North European countries, due to the small populations of these countries North Europe is the lowest gastric cancer incidence area in Europe. Actually the neighboring countries in the region as Estonia and Finland (30.5 vs. 9.6) and the countries located in a small distance across the Baltic Sea - Latvia and Sweden (24.6 vs. 8.0) have got substantially different standardized incidence of the disease in males, estimating on 100 000 world standard population [2].

Gastric cancer incidence estimates in the European countries for the year 2006 have been estimated by J.Ferlay et al. [15]; chart 3 is reflecting the comparison between the European countries with more than 20 cases per 100 000 standard European population.

The definition for 'European' countries differs among studies, and therefore this is important to understand which countries are included to the particular analysis. Depending on the above, the cancer statistics European data can be substantially differing.

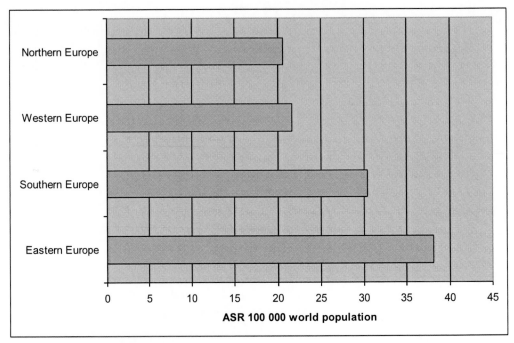

Source: GLOBOCAN 2002.

Chart 2. Gastric cancer incidence in different areas of Europe (ASR world standard).

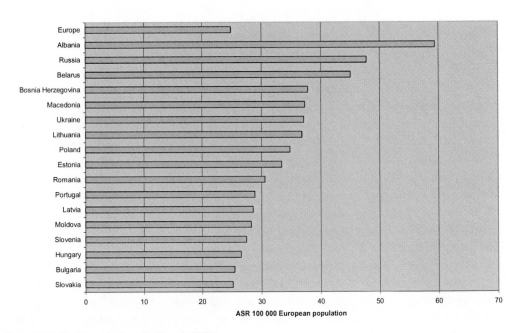

Source: Ferlay J. et al. Annals Oncol. 2007.

Chart 3. Gastric cancer incidence in males of high-incidence countries in Europe (estimated, ASR European standard).

Number of previous publications has analyzed European data considering the 15 EU countries before the enlargement of the Union; these were including Western and Southern Europe with generally low or medium gastric cancer incidence, and therefore the incidence and the mortality data are different, after the EU was extended by 10 countries in Central Europe joining the Union (EU25) in 2004, or, finally, when Romania and Bulgaria were joining in 2007 (EU27). From the epidemiology considerations this is logical to consider together the countries within the European Economic Area (EU countries plus Norway and Iceland) as well as Switzerland. European population in a wider sense should be considered by adding the following countries to the above: Albania, Belarus, Bosnia Herzegovina, Croatia, Macedonia, Serbia and Montenegro and Ukraine although actually a significant proportion of the Russia population is located in Asia. This approach has been used by J.Ferlay et al. [15] in estimating the cancer incidence and mortality in Europe as for 2006.

Gastric cancer is still remaining its importance in Europe (in wider sense). Altogether 159 900 estimated new cases are diagnosed annually as per 2006 [15], out of these 80 100 cases are occurring in EU25, but 81 600 in EEA countries. From the total number of cancer cases (but nonmelanoma skin cancer) per anum in male (1.7 million) stomach cancer (96 100 cases) is taking the 4th place in frequency following prostate, lung and colorectal cancers. Correspondingly in female (total number cancer cases 1.49 million) gastric cancer with 63 800 cases is in the 5th place in incidence following breast, colorectal, uterus and lung cancer [15].

The proportion of gastric cancer (cases and deaths) from the total number of cancer cases but nonmelanoma cancer is given in Table 2.

Table 2. Importance of gastric cancer compared to other gastrointestinal cancers (% of all cancers but nonmelanoma skin cancer) source: *Ferlay J. et al. Annals Oncol. 2007*

Cancer	Cases			Mortality		
	Europe	EEA	EU25	Europe	EEA	EU25
Esophagus	1.40%	1.40%	1.40%	2.30%	2.40%	2.40%
Stomach	5.00%	3.50%	3.50%	6.90%	4.90%	4.90%
CRC	12.90%	13.10%	13.00%	12.20%	12.00%	12.00%
Liver	NA	2.10%	2.10%	NA	3.60%	3.70%
Pancreas	NA	2.50%	2.50%	NA	5.50%	5.50%

CRC – colorectal cancer; NA – data in respect to wider Europe not available.

There is gastric cancer incidence differences present also in the high-incidence areas of Russia. All the territory of Russia is not covered by reliable cancer registration, and therefore the estimates may not be very exact. High incidence areas are not equally distributed over the country, and are found in either European or Asian part of the country; the highest incidence areas (ASR, world population) are in Tuva, Novgorod, Kostromsk and Vologradsk regions, but the lowest in the North Caucasus and Altai regions [16]. Although also in this country the cancer incidence has decreased, it is still steadily taking the 2nd place. In the neighboring to Russia countries – Uzbekistan, Tajikistan, Kyrgyzstan and Turkmenistan (localized in South-Central Asia) gastric cancer is still the leading cancer in incidence [2].

A study from Archangelsk region in the North European part of Russia and the comparison of the obtained data to neighboring Norway has revealed substantial differences between these two territories in respect to the gastric and colorectal cancer incidence; the authors have found that this area, where the incidence of gastric cancer is characteristic to the situation in Russia in general is quite similar to the situation that was present in Norway 30-40 years before [17].

Africa

High prevalence of *H.pylori* infection, but low incidence of the traditional bacteria related diseases, including gastric cancer and low surgery rate for peptic ulcer disease has been considered a condition difficult to interpret and is known in the literature as "African enigma". Different explanations have been suggested for this condition.

Like in the high risk areas most of the gastric cancers in Africa are localized in the antral part of the stomach, are of intestinal type, are more common in male and are occurring in individuals over 50 years of age [18]. At the same time the life expectancy in number of African countries is below 50.

Although the disease is rare in Southern and Eastern Africa, but in Central (Middle) Africa the incidence is not very low (see Chart 4), and is similar to many countries in Central Europe, i.e. ASR in male is 13.4, but in female 12.6 per 100 000 (the latter corresponding to the corresponding incidence figure of Eastern Europe).

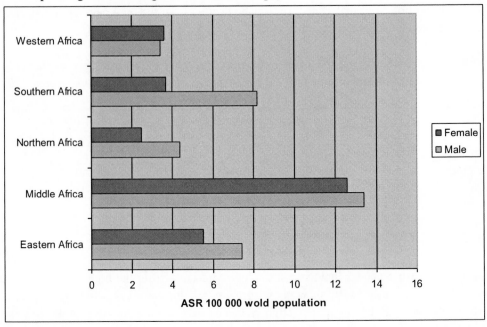

Source: GLOBOCAN 2002.

Chart 4. Gastric cancer incidence in different regions of Africa (ASR world standard).

Lifestyle factors, including alcohol and smoking [19] as well as low socioeconomic status [20], differences in *H.pylori* virulence factors [21] and even shift of immune response caused by enteric helminths [22] have been suggested to be responsible for the lower gastric cancer incidence in Africa.

The recent review by A.Agha and D.Graham [23] based on systemic analysis of 40 prospective endoscopic studies performed in 17 African countries and involving altogether 20 531 patients has suggested that the African enigma as such does not exist, and that the clinical outcomes associated to *H.pylori* infection in Africa are similar to those seen in industrialized countries, but the low gastric cancer incidence is mainly the result of poor diagnostic availability and early mortality. The prevalence of gastric cancer that was identified at endoscopy in Africa (3.4%) exceeded the frequency seen in developed countries in symptomatic individuals (below 2%) [23]. At the same this is difficult to analyze whether the symptoms in patients undergoing endoscopy in Africa have not been more severe than in upper endoscopy undertaking population in the West.

Asia

Approximately 56% of the newly diagnosed gastric cancer cases arise in East Asia, of these 42% are diagnosed in China and 12% in Japan [2,24].

Areas of Asia, including Japan and Korea are known to be the highest gastric cancer incidence areas globally, and the cancer is diminishing with the decline in prevalence of *H.pylori* infection. At the same time in other countries like India, Bangladesh, Pakistan and Thailand the infection is very common, it is obtained early in the life, and most of the adult population is infected; at the same time the incidence of gastric cancer in these countries is low, and lower than in the industrialized Asian countries with high cancer incidence like Japan [25]. The difference in incidence figures between high and low incidence areas is even 40-fold [2,24]. Likewise Africa this "controversy" is described as "Asian enigma".

In Japanese (Hisayama region) males, the prevalence of *H.pylori* infection in general population over the age of 40 is 71.5% [26], but the overall standardized gastric cancer incidence 62.1 per 100 000 [2]; in Korea *H.pylori* is infecting 54%-75% of the population [27], and gastric cancer incidence is 69.6 per 100 000 [2]. Contrary in Thailand the estimated prevalence of *H.pylori* is similar to Korea, i.e. 53.7%-74% [27], but the incidence of gastric cancer is only 4.3 per 100 000 [2]. In Bangladesh the infection is found in 92% [28], but gastric cancer standardized incidence is 1.6 per 100 000 [2]; in India correspondingly 67-81% [29,30] and 5.7 [2]. Also in many areas of Asia the statistics on the cancer incidence may not be very accurate due to poor diagnostic techniques, different reporting systems, and limited access to medical care, especially in the poorer, developing countries [27].

In general, the differenced between areas in Asia do exist objectively; the countries in East Asia have substantially higher gastric cancer incidence than the countries localized in South-Eastern and South-Central Asia.

Significant differences in gastric cancer incidence do exist also within particular countries in Asia. 5-fold difference in the incidence and 10-fold difference in the mortality caused by gastric cancer is found in two South regions of China – Changle of Fujian county and Hong Kong; study addressing these differences has suggested different prevalence of *H.pylori* being responsible for the differences [31].

Another area of high gastric cancer incidence in China is Linqu county in the Shandong Province with the incidence as high as 70 per 100 000 in males and 25 per 100 000 in females [32].

In Taiwan, the population of a small island of Matzu (population of 3500) has 4-fold higher mortality rate from gastric cancer than the population of Taiwan [33]. The factors found responsible for the progression of the disease towards pre-malignant lesions and cancer of the stomach were not different from other geographical areas, i.e. they were *H.pylori* infection, atrophy in the corpus mucosa, family history of gastric cancer and personal history of upper gastrointestinal disease [34].

Differences in gastric cancer-related mortality are observed also in the high cancer incidence area of Japan. There is more than 2.4 times higher gastric cancer caused death rate in Fukui, a typical rural prefecture located on the central Japanese mainland (Honshu) than in Okinawa, consisting of islands in the South-western part of Japan, and having history and food culture different from those of other parts of Japan [35]. These differences have been explained by different CagA type pf *H.pylori*, being identifies as Eastern (more related to gastric cancer) and western type CagA [24, 35].

MORTALITY AND 5-YEAR SURVIVAL

Gastric cancer was the main cause of mortality among malignant diseases in 1930-ies either in Europe or in the United States, and even now it is the second most frequent cause of mortality among the malignant diseases. In general poor survival and significant proportion of the cancers being diagnosed at late stages are responsible for such mortality figures, indicating the possible space of improvement.

In Europe (wider sense), the disease is responsible for 118 200 estimated annual deaths, of which 57 500 are occurring in 25EU, but 58 400 in EEA countries [15]. Therefore from all the gastric cancer related deaths in Europe only 49.4% are occurring in the EEA countries, while the majority of the cases are taking place outside the EEA (50.5%). The major proportion of gastric cancer caused deaths in the European countries outside the EU is coming from Russia (estimated cases 44 700 for 2002), Ukraine (12 500 cases) and Belarus (more than 3000). In absolute case numbers the following EU countries do have the highest estimated numbers of gastric-cancer caused deaths – Germany (13 800), UK (7100), Spain (6400), Poland (6200), France (5500), Romania (4000) and Portugal (2600) [2].

The overall prognosis of the disease is remaining poor. The survival is closely related to the extent of the disease. If the disease is diagnosed an advanced stage, the survival is in general low. If an early cancer is diagnosed confined to the inner lining of the stomach wall, 95% 5-year survival could be reached [36]; such results are mainly reported from Japan.

Overall the 5-year survival in the case of gastric cancer is low with the exception of Japan, where the survival rate is 52% [3]. This could be explained by substantially more aggressive diagnostic strategy and early diagnostics of the disease. Different definition from the Western countries and potentially different biology of the disease also may contribute. The influence of mass-screening by photofluoroscopy started in 1960s and involving over 6 million people annually is less convincing, yet is believed to reduce the mortality [37]. In screening photofluoroscopy detected gastric cancers the 5-year survival rate is 15%-30% better thank in symptom-diagnosed cases [37]. In the individuals undergoing annual endoscopy investigations for preventive purpose 91% of the gastric cancers identified are in early stage, but 9% - in advanced [38]. Recently other strategies, including upper endoscopy and biomarker screening has started their way towards mass screening, still so far they are not officially accepted as screening tools, and their use was not able to improve the survival on a national scale.

Relatively good 5-year survival rate is also in the United States where the standardized 5-year survival is about 40% [3] probably due to the good availability of endoscopy and related to large number of endoscopies performed in patients with upper gastrointestinal symptoms (mainly in screening for Barrett's and in patients with alarm symptoms).

Among the 18 registries representing European countries (15EU plus Switzerland, Poland, Slovenia, not Portugal) within the EUROCARE-4 study [39] for the period of 2000-2002 the relative mean 5-year survival of patients with gastric cancer was 24.9% within the frames from 16.6% for Scotland and 16.9% for England up to 33.2% for Italy, 32.7% for Belgium, 31.8% for Spain and 31.4% for Germany.

Substantially worse 5-year survival is reported from areas like sub-Saharan Africa, where it is as low as 6% [3].

TIME TRENDS

Either the incidence and mortality of gastric cancer in standardized indicators has steadily declinined over the period of at least 50 years, and this trend is present not only in developed, but also developing countries [40] although the mortality rates in high-incidence countries currently are on the level low-incidence countries had 40-50 years ago [17]. This convincing decline has started substantially before the discovery of *H.pylori* in 1984 and therefore other factors than the microorganism has the major importance in decreasing mortality.

Globally, in 2002 the incidence of 22 per 100 000 in male and 10.3 per 100 000 in female was about 15% lower than in 1985 [41,42]. In Russia, during a 10-year period between 1990 and 2000 the standardized incidence rates of gastric cancer have declined for close to 30% [16].

In EU gastric cancer mortality has been declining since several decades, and this trend is continuing. Since steady reduction of gastric cancer mortality is observed in middle age population, it can be considered that the decline will be continuing also in near future [43].

C.Bosetti et al. [43] has compared the age-adjusted (world population) mortality rates per 100 000 men and women aged 35-64 in the EU (27) within the last two decades, i.e. between 1982 – 1992; and 1992 – 2002. In males, the decrease in the gastric cancer mortality was 24.9% for the first period, and 31.7% for the consecutive one; in females the corresponding figures were 23.79% and 28.31%.

In Lithuania [44] during the time period 1993-2004 gastric cancer related mortality was also declining, and more rapid decline was present in urban than rural inhabitants. The annual decrease was 3.78% for urban and 2.06% for rural males and correspondingly 2.83% and 2.15% for urban and rural females.

More rapid decline could be observed in developed countries. A population-based study in Sweden has suggested the incidence decline rate of non-cardia gastric cancer to be 9% per year [45].

IMPACT OF THE AGING POPULATION

The aging western populations are expected to reflect in higher number of cancer-related deaths in these regions. Demographically the oldest-aged nations of the world are northern, southern and eastern regions of Europe as well as the United States [46]. In the United States, the population over the age of 65 years will double within the next 25 years [47, 48]. Italy ranks the oldest country in the world, and the trend is constantly continuing. If in 2000 18% of the population was over the age of 65, then this proportion of the population will increase up to 27% by 2030, and will compile a quarter of all the population [48].

In Europe, altogether 159 900 cancer related deaths are estimated as per 2006. European population is steadily aging, and between 2000 and 2015 there will be a 22% increase in the population older than 65 years and 50% increase in the population over 80 years. For cancers with stable age-standardized rate it is expected that there will be a 25% increase in absolute incidence between the years of 2007 and 2015 [15, 43].

Since the age-standardized rate for gastric cancer is declining, this increase in absolute incidence and mortality figures will not be so steep. Considering the decline in the standardized incidence rates as per 2002 and the connected continuation of the secular decline, but the aging global population, the expected number of new gastric cancer cases in 2010 is estimated to be around 1.1 million. This estimate is made considering that the increase in the risk-age population will be 21%, but the decreasing standardized rate will lower this increase to 19% [3]. In any case, increase, not decrease in absolute figures of both incidence and mortality is expected for the coming years.

MALE – FEMALE RATIO

Gastric cancer is significantly more predominant in male population although this predominance is less evident in diffuse type cancer. The male to female ratio is ranging from 1.5 to 3, but proportionally following the incidence trends in male [2,3,49].

At the same time the review on the prevalence of atrophic gastritis in different parts of the world by M.N.Weck and H.Brenner [50] did not reveal sex differences in the prevalence of atrophy between the sexes. Moreover, the EUROGAST study group [51] results indicate higher prevalence of atrophy in female, although this difference might at least partly explained by the differences in the body weight, and disappeared after adjusting for the factor.

Study based on the data from Finnish cancer registry in patients with pre-malignant lesions (atrophic gastritis in the antrum and/or corpus) revealed a significantly higher risk of cancer development in male if compared to female populations [52].

P.Sipponen and P.Correa [53] by analyzing data from 18 cancer registries worldwide and consecutive case data from Finland have found that the male : female ratio for gastric cancer is not stable over the time, but is rising and reaching its peak by the age of 60, but then – decreasing. The authors were suggesting that the intestinal type gastric cancer in female has similar biology than in males, but only with some 10-15 years delay in onset. They speculated that estrogens may protect women from gastric cancer development, but this protection is lost at the time of menopause when the proportion of intestinal type gastric cancers in women is increasing.

AGE AT ONSET

The age of onset for the disease is important in setting strategies for investigating individuals with dyspeptic symptoms, but without alarm symptoms to rule out the malignancy of the stomach. Since the proportion of early cancer onset differs in different areas, also this strategy should be adopted accordingly [54]. If a screening strategy is set up, the age at increasing risk is of importance to choose the appropriate target group.

Diffuse type cancer is found at comparatively early age than intestinal type. In more details this is described in another section.

In general, the disease is rare between the age of 40; the major increase is seen starting from the age of 50. Proportion of cancers diagnosed in very early age hereditary, linked to germline mutations in E-cadherin (CDH1) [55], yet this is a small number of the total. Cancers below the age of 30 are of diffuse type [45].

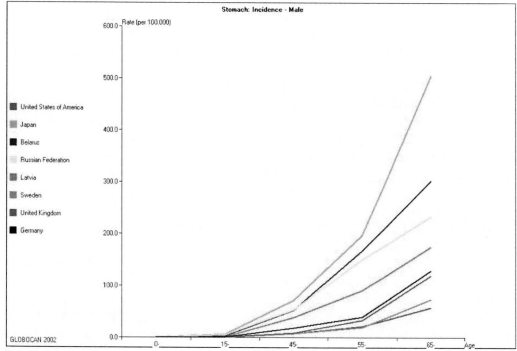

Source: GLOBOCAN 2002.

Chart 5. Gastric cancer incidence in different age groups of men, countries with significant differences in the incidence (ASR world standard).

The age-related trend is similar for high and low gastric cancer prevalence areas (see the Chart 5).

ADENOCARCINOMA OF THE ESOPHAGOGASTRIC
JUNCTION / CANCER OF THE CARDIA

Cancer of the cardia region can be arising from either the stomach or esophagus, and in about half of the cases these cancers are occurring in patients with the presence of Barrett's metaplasia in the esophagus [56].

Either from the epidemiology considerations or because of different underlying conditions this is important to distinguish between adenocarcinoma originating in either the stomach or esophagus, still in many cases this is impossible to extract these original locations of the tumor from the registries (morphologically the two adenocarcinomas are identical).

In many western populations gradual increase of incidence of adenocarcinoma of the esophagus and/or gastric cardia has been observed starting from 1970-ies; this trend was confirmed in countries as the United States, Australia, New Zealand and several West-European countries [57,58]. In the United States this increase was seen most evidently with close to 10% increase rate per year [59,60], and was observed in all the age groups.

A.A.M. Botterweck et al. [58] has analyzed the time-trends of age-standardized incidence of adenocarcinoma of the esophagus and gastric cardia in several areas of Europe between 1968 and 1995 based upon 11 population-based cancer registries from 10 countries in Europe by using the Eurocim database. The study revealed differences between the incidence of this cancer type in Europe; the highest incidence was found in males (ASR European population 9.7 per 100 000 person-years) and female (2.9) from Scotland but the lowest in male from Slovakia (3.5) and females from France, Bas-Rhin region (0.4). The proportion of this type of the cancers versus all cancers of the stomach among males was the lowest in Slovakia (9.3%), but highest in Denmark (41.8%), followed by Scotland (34.6%) and Switzerland (30%). Still this has to be considered that Slovakia is not the highest gastric cancer incidence country in the Eastern Europe, therefore the proportion between these two cancers is expected to be even higher. Additionally the period of data collection has started 40 years ago, therefore the current proportion between different European countries would be more pronounced as for today.

During the period of the 28 years the rise in incidence of adenocarcinoma of the esophagus and gastric cardia was demonstrated in nearly all the studied regions of Europe; in some areas there was not an evident increase seen, but these registries have covered smaller populations (e.g. Iceland, Switzerland, Basel and some other) [58]. The countries (England and Wales, Italy, Scotland, Slovakia) with the highest increase in the incidence within 12 year period (from 1981-1983 to 1990-1992) were showing up to 46-81% increase of this type of the cancer [58].

Over a 15-year period (1989-2003) in the Netherlands the esophago-cardia localized adenocarcinomas have increased for 34% in males, 25% in females, and by 33% for both the sexes combined [61]. Still when looking at the cancers of the different localizations separately, the increase was convincingly coming from the adenocarcinomas localized in the esophagus, but the incidence of cardia localized cancers was actually decreasing by the annual rate of 1.7% in males and 1.2% in females [61].

According to the data from Swedish cancer registry the incidence of adenocarcinoma in gastric cardia in this country had increased twice between 1970-1974 and 2000-2004 time periods, giving the annual increase rate 2.3% in males and 2.1% in females [62].

At the same time this should be mentioned that data retrieved from cancer registries may lack the sufficient accuracy for epidemiological studies in respect to the cancer of the cardia. Ekstrom et al. [63] have conducted a study by comparing their population-base identified patients to the data of the Swedish cancer registry, which is considered among the best worldwide. Altogether 178 cancers of the cardia were identified by the authors, yet the register failed to identity a significant proportion of these cancers. The authors conclude that the true cardia cancer incidence could be up to 45% higher or 15% lower than reported in the Cancer Registry. With such potential registration errors the validity of many registry-based studies, including the one cited above from Sweden demonstrating the increase in the cardia cancer could be questioned.

Moreover A.M.Ekstrom et al. [45] have conducted a well-designed prospective study in five counties of Sweden between 1989 and 1994; and what they found was that the incidence of cardia cancer has been stable, but not increasing in this area of Sweden during the study period.

In summary, there are sufficient data to consider that the adenocarcinoma of the esophago-cardia location is increasing substantially, yet mainly due to adenocarcinoma in the esophagus. The epidemiological studies based on cancer registries may fail to give exact data on the real changes in the incidence. Considering that significant attention has been paid to the cancer of the cardia during the recent two decades, we could expect that cancers previously been misclassified as gastric cancers lately are entered in the registries as cancers of the cardia; this could result in more rapid increase indication than it is in the reality.

DIFFERENCES BETWEEN THE INTESTINAL AND DIFFUSE TYPE GASTRIC CANCER EPIDEMIOLOGY (ACCORDING TO THE LAUREN CLASSIFICATION)

There are limited possibilities to evaluate the global distribution between the intestinal and diffuse type of gastric cancers since most of the cancer registries do not collect data on the cancer distribution between these two types (the ICD-10 classification considers the localization, but not the morphological type of the cancer). Most of the available data are reported from regional or comparative studies with only few well-designed population-based studies.

Intestinal type cancers are more frequent in males, in particular elderly populations with pre-existing premalignat lesions, including atrophic gastritis and intestinal metaplasia. In the population of the Unites States intestinal type cancer is more common in African-Americans than in whites [64]. In Sweden the intestinal type cancer is significantly more predominant in the cardia region than in the rest of the stomach (75% vs. 58%); the male : female ratio for intestinal cancer type is 3 : 1 for the non-cardia location and 4 : 1 for cardia located cancer [45].

Diffuse cancer type is more frequent in relatively younger individuals and females. In the prospective population-based study in Sweden [45] diffuse type cancer was significantly more common before the age of 50: this type cancer was responsible for all the gastric cancer cases below the age of 30 and for 56% of the cases in 45-50 years old age group. Diffuse type was compiling 40% of all the adenocarcinoma in female, but only 25% - in male. The male :

female ratios for diffuse type cancer was 1.2 : 1 in non-cardia, and 2.5 : 1 in cardia location [45].

In general, most of the cancers in the East are of intestinal type, but higher proportion of diffuse type cancers are seen in the West.

In the series from Japan approximately two-thirds are intestinal type, but one third – diffuse type cancers [38,65].

In a cohort from altogether 10 west and south EU countries 344 gastric adenocarcinomas have been analyzed within the validation study of the EPIC/EUR-GAST study [7]. The majority of the cases were non-cardia cancers (48%), while cancers of the cardia constituted a substantial proportion (29%), while the remaining 23% cases were of unknown location. In this cohort the proportion of intestinal and diffuse type cancers were close to equal with shift towards diffuse cancer type (intestinal 33%, diffuse 34%, mixed 1%, unclassified or unknown 32% from all the adenocarcinomas of the stomach and correspondingly 35%, 39%, 1% and 15% from the subgroup of non-cardia adenocarcimomas [7]. This has to be mentioned that the study was not population-based, moreover none of the new-EU countries with high gastric cancer incidence were included. The majority of the cancer cases in this study were from the Northern countries; at the same time the reported proportion between the intestinal and diffuse type cancers is contradicting to other studies performed in Sweden, in particular to the well-defined Swedish population-based series of 1337 gastric cancers from five counties (with all the cases been analyzed by a single pathologist efforts having been made to miss any cancer in the target population) where 59% cancers were intestinal, 30% diffuse and 6% mixed type [45]; therefore also in the Western European countries the proportion between the intestinal and diffuse cancer types is quite similar to Japan.

Traditionally there has been a belief that intestinal cancer is declining, but the diffuse is not [66]. Decline of intestinal type cancer, but increase in diffuse type between 1973 and 2000 has been reported in the United States [64]. In contrast, a consistent increase of diffuse type gastric cancer was observed from 0.3 to 1.8 cases per 100 000 persons. The increase was observed in both the sexes and either African Americans or whites; morphologically signet ring cell type cancer was mainly responsible for the increase.

The analysis performed on the data from Gastric Cancer Registry in Japan [65] (161 067 cases) between 1975 and 1989 suggested decreasing trend of the intestinal type, but stable trend of the diffuse type gastric cancer; tubular (moderately differentiated type), poorly differentiated adenocarcinomas and signet ring cell carcinoma were found to be statistically stable during the period.

Two epidemiology studies on gastric cancer involving both the histological subtypes have been published based on the data from Sweden. A study from a single Swedish county (Ostergotland) has compared adenocarcinoma or the stomach (1161 cases) according to the Lauren classification and localization between the time periods 1974-1982 (period 1) and 1983-1991 (period 2) [67]. The authors suggested slight increase in the proportion of diffuse type gastric adenocarcinoma (from 27% to 35%), while the proportion of intestinal type cancer was remaining stable (the proportion of mixed type gastric cancer was declining). Also the proportion of tumors located in the proximal two-thirds of the stomach increased (from 32% to 42%).

Another prospective perfectly designed study in a well-defined population of 5 Swedish counties was carried out by Ekstrom et al. [45] within the time period 1989-1994. The thorough design of the study ensured that there was practically no possibility to miss cancers in the target population; altogether 1337 gastric cancer cases were identified. Highly significant decline of both the histologic types of non-cardia location was identified during the study period, whereas the intestinal type cancer declined, on average, by 9% (95% CI 4-14%), but the diffuse type by 8% (95% CI 3-15%) annually. No similar trend for either intestinal or diffuse type cancers of cardia localized cancers were seen [45].

DIFFERENCES IN WESTERN AND JAPANESE SERIES

In Japan, the three most frequent and stable types of gastric cancer are moderately differentiated adenocarcinomas, poorly differentiated adenocarcinomas, and signet-ring cell carcinoma [65]; these are common morphological cancer types also in other parts of the world.

Considering wide screening for asymptomatic patients in Japan, the proportion of early gastric cancers is high, ranging 30-50% [68,69], while in the Western countries 16-24% [4,70,71], having substantially better survival results. Substantial proportion of these early gastric cancers is limited only to mucosa layer (in the series of Ohata and colleagues [38] – 76%). According to the Western pathologists these may be defined high-grade adenoma/dysplasia (intraepitheal neoplasia) [72].

This may be causing some discrepancies of gastric cancer incidence between East and West, yet cannot be very substantial because high-grade intraepitheal neoplasia is also not a frequent diagnosis in the West. A study of G.M.Naylor et al. [73] was comparing gastritis in two matched dyspepsia patient populations from Japan and UK. The Japanese patients were found to have gastritis more often (12.5% difference in the prevalence), gastritis among these patients was more severe, was present at earlier age, and was more likely to be corpus predominant or pangastritis [73].

FACTORS ASSOCIATED TO THE CANCER

Factors Increasing the Risk

H.pylori Infection

About half of the global population is infected with *H.pylori*. The prevalence of *H.pylori* infection is about 30% in Western populations and 60-88% in Asian populations [74].

The prevalence of *H.pylori* infection in Europe well correlates to the incidence of gastric cancer, and follows the birth cohort-related phenomenon. In cohorts born in the beginning of the century the prevalence of the infection alien with gastric cancer and *H.pylori* related complications is high, with decline over the time in later birth cohorts [75]. Back in 1994 IARC (International Agency for Research on Cancer) has placed *H.pylori* in the class I or definitely proven carcinogen in humans in respect to the development of non-cardia gastric cancer [76]. The currently available data support the correlation of both the histological types – not only intestinal, but also diffuse type cancer to the infection. *H.pylori* is a common risk actor for both – intestinal and diffuse type gastric cancer, but the association is stronger for the intestinal type [38].

The landmark study having demonstrated the role of *H.pylori* and other factors in the development of gastric cancer was conducted in Japan by N.Uemura et al. [77] stating that *H.pylori* infected, but not uninfected individuals are developing this type of cancer.

Out of all the *H.pylori* infected individuals developing chronic active gastritis approximately half is developing atrophy of the mucosa, 40% - intestinal metaplasia, 8% dysplasia, but 1% [78].

Number of studies has addressed the magnitude of risk increase to develop gastric cancer due to *H.pylori*. The initial studies have been resulting in underestimate of the risk because at the late stages of premalignant lesions, e.g. advanced atrophy *H.pylori* is gradually disappearing even if not intentionally having been eradicated, and therefore case-control studies in gastric cancer patients may result in underestimating the prevalence of the prevalence of *H.pylori*.

In 2001, the Helicobacter and Cancer Collaborative Group has summarized the available evidence [79] from case control studies, and concluded that *H.pylori* is increasing the risk for non-cardia, but not for cardia gastric cancer, and that the microorganism increased the risk for about 6-fold (OR 5.9; 95% CI 3.4-10.3), if the blood samples for *H.pylori* serology were collected at least 10 years prior to the diagnosis of the cancer. Even this is likely to be an underestimate, because does not exclude the presence of the microorganism earlier in life. By using Western blot analysis in a case-control study to test for past *H.pylori* infection in those that would have been reported the infection-negative according to the serology test, the odds ratio for non-cardia gastric cancer was increasing from 3.7 (95% CI 1.7-7.9) to 18.3 (95% CI 2.4 -136.7) for any *H. pylori* infection and from 5.7 (95% CI 2.6-12.8) to 28.4 (95% CI 3.7-217.1) for CagA-positive *H. pylori* infections [80]. In a larger study of similar design from Sweden [81] adding past to the present *H.pylori* infection increased the odds ratio from 2.1 (95% CI 1.4-3.6) to 21 (95% CI 8.3-53.4). Therefore this is more likely that *H.pylori* infection is increasing the risk for no-cardia cancer in the range between 18 and 28 times.

Different subtypes of *H.pylori* (different virulence factors) possess variable level of carcinogenesis, what could be at least partly explaining the geographical differences. The epidemiology of the subtypes will not be detailed in this chapter.

H.pylori does not seem to increase or otherwise influence the risk of cancer of the cardia. In the metaanalysis by Helicobacter and Cancer Collaborative Group in respect to the cancer of the cardia odds ratio was clearly unchanged (OR 1.0; 95% CI 0.7-1.4) [79]. At the same time some researchers have hypothesized that diminishing *H.pylori* infection may be linked to increasing incidence of cardia cancer [82].

Atrophic Gastritis

Atrophic gastritis develops in a proportion of patients with *H.pylori* infection, some degree of atrophy can be present even in each second patient with uncured infection [78]. The other cause for developing atrophy is autoimmune gastritis, which is more commonly found in North European populations. Still *H.pylori* infection is found to be the most frequent cause of atrophy [83-85].

In clinical practice frequently the presence of atrophy is under evaluated since far from all patients undergoing upper endoscopy are biopsied according to the recommendations [86]. Methods of indirect detection of atrophy by detecting pepsinogens and gastrin-17 in blood have been suggested, but their wide usage in population settings has to be still proven.

According to the data from the study in Japan by Uemura et al. [77] severe atrophy increased the risk of the stomach close to 5-fold (OR 4.9; 95% CI 2.8–19.2), while the authors were reporting significantly higher risk for corpus predominant gastritis or gastritis of "cancer type" (OR 34.5; 95% CI 7.1–166.7) [77]. Still this has to be stated that the detection of "corpus predominant" gastritis is somewhat controversial. According to the estimates made by P.Sipponen et al. [52] severe pan-gastritis, i.e. severe gastritis in both – corpus and antral part of the stomach may increase the risk up to 90-fold.

Even moderate atrophy could substantially increase the risk of the cancer [87]. A recent study from Japan by histopathological re-evaluation of gastric carcinoma cases was suggesting that most of differentiated adenocarcinomas develop in mildly to moderately atrophic mucosa with ongoing *H.pylori* infection rather than severely atrophic mucosa [88].

M.N.Weck and H.Brenner [50] have reviewed studies addressing the prevalence of atrophic gastritis in different parts of the world, most of the studies have been based on biomarker screening for pepsinogens. Relatively high prevalence of atrophy was found in elderly populations of different countries; high prevalence of atrophy has been demonstrated in areas with high gastric cancer prevalence, including East Asia (China, Japan) and South America. At the same time considerable proportion of patients with atrophy was revealed also in countries with low gastric cancer incidence, e.g. Sweden (36% in 65-74 old individuals and 56% in individuals over 75 years) and Australia (39% in individuals over the age of 50). Interestingly that between the two neighboring countries with different gastric cancer incidence the prevalence of atrophy was higher or at least not lower in Finland if compared to Estonia, the latter having substantially higher gastric cancer incidence; although this has to be considered that the study in Finland was performed some 10-13 years prior to the one in Estonia.

Also an earlier study by EUROGAST study group [51] by investigating low pepsinogen I levels in 17 populations worldwide revealed lower pepsingen levels characteristic for atrophy in areas with high gastric cancer incidence. Random population sampling was performed within the study. In none of the countries in the age group 55-64 years the prevalence of atrophy detected indirectly by the method exceeded 20%; the highest prevalence in male in this age group was present in Japan (10.2-17.8%), while in most of the investigated groups atrophy was less prevalent than 10% in this age group.

Intestinal Metaplasia

Although intestinal metaplasia is an important segment of so Correa cascade of gastric cancer development [89], the role of it in the development of gastric cancer is still somewhat controversial.

Limited number of previous studies has succeeded to indicate the role of intestinal metaplasia in gastric cancer development; only type III intestinal metaplasia in a study from Slovenia was revealed to have mild correlation to gastric cancer development [90], yet the study has been criticized in respect to the methodological issues.

M.Stolte's group in Germany [10] consider that a substantial sampling error may be present in detecting intestinal metaplasia based on the recommended biopsy sampling approaches, and that the presence or absence of intestinal metaplasia in the biopsies from the corpus mucosa is a very unspecific marker, and therefore cannot be used to identify the group at increased risk for developing gastric cancer, nor for the surveillance of these patients. Similarly a recent histopathology study from Japan on gastric cancer series did not confirm the importance of intestinal metaplasia in the development of gastric cancer, therefore supporting the suggestion of M.Stolte's group that intestinal metaplasia is not a pre-cancerous, but rather a para-cancerous lesion [88].

Contrary results have been revealed in a nation-wide Dutch study based upon the data of national histopathology registry, suggesting that patients with intestinal metaplasia progress faster to gastric cancer than patients with atrophy (but slower than patients with dysplasia) [91]. The annual incidence of gastric cancer was 0.1% for patients with atrophic gastritis, 0.25% for intestinal metaplasia, 0.6% for mild-to-moderate dysplasia, and 6% for severe dysplasia within 5 years after diagnosis, and the authors suggest surveillance of these patients [91].

Hyperplastic Polyps

Out of the number of histological types of polyps that are found in the stomach, hyperplastic polyps are the most common [92], and earlier have been considered to increase the risk of gastric cancer. A recent review of literature in respect to the role of hyperplastic polyps in gastric cancer development state that the risk of carcinoma developing in a hyperplastic polyp is extremely low, and suggest that hyperplastic polyps *per se* do not lead to the cancer, but rather the association to chronic gastritis and mucosal atrophy [93].

Point-of-no-return

If gastric cancer is following the traditional Correa's cascade, there should be a break-point in this cascade, where the changes become irreversible. Issue on the point-of-no-return in the carcinogenesis of stomach cancer is still remaining an unresolved issue of high importance.

The available data indicate that dysplastic changes in the gastric mucosa are irreversible [94,95], still more controversial is the question of atrophy and intestinal metaplasia reversibility.

The current international guidelines list atrophy of the mucosa among unquestionable indications for *H.pylori* eradication [54], while the recent Asia-Pacific consensus guidelines on gastric cancer prevention [96] recommend eradication prior to the development of atrophy. The question is still remaining on whether this is not too late to have the eradication performed in a patient of advanced atrophy, and how such patients should be followed-up. In a prospective, randomized, placebo-controlled, population-based study from China [97] after *H.pylori* eradication no gastric cancers were diagnosed in patients without premalignant lesions (atrophy, intestinal metaplasia, dysplasia) at the time of inclusion, yet there were several cases of cancers developing in the group with successful eradication, but with pre-malignant lesions at the inclusion.

Number of experimental and clinical studies has been addressing the reversibility of atrophy and intestinal metaplasia, and the results have not been homogeneous.

By using an animal model of gastric cancer development by infecting mice with *Helicobacter felis*, a relative to human *H.pylori* causing similar changes in the mucosa in these animals X.Cai et al. [98] have demonstrated the reversibility of inflammation, intestinal metaplasia and even dysplasia, if the eradication therapy was given early enough.

Some researchers have suggested intestinal metaplasia to be the point-of-no-return, still there are no string data available to support thys hypothesis. J.Watari et al. [99] has recently summarized studies reporting the improvement of histological grade of gastric intestinal metaplasia following the eradication and studies not finding any change.

The cotroversies are remaining in respect to whether intestinal metaplasia is a consequence of atrophy in the clearly defined Correa's model of pathogenesis or still a parallel condition to atrophy [10]; additionally – how to identify the point-of-no-return in the pathogenesis of diffuse type gastric cancer without clear pre-malignant lesions. Therefore we are still lacking the criteria for the point-of-no-return.

Post-surgery

Partial gastrectomy with Billroth I or Billroth II reconstructions increase the risk for gastric cancer after 15 year period from the operation [100]. A risk increase of 28% for each successive five-year interval after operation has been calculated based on the results of a large cohort study by using the data from the Swedish Cancer registry [101].

Factors Diminishing the Risk

Helminths

Experimental work on mice by J.Fox et al. [22] has suggested that in mice with concurrent helminth infection *H.pylori* associated atrophy of the gastric mucosa was considerably reduced despite the presence of chronic inflammation and intensive *H.pylori* colonisation. This is suggested that parasite invasion could be shifting the immune response from Th1 to polarized Th2 response resulting in lower production of pro-inflammatory cytokines (such as IFN-γ, TNF-α and IL-1β), but stimulation of anti-inflammatory Th2 cytokine production (such as IL-4 and IL-10).

The hypothesis was supported by a study in Columbian children [102] where children in lower gastric cancer incidence area were found to be more infected with helminths, had higher serum IgE levels, and had higher Th2-associated IgG1 subclass responses to *H. pylori*.

Impact of Lifestyle Factors

There are limitations to interpret the role of a particular factor in respect to the gastric cancer carcinogenesis since significant overlap and relations could be found between many of the factors. High intake of salted food is closely inversively related to the use of refrigeration, lower socieconomic status – with minor intake of fresh fruit and vegetables, and therefore – antioxidants, but higher prevalence of *H.pylori* infection, etc.

Smoking

The meta-analysis of 40 studies by J.Tredaniel et al. [103] back in 1997 already clearly stated the positive association between gastric cancer and smokig; the relative risk was estimated 1.5-1.6 times higher than in non-smokers. This has been more recently confirmed also by IARC [104]; this relation was confirmed also by later studies. Smoking was found to correlate with low gastrin I levels characteristic for atrophy in the study in 17 centers in 13 countries by the EUROGAST study group [51].

Differences might be present on whether smokings and tabacco influences most significantly adenocarcinoma of the cardia or similar impact is present also in respect to the non-cardia gastric cancer. The European Prospective Investigation Into Cancer and Nutrition (EPIC) identified smoking as a risk factor for both – cardia and non-cardia gastric cancer; the the hazard ratio (HR) for ever smokers was 1.45 (95% CI 1.08-1.94). Smoking was found to increase the risk for both the sexes. The HR increased with the intensity and duration of smoking. The risk was higher in respect to the cancer of cardia (HR = 4.10) than for distal cancer (HR 1.94) [105]. In a data-set from the United States published a decade ago smoking has been suggested to be associated with up to 40% cases of the esophageal and gastric cardia adenocarcinoma cases [106].

In a large prospective cohort study in Japan [107] with 10 years follow-up and 293 cancer cases by the end of the sudy smoking was associated with an increased risk of the differentiated type distal gastric cancer; compared to the group who never smoked, the adjusted rate ratios of gastric cancer for past and current smokers were 2.0 (95% CI 1.1-3.7) and 2.1 (95% CI 1.2-3.6), respectively. There was no association found between cigarette smoking and the risk of undifferentiated type distal gastric cancer; but a trend was observed in respect to the association with cardia cancer [107].

In Russia, smoking was found to increase the risk of developing gastric cancer in men, but not in women; this correlation was found to be dose-dependent (p = 0.03), as well as related to pack-years of cigarettes smoked (p = 0.01) and duration of smoking (p = 0.08) in respect to the risk of cancer of gastric cardia [108].

The risk to develop cancer is diminishing after stopping smoking, still the period in which the risk decline is significan ir reported different by different studies. In Poland, a high gastric cancer incidence area ex-smokers did not have increased risk in general, the increased risk was declining soon after quitting smoking [109]. In the EPIC study in European population decreased risk was observed after 10 years of quitting smoking [106], in Japanese cohorts, - up to 14 years [110], but un the United States up to 30 years after the cessation [106].

Diet

As described beforehand, the decline of the gastric cancer incidence was observed years before the discovery of *H.pylori* took place, and therefore long before intentional eradication of this microorganism could reflect in lowering the incidence of this type of cancer. Although also the prevalence of *H.pylori* could be decreasing even before we knew about the bacteria due to better socioeconomic factors and hygene, other even more important factors, including the food have left the major impact upon the decreasing incidence and mortality caused by gastric cancer. There has been an indication from case-control studies in general that good meal habits were protective factors against gastric cancer, and vice versa [111] as well as the lack of refrigeration at home or use of leftover gruel is related to increased risk of the disease [112]. Appearently these facto●●re closer linked to the socioeconomic class than preferrence of particular food type.

Alcohol

Also regular alcohol use is frequently associated to a lower socioeconomic class, and therefore this is difficult to evaluate the impact of this factor isolated [106].

A cohort study in Japan was suggesting that only cardia cancer of any histologic type could have the relationship to increased alcohol intake, yet the relationship failed to reach significance [107].

In the capital of Russia (a case control study eith 448 cases and 610 controls) hard alcohol, particularly vodka consumption was found to increase the risk of gastric cancer; the effect was stronger in men for cardia cancer (OR 3.4; CI 1.2-10.2), while in women the effect was stronger for cancer of sites other than gastric cardia (OR 1.5; CI = 1.0-2.3) [108].

Beer may be increasing the risk of gastric cancer not only due to the content of alcohol, but also N-nitroso compounds in it. A prospectice cohort study of women attending mammography in Sweden has suggested that the the use of medium-strong/strong beer was associated with a statistically significant increased risk of gastric cancer [113], still the total alcohol intake was not significantly associated with risk of gastric cancer. Systemic analysis by P.Jakszyn et al. [114] has identified that 6 out of 7 case control studies have suggested the negative effect of beer, yet only one reached statistical significance.

The potential impact of wine consumption is somewhat controversial. In Mexico, consumption of at least 10 glasses of wine per month yealded in significant risk increase (OR2.93; 95% CI 1.27-6.75) [115], whereas wine-drinking seemed to have a protective effect in respect to gastric cancer in Denmark – when compared to non-wine drinkers those who drank 1-6 glasses of wine had a relative risk ratio of 0.76 (95% confidence interval (CI) 0.50-1.16), whereas those who drank >13 glasses of wine per week had a relative risk ratio of 0.16 (95% CI 0.02-1.18), and the linear trend test showed a significant association with a relative risk ratio of 0.60 (95% CI 0.39-0.93) per glass of wine drunk per day [116]. Also in the United States the risk for esophageal and cardia adenocarcinoma was reduced in wine-drinkers (OR 0.6; 95% CI 0.5-0.8), in difference for consumers of other alcohol [106].

A meta-analysis by V. Bagnardi et al. [117] has suggested that 50 g/day alcohol intake resulted in 1.15 (95% CI 1.09-1.22) relative risk increase, but 100 g/day intake – in 1.32 (95% CI 1.18-1.49), respectively.

Tea consumption. Data from animal experiments suggest that several epicatechin derivatives (polyphenols) present in green tea have anticarcinogenic activity, the most active being epigallocatechin-3-gallate [118]. It has been suggested that tea, in particular green tea is protective against gastric cancer in humans. Nevertheless most of the prospective studies have failed to demonstrate this inverse relation with an exception of one [119] that was able to demonstrate an inverse association to distal gastric cancer in women.

Coffee consumption has been considered unrelated to gastric cancer. Based on 23 studies from the United States and South America as well as Japan and Europe L. Botelho et al. [121] have published a meta-analysis that did not reveal any associated of coffee to gastric cancer. There have been other studies suggesting positive or borderline correlation of the cancer to heavy coffee consumption [122,123], yet the results have not given a conclusive evidence.

High salt diet in has been traditionally believed to be directly linked to increased incidence of gastric cancer.

A review on descriptive epidemiology and ecological studies from Japan and international studies [124] is stating that the majority of the geographical variation in gastric cancer mortality worldwide and in Japan at the population level is correlating to the daily salt intake level. Many, but not all of the case-control studies have shown a positive association between high-salt containing products, such as salted fish, cured meat, salted vegetables or table salt and gastric cancer [124,125]. Positive association between the use of preserved fish and preserved vegetable intake and gastric cancer has been confirmed by the recent review [114]. A more cecent case-control study from Lithuania (the previous review was not including any East-European country) including 379 cancer cases and 1137 controls has confirmed the association berween the use of salty meat and gastric cancer (OR1.85, 95% CI 1.12-3.04, for the use of salty meat 1-3 times/month vs. almost never; and OR2.21, 95% CI1.43-3.42, for 1-2 times/week or more vs. almost never) [126].

The potential correlation of salt intake and cured meat consumption as well as refrigerator use was analyzed in respect to the gastric cancer incidence in a prospective cohort study in Netherlands [127]. The obtained results suggested that energy-adjusted intake of dietary salt was associated to increased risk for gastric cancer, but the results were lacking consistency. Adding of salt to hot meal during cooking was inversively associated with the risk; and there was no association between salt added to home-made soup, use of salt at the table, salt preference and the cancer. Also the duration of refrigeration use or the use of a freezer was not found to be related to gastric cancer in this study population. At the same time high intake of bacon and other sliced cold meat was associated to increased cancer risk.

The way of food preservation is closely linked either to the salt intake with the preserved food or the intake of N-nitroso compounds being used in the quality of meet and fish preservatives. The use of high amounts of salt is closely inversively related to the use of refrigerated food, higher consumption of fresh vegetables and fruit, and even directly related to lower socio-economic class.

Therefore this is difficult to prove that salt itself is involved in gastric cancer pathogenesis, and there are no grounds to believe that reduction of daily salt intake in the Western diet would have any effect on the risk of developing any form of cancer, including the gastric cancer [128].

Meat intake. Within the European Prospective Investigation Into Cancer and Nutrition (EPIC) study with data originating from 10 European countries association was found that the use of red and processed meat were associated with an increased risk of gastric non-cardia cancer [129]; this association was more pronounced in *H.pylori* infected individuals.

The mentioned as well 9 other cohort studies and 19 case-control studies were included included in the meta-analysis by S.C.Larson et al. [130] on processed meat consumption and the risk for gastric cancer. This meta-analysis revealed association between the consumption of processed meat (bacon, sausage, hot dogs, salami and ham) and increased risk for the gastric cancer, still could not exclude the influence of other confounding factors (including *H.pylori*, and N-nitroso compounds) upon the results. The relative risks for gastric cancer for 30 g/day (approx. ½ of an average serving) increase in processed meat consumption were 1.15 (95% CI 1.04-1.27) for cohort studies and 1.38 (95% CI 1.19-1.60) for case-control studies.

Pickled food. Studies from different parts of the world [120, 131] have reported increased gastric cancer risk among individuals frequently consuming pickled food, including vegetables. This type of food may be containing N-nitroso compounds and benzopyrenes [120].

Smoked, fried, grilled food. During incomplete combustion of organic material, what can take place also while smoking or frying foodstaff over an open fire, polycyclic aromatic hydrocarbons are formed; many of them are regarded carcinogenic in humans [120].

All the three case-control studies addressing the relation of gastric cancer to smoked food that were included in the systemic review by P.Jakszyn et al. [114] have indicated positive relation between the above.

Several more recent studies not included analysis have supported this association [111,126,132]. A case control study from hight gastric cancer incidence area in India, where the food habits are different from the major part of this country has revealed that frequent consumption of smoked dried salted meat and fish increased the risk for gastric cancer signidicantly (OR 2.8 and 2.5, respectively).

The effect of grilling, broiling and flying seem to be more controversial.

Broiling and grilling have been reported to increase the disease risk in some studies [112,133], but not in the others [134].

Similarly there is no common agreement in respect whether frying itself is linked to gastric cancer. Controversial data from case control studies are available even from the same geographical area. In Shanhai urban inhabitants frying was identified a risk factor aline with smoking and pickling [111], while in Korea frying tended to decrease the risk [135].

Fruit and vegetables. In 1997 World Cancer Research Fund – American Institute for Cancer Research international expert panel stated that there is convincing evidence that high intake of vegetables, particularly raw and allium vegetables, reduces the risk of gastric cancer [136]. Similarly also high fruit consumption is considered to have a beneficial effect. This protection of the plant foods have been attributed to their high concentrations of antioxidant substances, notably carotenoids, vitamin C and vitamin E compounds [120].

A more recent meta-analysis [137] also supported the overall positive effect of fruit and vegetables (the overall relative risk was 0.81; 95% CI 0.75-0.87 of vegetables and 0.74; 95% CI 0.69-0.81 for fruit; calculated for 100 g daily intake each), yet the effect was more pronounced in case-control than cohort studies possibly related to recall and selection biases in case-control studies.

However the recent European multinational cohort within the EPIC study with data collected from 10 European countries [138] in overall failed to find the protective role of vegetables and fruit in respect to gastric cancer. A negative, but non-convincing association was found only for intestinal type cancer and total vegetable, onion and garlic intake. A negative, but not-significant association was found between citrus fruit intake and the cardia site cancer.

A recent case-control study in Canada [139] involving 1169 gastric cancer cases and 2332 controls revealed that increased consumption of fruits, vegetables, and fish were associated with lessened risk, but dietary patterns characterized by Western features (soft drinks, processed meats, refined grains, and sugars) were associated with increased risk of gastric adenocarcinoma.

Several case-control studies from Asia have indicated that increased use of beans, including soybeans in the food-stuffs correlate to lower risk for gastric cancer development [111,112,133].

N-nitroso compounds (NOCs) are found to be carcinogenic in multiple organs in animals, and also there are indications that these compounds are carcinogenic in humans, first of all, in relation to the gastric cancer. The major source of NOCs in humans is food – processed meats, smoked preserved foods, picled and salty preserved foods, foods dried at high temperatures (such as constuents of beer, whisky, and dried milk), tobacco smoke and drinking water, but typically at least half of NOCs come from endogenous synthesis

[120,140]. In western countries the amount of volatile N-nitrosamines declined in recent years; higher concentrations of nitrosamines are found in Asian than western foods [141]. A study in Kashmir, India indicated that the major sources of N-nitrosamines in this area were smoked fish, sun-dried spinach, sun-dried pumpkin, and dried, mixed vegetables [142].

Large proportion (typically over 50%) of nitrosamines is formed endogenously from nitrate and nitrite. The main source for nitrates is vegetables and water.

Nitrites are either ingested with food or produced endogenously. Sodium nitrites are food preservatives, mainly used to preserve meet. Although the use of the preservatives have declined over years, they are still widely used preservatives. Endogenous nitrites are produced by the reduction of salivary nitrates in the presence of the oral microflora.

When the nitrite in saliva encounter gastric juice, nitrous acid and nitrosating species, including nitric oxide are produced [143,144]. By reacting to thiocyanate from saliva nitric oxide forms potent nitrosating species that are are able to react with variety of organic nitrogenous compounds to generate NOCs [143,144].

In Thailand with low incidence of gastric cancer, in general there is significantly higher incidence of this cancer North and Northeast Thailand, and a recent study [145] has suggested linkage to increased daily dietary intake of nitrate, nitrite, and nitrosodimethylamine in these areas.

It has been suggested that higher concentrations of NOCs are found in gastric juice in patients with pre-malignant lesions for gastric cancer, in particular – in the presence of dysplasia [114,146], but this has not been proved in other studies [147].

Systemic analysis by P.Jakszyn and A.Gonzales [114] has confirmed the positive association between nitrite and nitrosamine intake and gastric cancer, still the authors consider that this association still is not conclusive. Five of seven case controled studies on nitrates and 4 of 5 on nitrosamines showed the possitive association, while statistical significance was reached in 3 studies in each of the groups [114].

Considering the potential negative impact of increased food nitrate and the protective effect of antioxidants, H.J. Kim et el. [148] have suggested that decrease in the intake of nitrate relative to antioxidants may have more effect on preventing gastric cancer than either a lower absolute nitrate or higher intake of antioxidant vitamins alone.

Antioxidants and phytochemicals are inhibiting the intragastric formation of N-nitroso compunds, and through this mechanism are suggested to be protective against gastric cancer [149,150]. The key factor protecting against the process of NOCs production by the nitrosating species is ascorbic acid that is secreted in the gastric juice [151].

Two of the studies – one from South America, the other from China favour antioxidant treatment. A study by P.Correa [152] in Columbia demonstrated significant regression or atrophy and intestinal metaplasia in patients receiving ascorbic acid and ß-carotene. The regression was similar to the one seen in patients having received *H.pylori* eradication therapy. At the same time this was confusing that the combination of antioxidants and eradication therapy did not provide any further benefit to the patients. A study from China [153] was suggestive for the protective role of ß-carotene, vitamin E and selenium may have role to reduce cancer-related mortality, including in respect to the stomach cancer. Close to 30 000 adult individuals were asigned for one of four treatment arms, still there was no pacebo-controlled arm in this study.

A relatively small randomized placebo-controlled study [154] on 216 patients with atrophic gastritis was conducted in China to evaluate the protective effect of folate, natural ß-carotene and synthetic beta-carotene in preventing gastric cancer over the follow-up period of 7 years. The study failed to reach statistical significane in respect to preventing gastric cancer, if the treatment groups were analysed separately, still patients having received folic acid reversed atrophy and inflammation, and even displasia.

Contrary to the above number of other interventional studies failed to reproduce the data on the protective effect of most frequesntly used antioxidants for gastric cancer development.

In a randomised, double blind, placebo-controlled study with ß-carotene in more than 11 000 US male physicians [155] in each of the groups and follow-up for a 12 year period, there was no effect of ß-carotene supplementation seen in preventing gastric, nor other malignant neoplasms. In a similar size randomised controlled trial in Finland α-tocopherol and ß-carotene in 5-8 year treatment were not found to have protective effect in respect to gastric cancer among male smokers [156,157].

Negative results were obtained in a placebo-controlled randomised trial in a high gastric cancer incidence area – Linqu County, Shandong Province of China, where neither vitamin C and vitamin E, nor garlic extract or garlic oil within 7.3 years showed beneficial effect on the prevalence of precancerous gastric lesions or on gastric cancer incidence [94].

Another placebo-controlled study in a high-risk population of Venezuela was addressing the protective effect of vitamin C, vitamin E and ß-carotene on the status of precancerous gastric lesions [158]. The majority of the study population had pre-malignant lesions at the inclusion, i.e. 44% of the patients were with multifocal atrophic gastritis, 31% had intestinal metaplasia, but 1% - dysplasia. The obtained results after a 3 year treatment from 678 individuals having completed the active treatment and 705 individuals in the placebo arm did not support the beneficial effect of the tested antioxidants upon the regression of precancerous lesions.

In summary, the present evidence does not support the benefit of the most widely used and available antioxidants (ascorbic acid, α-tocopherol and ß-carotene) in preventing gastric cancer. This does not exclude the potential beneficial effect of these antioxidants, if used for a longer duration, or the beneficial effect of other antioxidants.

Socioeconomic Factors

Lower social class and worse economic conditions, in particular in childhood have been attributed to increased risk of gastric cancer development. Since these factors are oftain related lo worse hygene in the families, the impact of these factors to a great extend may be related to better transmission possibilities for *H.pylori* infection.

In the EPIGAST [159] study incolving patients from West and South European countries educational level was used to characterize the socioeconomic position. Higher education was significantly associated with a reduced risk of gastric cancer when compared to individuals with lower education (hazard ratio (HR) 0.64, 95% CI 0.43-0.98, and this effect was more pronounced for cancer of the cardia: HR 0.42; 95% CI: 0.20-0.89 and for intestinal rather than diffise histological subtype). When the results were adjusted for *H.pylori* infection in a nested case-control study, inverse but statistically non-significant associations were found [159].

In a multicenter, population-based study in the United States [106] either the level of education or the yearly income level were used to describe the socioeconomic level. Either for the cancer in gastric cardia or for non-cardia stomach cancers the trend was present that individuals with higher education and higher income had lower risk of both cancer types. Similar results were obtained in a prospective cohort study in the Netherlands [160], where men with the highest attained level of education were found to have lower risk for either the cardia or non-cardia cancers.

A prospective study in Norway [161] has found the link between the childhood socioeconomic position desribed by parients' occupational classs and income, and gastric cancer caused mortality between the age of 41 and 61; more frequent gastric cancer was the cause of death in families with father performing manual work, this was more evident in men. The role of the childhood socioeconomic conditions in respect to the gastric cancer caused mortality on a population level has been addressed in a study within 7 Europeans countries with substantial differences in the mortality rates. The trends in the mortalily, althogh declining in general, have been well related to infant mortality rate and gross domestic product (GDP) at the time of birth [162]. Similar results have been obtained also in other studies [163,164]. Additionally to the above, data from Finland suggest that in Europe the gastric cancer incidence over time has decreased in both the genders and in all social classes, still sustaining the large differences between social classes [165].

Migrations

In the persons from high risk areas having emigrated to low risk areas the cancer development risk is still remaining increased, still in consecutive generations the risk is diminishing. Immigration of populations with high incidence of stomach cancer could be an important aspect that has to be considered in areas to low incidence areas since different management and follow-up strategies might be required in these populations.

The above has been demonstrated in Japanese populations having emigrated to the America continent [166,167], Koreans emigrating to the United States [168] as well as in some European populations.

An interesting and not fully understood trend has been explaind in Inuit populations (originally living in Arctic, Greenland) having immigrated to Denmark [169]. Those Inuits having lived in Denmark for less than 20 years were found to have substantially higher gastric cancer incidence than the ones never having lived in Greenland (and the authors consider that this is not linked to the availability of endocospy services); still for the individuals having lived in Denmark for more than 20 years, the gastric cancer incidence was lower [169].

Although the total cancer caused mortality was lower in migrants to the Netherlands, gastric cancer was one of the cancers that was causing higher mortality among the first-generation immigrants (relative risk 1.16; 95% CI 0.96-1.40) [170]. In Germany even larger mortality difference was found between the German population and immigrants from former Soviet Union, mostly Russians [171]. In 2002 Russian males had 2.95, but females 2.24 higher risk to develop gastric cancer if compared to the German population.

Occupational and Toxic Exposure

Several studies have been addressing professional or other toxic exposures as the potential risk factor for gastric cancer.

A large cohort (n = 413,877) of female workers born 1906 through 1945 was followed in Finland, and the incident cancer cases were explored during 1971 to 1995. Association with exposure to *electromagnetic fields* (RR at the medium/high level of exposure 1.44, 95% CI 1.01-2.05) and *man-made vitreous fibres* (p trend 0.03) was reported in respect to the gastric cancer (altogether 1881 cases) [172].

K.Steenland and P.Boffetta [173] have reviewed the *lead* exposure impact to cancer mortality; eight studies of cancer mortality or incidence among highly exposed workers were included, most being cohort studies on lead smelter or battery workers exposed decades ago. Relative risk increase of 1.34 (OR 1.14-1.57) was reported by this meta-analysis in respect to the gastric cancer. The authors conclude that the data are suggestive, but not conclusive. Furthermore the study of M.C. Rousseau and colleagues reported correlation of gastric cancer either to organic lead or exposure to lead in gasoline emissions, yet no association with inorganic lead [174].

Controversial results in respect to lead exposure as the risk for gastric cancer are available from case-control studies. A cohort analysis of 4,518 workers at lead battery plants and 2,300 at lead smelters in the United States [175] indicated significant increase of gastric cancer caused mortality in this group when compared to the expected figures, at the same time, based on the analyses in the cohort study and the nested case-control study, the authors failed to prove that this increase was related to lead exposure. Cocco et al. [176] found a significant (60%) increase in the risk for cardia cancer in males having had exposure to high levels of lead. Some other case-control studies also suggest a positive association [177,178].

The exposure to *benzopyrene* in the aluminium industry in Canada has been reported to be related to gastric cancer [179].

A study in Japan has indicated increased risk of gastric cancer (age and smoking adjusted OR 1.22; 95% CI 0.74-2.01) being related to silica exposure at work [180].

By studying altogether 4 552 male workers in Sardinia, Italy having been exposed to dichlorodiphenyltrichloroethane (*DDT*) during antimalarial operations between 1946 and 1950, a two-fold increase of gastric cancer caused mortality (relative risk, 2.0; 95% confidence interval, 0.9-4.4) was revealed, but no exposure-response trend was observed [181].

A study involving considerable number of gastric cancer cases (443) addressing the risk of gastric adenocarcinoma by grouped occupations and industries, as well as by some specific occupational exposures has been conducted in Poland [182]. Only few occupations and industries were associated with significantly increased risks of stomach cancer, out of which the highest risk was found in *leather industry* (OR 5.1; 95% CI 1.0-25.0 in males and OR 3.1; 95% CI 0.7-14.9 in females), but also the risk was significantly higher among men working in fabricated metal production and among women ever employed as managers and governmental officials. On the other hand, 10 or more years exposure to asbestos, metal dust, and nitrosamines did not increase the risk of gastric cancer in male.

Dry cleaners, in particular during the period tetrachloroethylene was extensively used have been suggested to be at increased risk for upper digestive system, still the data are conflicting. Data based on the records of the Swedish Cancer register [183] suggest that gastric cancer incidence may be increased among cleaning, laundry and ironing male workers (RR 1.80,95% CI 1.05-3.11). This was not confirmed by another study, also in the Nordic area [184] that did not reveal increase in gastric cardia cancers.

Industrial dust has been suggested to be related not only to cancers of respiratory system, but also gastric cancer. In a prospective cohort study of 256,357 in Sweden contributing 5,378,012 person-years at risk, altogether 948 noncardia gastric cancers were identified [185]; increased risk for the cancer (incidence rate ratios (IRR) and 95% confidence intervals) was found among workers exposed to cement dust (IRR 1.5; 95% CI 1.1-2.1), quartz dust (IRR 1.3; 95% CI 1.0-1.7) and diesel exhaust (IRR 1.4; 95% CI 1.1-1.9); these correlations were dose-dependent. Silicon carbide fibres in the industrial dust may also be attributed to increased risk of gastric cancer [186].

A meta-analysis of cohort studies to determine whether there was excessive risk of cancer among workers exposed to *chrysotile asbestos* was performed by L.Li et al. [187], who found significantly increased risk of gastric cancer among asbestos product manufacturers (pooled standardized mortality ratio 1.49, p<0.05). Asbestos may also be injected with drinking water contaminated with asbestos from natural sources or asbestos-cement containing water pipes. K. Kjaerheim et al. [188] has observed increased gastric cancer incidence in individuals with asbestos exposure with drinking water in Norway. Contrary a study from Australia did not confirm that past exposure to crocidolite (blue asbestos) is related to gastric cancer or other gastrointestinal cancers [189].

Several studies have reported increased incidence and mortality of gastric cancer among *rubber industry* workers. In the United Kingdom rubber industry workers were not found to have increased risk for gastric cancer development [190]. The study performed in Germany did not identify increased gastric cancer risk in rubber industry workers with exposure to high concentrations of nitrosamines [191], but considered talc and asbestos combined dust to be responsible for increased risk of gastric cancer among this profession (RR 1.8, 95% CI: 0.9, 3.8 for medium exposure; RR 2.7, 95% CI: 1.0, 7.1 for high exposure) [192].

Also *road-paving workers* in France had increased trend to have higher mortality of gastric cancer (RR 2.8, 95% CI (0.7-11.4) [193], yet there was no significant gastric cancer incidence revealed among this profession in the Nordic countries [194].

Nickel exposure has not been confirmed to be related to gastric cancer in male workers, moreover mortality was only 50% (observed 8, expected 16.0) of the expected in respect to this type of cancer [195]. *Cadmium* exposure also is also considered equivocal in respect to development of gastric cancer [196].

A nested case-cohort study has been conducted among textile-industry workers in China [197], 646 workers with incident stomach cancer were enrolled in the group. The authors report that the cumulative exposure to *endotoxin*, a contaminant of cotton dust, was inversely related to risk of gastric cancer (p-trend < 0.001) when exposures were lagged 20 years, and suggest further study on the potentially protective role of endotoxin.

According to the results of meta-analysis in 350,000 workers from several western countries, no mortality increase of digestive cancers, including gastric cancer has been observed in *petroleum industry*. Exposure to *ethylene oxide* [198] or *polychlorinated biphenyls* (PCBs) [199] has not been proven to correlate to gastric cancer.

Number of publications have addressed potentially increased risk of the cancer also among woodworking industry related professions [200], dye and resin manufacturers [201], in pulp and paper-mill workers [202] and capacitor manufacturing workers [203].

In Sweden manual workers and farmers have been found to be at increased risk for gastric cancer [204]. Also other studies have indicated that farm workers may be at increased risk of gastric cancer. The agricultural workers may be exposed to potentially toxic chemicals. P.K.Mills and R.C.Yang have reported the association of gastric cancer with the use of the acaricide propargite and the herbicide triflurin (OR 2.86; 95% CI 1.56-5.23 and 1.69; 95% CI 0.99-2.89, respectively) in Hispanic farm workers in California [205].

Therefore several occupational exposures with either dust or inorganic and organic substances are reported to be related to some, but not major increase in gastric cancer incidence and mortality. The incidence and mortality in many of the studies have been compared to the corresponding parameters of the respective populations or unexposed individuals of the region. Still the influence of other factors cannot be excluded in many cases, in particular – the influence of socioeconomic factors.

This should be considered that there might be situations, when the lifestyle rather than exposure to toxic factors may be the cause for increased gastric cancer risk among several professions. In the case-control analysis by P.Cocco [176] in the United States the occupation with the highest risk for cancer of the cardia among males was found to be financial managers (OR 6.1; 95% CI: 1.3-28.8), but in Poland the professions at increased risk for gastric cancer among female were managers and governmental officials [182].

REFERENCES

[1]   World Health Organization Statistical Information System. WHO Mortality data base. 2007; accessed November 15, 2008. Web Page.

[2]   Ferlay J, Bray F, Pisani P, Parkin DM. GLOBOCAN 2002. Cancer incidence, mortality and prevalence worldwide. *IARC CancerBase, No.5, Version 2.0. Lyon: IARCPress, 2004*. Notes: (http://www-depdb.iarc.fr/globoscan2002.htm)

[3]   Parkin DM, Bray F, Ferlay J, Pisani P. Global cancer statistics, 2002. *CA Cancer J Clin.* 2005;55:74-108.

[4]   Hamilton SR, Aaltonen LA. *Tumours of the Digestive System. Pathology & Genetics.* Lyon: IARC Press; 2000.

[5]   Lauren P. The two histological main types of gastric carcinoma: diffuse and so-called intestinal-type carcinoma. An attempt at a histo-clinical classification. *Acta Pathol Microbiol Scand.* 1965;64:31-49.

[6]   Lee KH, Lee JH, Cho JK, et al. A prospective correlation of Lauren's histological classification of stomach cancer with clinicopathological findings including DNA flow cytometry. *Pathol Res Pract.* 2001;197:223-9.

[7]   Carneiro F, Moutinho C, Pera G, et al. Pathology findings and validation of gastric and esophageal cancer cases in a European cohort (EPIC/EUR-GAST). *Scand J Gastroenterol.* 2007;42:618-27.

[8]   Hattori T. Morphological range of hyperplastic polyps and carcinomas arising in hyperplastic polyps of the stomach. *J Clin Pathol.* 1985;38:622-30.

[9]   Bamba M, Sugihara H, Kushima R, et al. Time-dependent expression of intestinal phenotype in signet ring cell carcinomas of the human stomach. *Virchows Arch.* 2001;438:49-56.

[10]   Meining A, Morgner A, Miehlke S, Bayerdorffer E, Stolte M. Atrophy-metaplasia-dysplasia-carcinoma sequence in the stomach: a reality or merely an hypothesis? *Best Pract Res Clin Gastroenterol.* 2001;15:983-98.

[11] Carneiro F, Seixas M, Sobrinho-Simoes M. New elements for an updated classification of the carcinomas of the stomach. *Pathol Res Pract.* 1995;191:571-84.

[12] Japanese Gastric Cancer Association. Japanese Classification of Gastric Carcinoma - 2nd English Edition -. *Gastric Cancer.* 1998;1:10-24.

[13] Schlemper RJ, Riddell RH, Kato Y, et al. The Vienna classification of gastrointestinal epithelial neoplasia. *Gut.* 2000;47:251-5.

[14] Misumi A, Murakami A, Harada K, Baba K, Akagi M. Definition of carcinoma of the gastric cardia. *Langenbecks Arch Chir.* 1989;374:221-6.

[15] Ferlay J, Autier P, Boniol M, Heanue M, Colombet M, Boyle P. Estimates of the cancer incidence and mortality in Europe in 2006. *Ann Oncol.* 2007;18:581-92.

[16] Aksel EM, Davidov MI, Usakova TI. (Malignant tumours of gastrointestinal tract: the main statistical indicators and trends). *Sovremennaja Onkologia (in Russian).* 2001;3:http://www.consilium-medicum.com/media/onkology/01_04/141.shtml.

[17] Vaktskjold A, Lebedintseva JA, Korotov DS, Tkatsjov AV, Podjakova TS, Lund E. Cancer incidence in Arkhangelskaja Oblast in northwestern Russia. The Arkhangelsk Cancer Registry. *BMC Cancer.* 2005;5:82.

[18] Segal I, Ally R, Mitchell H. Gastric cancer in sub-Saharan Africa. *Eur J Cancer Prev.* 2001;10:479-82.

[19] Lunet N, Barros H. Helicobacter pylori infection and gastric cancer: facing the enigmas. *Int J Cancer.* 2003;106:953-60.

[20] Correa P, Piazuelo MB. Natural history of Helicobacter pylori infection. *Dig Liver Dis.* 2008;40:490-6.

[21] Bravo LE, van Doom LJ, Realpe JL, Correa P. Virulence-associated genotypes of Helicobacter pylori: do they explain the African enigma? *Am J Gastroenterol.* 2002;97:2839-42.

[22] Fox JG, Beck P, Dangler CA, et al. Concurrent enteric helminth infection modulates inflammation and gastric immune responses and reduces helicobacter-induced gastric atrophy. *Nat Med.* 2000;6:536-42.

[23] Agha A, Graham DY. Evidence-based examination of the African enigma in relation to Helicobacter pylori infection. *Scand J Gastroenterol.* 2005;40:523-9.

[24] Nguyen LT, Uchida T, Murakami K, Fujioka T, Moriyama M. Helicobacter pylori virulence and the diversity of gastric cancer in Asia. *J Med Microbiol.* 2008;57:1445-53.

[25] Singh K, Ghoshal UC. Causal role of Helicobacter pylori infection in gastric cancer: an Asian enigma. *World J Gastroenterol.* 2006;12:1346-51.

[26] Yamagata H, Kiyohara Y, Aoyagi K, et al. Impact of Helicobacter pylori infection on gastric cancer incidence in a general Japanese population: the Hisayama study. *Arch Intern Med.* 2000;160:1962-8.

[27] Miwa H, Go MF, Sato N. H. pylori and gastric cancer: the Asian enigma. *Am J Gastroenterol.* 2002;97:1106-12.

[28] Ahmad MM, Rahman M, Rumi AK, et al. Prevalence of Helicobacter pylori in asymptomatic population--a pilot serological study in Bangladesh. *J Epidemiol.* 1997;7:251-4.

[29] Graham DY, Adam E, Reddy GT, et al. Seroepidemiology of Helicobacter pylori infection in India. Comparison of developing and developed countries. *Dig Dis Sci.* 1991;36:1084-8.

[30]   Gill HH, Majmudar P, Shankaran K, Desai HG. Age-related prevalence of Helicobacter pylori antibodies in Indian subjects. *Indian J Gastroenterol.* 1994;13:92-4.

[31]   Wong BC, Lam SK, Ching CK, et al. Differential Helicobacter pylori infection rates in two contrasting gastric cancer risk regions of South China. China Gastric Cancer Study Group. *J Gastroenterol Hepatol.* 1999;14:120-5.

[32]   You WC, Chang YS, Heinrich J, et al. An intervention trial to inhibit the progression of precancerous gastric lesions: compliance, serum micronutrients and S-allyl cysteine levels, and toxicity. *Eur J Cancer Prev.* 2001;10:257-63.

[33]   Chen SY, Liu TY, Chen MJ, Lin JT, Sheu JC, Chen CJ. Seroprevalences of hepatitis B and C viruses and Helicobacter pylori infection in a small, isolated population at high risk of gastric and liver cancer. *Int J Cancer.* 1997;71:776-9.

[34]   Liu CY, Wu CY, Lin JT, Lee YC, Yen AM, Chen TH. Multistate and multifactorial progression of gastric cancer: results from community-based mass screening for gastric cancer. *J Med Screen.* 2006;13 Suppl 1:S2-5.

[35]   Azuma T, Yamazaki S, Yamakawa A, et al. Association between diversity in the Src homology 2 domain--containing tyrosine phosphatase binding site of Helicobacter pylori CagA protein and gastric atrophy and cancer. *J Infect Dis.* 2004;189:820-7.

[36]   Crew KD, Neugut AI. Epidemiology of gastric cancer. *World J Gastroenterol.* 2006;12:354-62.

[37]   Tsubono Y, Hisamichi S. Screening for gastric cancer in Japan. *Gastric Cancer.* 2000;3:9-18.

[38]   Ohata H, Kitauchi S, Yoshimura N, et al. Progression of chronic atrophic gastritis associated with Helicobacter pylori infection increases risk of gastric cancer. *Int J Cancer.* 2004;109:138-43.

[39]   Verdecchia A, Francisci S, Brenner H, et al. Recent cancer survival in Europe: a 2000-02 period analysis of EUROCARE-4 data. *Lancet Oncol.* 2007;8:784-96.

[40]   Parkin DM, Bray FI, Devesa SS. Cancer burden in the year 2000. The global picture. *Eur J Cancer.* 2001;37 Suppl 8:S4-66.

[41]   Parkin DM, Pisani P, Ferlay J. Estimates of the worldwide incidence of eighteen major cancers in 1985. *Int J Cancer.* 1993;54:594-606.

[42]   Parkin DM. The global health burden of infection-associated cancers in the year 2002. *Int J Cancer.* 2006;118:3030-44.

[43]   Bosetti C, Bertuccio P, Levi F, Lucchini F, Negri E, La Vecchia C. Cancer mortality in the European Union, 1970-2003, with a joinpoint analysis. *Ann Oncol.* 2008;19:631-40.

[44]   Smailyte G, Kurtinaitis J. Cancer mortality differences among urban and rural residents in Lithuania. *BMC Public Health.* 2008;8:56.

[45]   Ekstrom AM, Hansson LE, Signorello LB, Lindgren A, Bergstrom R, Nyren O. Decreasing incidence of both major histologic subtypes of gastric adenocarcinoma--a population-based study in Sweden. *Br J Cancer.* 2000;83:391-6.

[46]   Kinsella K, Velkoff VA. An Aging World: 2001. *U.S. Census Bureau, Series P95/01-1, U.S. Government Printing Offica, Washington D.C.* 2001.

[47]   Kent MM, Mather M. What Drives U.S. Population Growth? *Population Bull.* 2002;57:1-40.

[48] Yancik R. Population aging and cancer: a cross-national concern. *Cancer J.* 2005;11:437-41.

[49] Imamura Y, Yoshimi I. Comparison of Cancer Mortality (Stomach Cancer) in Five Countries: France, Italy, Japan, UK and USA from the WHO Mortality Database (1960-2000). *Jpn J Clin Oncol.* 2005;35:103-5.

[50] Weck MN, Brenner H. Prevalence of chronic atrophic gastritis in different parts of the world. *Cancer Epidemiol Biomarkers Prev.* 2006;15:1083-94.

[51] Webb PM, Hengels KJ, Moller H, et al. The epidemiology of low serum pepsinogen A levels and an international association with gastric cancer rates. EUROGAST Study Group. *Gastroenterology.* 1994;107 :1335-44.

[52] Sipponen P, Kekki M, Haapakoski J, Ihamaki T, Siurala M. Gastric cancer risk in chronic atrophic gastritis: statistical calculations of cross-sectional data. *Int J Cancer.* 1985;35:173-7.

[53] Sipponen P, Correa P. Delayed rise in incidence of gastric cancer in females results in unique sex ratio (M/F) pattern: etiologic hypothesis. *Gastric Cancer.* 2002;5:213-9.

[54] Malfertheiner P, Megraud F, O'Morain C, et al. Current concepts in the management of Helicobacter pylori infection: the Maastricht III Consensus Report. *Gut.* 2007;56:772-81.

[55] Bacani JT, Soares M, Zwingerman R, et al. CDH1/E-cadherin germline mutations in early-onset gastric cancer. *J Med Genet.* 2006;43:867-72.

[56] Clark GW, Smyrk TC, Burdiles P, et al. Is Barrett's metaplasia the source of adenocarcinomas of the cardia? *Arch Surg.* 1994;129:609-14.

[57] Powell J, McConkey CC. The rising trend in oesophageal adenocarcinoma and gastric cardia. *Eur J Cancer Prev.* 1992;1:265-9.

[58] Botterweck AA, Schouten LJ, Volovics A, Dorant E, van Den Brandt PA. Trends in incidence of adenocarcinoma of the oesophagus and gastric cardia in ten European countries. *Int J Epidemiol.* 2000;29:645-54.

[59] Blot WJ, Devesa SS, Kneller RW, Fraumeni JF Jr. Rising incidence of adenocarcinoma of the esophagus and gastric cardia. *JAMA.* 1991;265:1287-9.

[60] Kim R, Weissfeld JL, Reynolds JC, Kuller LH. Etiology of Barrett's metaplasia and esophageal adenocarcinoma. *Cancer Epidemiol Biomarkers Prev.* 1997;6:369-77.

[61] van Blankenstein M, Looman CW, Siersema PD, Kuipers EJ, Coebergh JW. Trends in the incidence of adenocarcinoma of the oesophagus and cardia in the Netherlands 1989-2003. *Br J Cancer.* 2007;96:1767-71.

[62] Falk J, Carstens H, Lundell L, Albertsson M. Incidence of carcinoma of the oesophagus and gastric cardia. Changes over time and geographical differences. *Acta Oncol.* 2007;46:1070-4.

[63] Ekstrom AM, Signorello LB, Hansson LE, Bergstrom R, Lindgren A, Nyren O. Evaluating gastric cancer misclassification: a potential explanation for the rise in cardia cancer incidence. *J Natl Cancer Inst.* 1999;91:786-90.

[64] Henson DE, Dittus C, Younes M, Nguyen H, Albores-Saavedra J. Differential trends in the intestinal and diffuse types of gastric carcinoma in the United States, 1973-2000: increase in the signet ring cell type. *Arch Pathol Lab Med.* 2004;128:765-70.

[65] Kaneko S, Yoshimura T. Time trend analysis of gastric cancer incidence in Japan by histological types, 1975-1989. *Br J Cancer.* 2001;84:400-5.

[66] Correa P, Chen VW. Gastric cancer. *Cancer Surv.* 1994;19-20:55-76.

[67] Borch K, Jonsson B, Tarpila E, et al. Changing pattern of histological type, location, stage and outcome of surgical treatment of gastric carcinoma. *Br J Surg.* 2000;87:618-26.

[68] Ohta H, Noguchi Y, Takagi K, Nishi M, Kajitani T, Kato Y. Early gastric carcinoma with special reference to macroscopic classification. *Cancer.* 1987;60:1099-106.

[69] Hisamichi S, Sugawara N. Mass screening for gastric cancer by X-ray examination. *Jpn J Clin Oncol.* 1984;14:211-23.

[70] Green PH, O'Toole KM, Weinberg LM, Goldfarb JP. Early gastric cancer. *Gastroenterology.* 1981;81:247-56.

[71] Carter KJ, Schaffer HA, Ritchie WP Jr. Early gastric cancer. *Ann Surg.* 1984;199:604-9.

[72] Dixon MF. Gastrointestinal epithelial neoplasia: Vienna revisited. *Gut.* 2002;51:130-1.

[73] Naylor GM, Gotoda T, Dixon M, et al. Why does Japan have a high incidence of gastric cancer? Comparison of gastritis between UK and Japanese patients. *Gut.* 2006;55:1545-52.

[74] Prinz C, Schwendy S, Voland P. H pylori and gastric cancer: shifting the global burden. *World J Gastroenterol.* 2006;12:5458-64.

[75] Sipponen P. Helicobacter pylori gastritis--epidemiology. *J Gastroenterol .* 1997;32:273-7.

[76] International Agency for Research on Cancer. Schistosomes, liver flukes and Helicobacter pylori. IARC Working Group on the Evaluation of Carcinogenic Risks to Humans. Lyon, 7-14 June 1994. *IARC Monogr Eval Carcinog Risks Hum.* 1994;61:1-241.

[77] Uemura N, Okamoto S, Yamamoto S, et al. Helicobacter pylori infection and the development of gastric cancer. *N Engl J Med.* 2001;345:784-9.

[78] Kuipers EJ. Review article: exploring the link between Helicobacter pylori and gastric cancer. *Aliment Pharmacol Ther.* 1999;13 Suppl 1:3-11.

[79] Helicobacter and Cancer Collaborative Group. Gastric cancer and Helicobacter pylori: a combined analysis of 12 case control studies nested within prospective cohorts. *Gut.* 2001;49:347-53.

[80] Brenner H, Arndt V, Stegmaier C, Ziegler H, Rothenbacher D. Is Helicobacter pylori infection a necessary condition for noncardia gastric cancer? *Am J Epidemiol.* 2004;159:252-8.

[81] Ekstrom AM, Held M, Hansson LE, Engstrand L, Nyren O. Helicobacter pylori in gastric cancer established by CagA immunoblot as a marker of past infection. *Gastroenterology.* 2001;121:784-91.

[82] Kamangar F, Dawsey SM, Blaser MJ, et al. Opposing risks of gastric cardia and noncardia gastric adenocarcinomas associated with Helicobacter pylori seropositivity. *J Natl Cancer Inst.* 2006;98:1445-52.

[83] Aromaa A, Kosunen TU, Knekt P, et al. Circulating anti-Helicobacter pylori immunoglobulin A antibodies and low serum pepsinogen I level are associated with increased risk of gastric cancer. *Am J Epidemiol.* 1996;144:142-9.

[84] Sande N, Nikulin M, Nilsson I, et al. Increased risk of developing atrophic gastritis in patients infected with CagA+ Helicobacter pylori. *Scand J Gastroenterol.* 2001;36:928-33.

[85]   Annibale B, Negrini R, Caruana P, et al. Two-thirds of atrophic body gastritis patients have evidence of Helicobacter pylori infection. *Helicobacter.* 2001;6:225-33.

[86]   de Vries AC, Haringsma J, Kuipers EJ. The detection, surveillance and treatment of premalignant gastric lesions related to Helicobacter pylori infection. *Helicobacter.* 2007;12:1-15.

[87]   Inoue M, Tajima K, Matsuura A, et al. Severity of chronic atrophic gastritis and subsequent gastric cancer occurrence: a 10-year prospective cohort study in Japan. *Cancer Lett.* 2000;161:105-12.

[88]   Kakinoki R, Kushima R, Matsubara A, et al. Re-evaluation of Histogenesis of Gastric Carcinomas: A Comparative Histopathological Study Between Helicobacter pylori-Negative and H. pylori-Positive Cases. *Dig Dis Sci.* 2009 Mar;54(3):614-20.

[89]   Correa P. A human model of gastric carcinogenesis. *Cancer Res.* 1988;48:3554-3560.

[90]   Filipe MI, Munoz N, Matko I, et al. Intestinal metaplasia types and the risk of gastric cancer: a cohort study in Slovenia. *Int J Cancer.* 1994;57:324-9.

[91]   de Vries AC, van Grieken NC, Looman CW, et al. Gastric cancer risk in patients with premalignant gastric lesions: a nationwide cohort study in the Netherlands. *Gastroenterology.* 2008;134:945-52.

[92]   Abraham SC, Singh VK, Yardley JH, Wu TT. Hyperplastic polyps of the stomach: associations with histologic patterns of gastritis and gastric atrophy. *Am J Surg Pathol.* 2001;25:500-7.

[93]   Jain R, Chetty R. Gastric Hyperplastic Polyps: A Review. *Dig Dis Sci.* 2009 Sep;54(9):1839-46.

[94]   You WC, Brown LM, Zhang L, et al. Randomized double-blind factorial trial of three treatments to reduce the prevalence of precancerous gastric lesions. *J Natl Cancer Inst.* 2006;98:974-83.

[95]   Srivastava A, Lauwers GY. Gastric epithelial dysplasia: the Western perspective. *Dig Liver Dis.* 2008;40:641-9.

[96]   Fock KM, Talley N, Moayyedi P, et al. Asia-Pacific consensus guidelines on gastric cancer prevention. *J Gastroenterol Hepatol.* 2008;23:351-65.

[97]   Wong BC, Lam SK, Wong WM, et al. Helicobacter pylori eradication to prevent gastric cancer in a high-risk region of China: a randomized controlled trial. *JAMA.* 2004;291:187-94.

[98]   Cai X, Carlson J, Stoicov C, Li H, Wang TC, Houghton J. Helicobacter felis eradication restores normal architecture and inhibits gastric cancer progression in C57BL/6 mice. *Gastroenterology.* 2005;128:1937-52.

[99]   Watari J, Das KK, Amenta PS, et al. Effect of eradication of Helicobacter pylori on the histology and cellular phenotype of gastric intestinal metaplasia. *Clin Gastroenterol Hepatol.* 2008;6:409-17.

[100] Tersmette AC, Offerhaus GJ, Tersmette KW, et al. Meta-analysis of the risk of gastric stump cancer: detection of high risk patient subsets for stomach cancer after remote partial gastrectomy for benign conditions. *Cancer Res.* 1990;50:6486-9.

[101] Lundegardh G, Adami HO, Helmick C, Zack M, Meirik O. Stomach cancer after partial gastrectomy for benign ulcer disease. *N Engl J Med.* 1988;319:195-200.

[102] Whary MT, Sundina N, Bravo LE, et al. Intestinal helminthiasis in Colombian children promotes a Th2 response to Helicobacter pylori: possible implications for gastric carcinogenesis. *Cancer Epidemiol Biomarkers Prev.* 2005;14:1464-9.

[103] Tredaniel J, Boffetta P, Buiatti E, Saracci R, Hirsch A. Tobacco smoking and gastric cancer: review and meta-analysis. *Int J Cancer.* 1997;72:565-73.

[104] International Agency for Research on Cancer; *Tobacco Smoke and Involuntary Smoking.* IARC Monogr Eval Carcinog Risks Hum; 2004;83:1: 1-1438.

[105] Gonzalez CA, Pera G, Agudo A, et al. Smoking and the risk of gastric cancer in the European Prospective Investigation Into Cancer and Nutrition (EPIC). *Int J Cancer.* 2003;107:629-34.

[106] Gammon MD, Schoenberg JB, Ahsan H, et al. Tobacco, alcohol, and socioeconomic status and adenocarcinomas of the esophagus and gastric cardia. *J Natl Cancer Inst.* 1997;89:1277-84.

[107] Sasazuki S, Sasaki S, Tsugane S. Cigarette smoking, alcohol consumption and subsequent gastric cancer risk by subsite and histologic type. *Int J Cancer.* 2002;101:560-6.

[108] Zaridze D, Borisova E, Maximovitch D, Chkhikvadze V. Alcohol consumption, smoking and risk of gastric cancer: case-control study from Moscow, Russia. *Cancer Causes Control.* 2000;11:363-71.

[109] Chow WH, Swanson CA, Lissowska J, et al. Risk of stomach cancer in relation to consumption of cigarettes, alcohol, tea and coffee in Warsaw, Poland. *Int J Cancer.* 1999;81:871-6.

[110] Koizumi Y, Tsubono Y, Nakaya N, et al. Cigarette smoking and the risk of gastric cancer: a pooled analysis of two prospective studies in Japan. *Int J Cancer.* 2004;112:1049-55.

[111] Fei SJ, Xiao SD. Diet and gastric cancer: a case-control study in Shanghai urban districts. *Chin J Dig Dis.* 2006;7:83-8.

[112] Takezaki T, Gao CM, Wu JZ, et al. Dietary protective and risk factors for esophageal and stomach cancers in a low-epidemic area for stomach cancer in Jiangsu Province, China: comparison with those in a high-epidemic area. *Jpn J Cancer Res.* 2001;92:1157-65.

[113] Larsson SC, Giovannucci E, Wolk A. Alcoholic beverage consumption and gastric cancer risk: a prospective population-based study in women. *Int J Cancer.* 2007;120:373-7.

[114] Jakszyn P, Gonzalez CA. Nitrosamine and related food intake and gastric and oesophageal cancer risk: a systematic review of the epidemiological evidence. *World J Gastroenterol.* 2006;12:4296-303.

[115] Lopez-Carrillo L, Lopez-Cervantes M, Ramirez-Espitia A, Rueda C, Fernandez-Ortega C, Orozco-Rivadeneyra S. Alcohol consumption and gastric cancer in Mexico. *Cad Saude Publica.* 1998;14 Suppl 3:25-32.

[116] Barstad B, Sorensen TI, Tjonneland A, et al. Intake of wine, beer and spirits and risk of gastric cancer. *Eur J Cancer Prev.* 2005;14:239-43.

[117] Bagnardi V, Blangiardo M, La Vecchia C, Corrao G. Alcohol consumption and the risk of cancer: a meta-analysis. *Alcohol Res Health.* 2001;25:263-70.

[118] Katiyar SK, Mukhtar H. Tea antioxidants in cancer chemoprevention. *J Cell Biochem Suppl.* 1997;27:59-67.

[119] Sasazuki S, Inoue M, Hanaoka T, Yamamoto S, Sobue T, Tsugane S. Green tea consumption and subsequent risk of gastric cancer by subsite: the JPHC Study. *Cancer Causes Control.* 2004;15:483-91.

[120] Hansson LE, Nyrén O, Bergström R, Wolk A, Lindgren A, Baron J, Adami HO. Nutrients and gastric cancer risk. A population-based case-control study in Sweden. *Int J Cancer.* 1994 Jun 1;57(5):638-44.

[121] Botelho F, Lunet N, Barros H. Coffee and gastric cancer: systematic review and meta-analysis. *Cad Saude Publica.* 2006;22:889-900.

[122] Galanis DJ, Kolonel LN, Lee J, Nomura A. Intakes of selected foods and beverages and the incidence of gastric cancer among the Japanese residents of Hawaii: a prospective study. *Int J Epidemiol.* 1998;27:173-80.

[123] Larsson SC, Giovannucci E, Wolk A. Coffee consumption and stomach cancer risk in a cohort of Swedish women. *Int J Cancer.* 2006;119:2186-9.

[124] Tsugane S. Salt, salted food intake, and risk of gastric cancer: epidemiologic evidence. *Cancer Sci.* 2005;96:1-6.

[125] Kono S, Hirohata T. Nutrition and stomach cancer. *Cancer Causes Control.* 1996;7:41-55.

[126] Strumylaite L, Zickute J, Dudzevicius J, Dregval L. Salt-preserved foods and risk of gastric cancer. *Medicina (Kaunas).* 2006;42:164-70.

[127] van den Brandt PA, Botterweck AA, Goldbohm RA. Salt intake, cured meat consumption, refrigerator use and stomach cancer incidence: a prospective cohort study (Netherlands). *Cancer Causes Control.* 2003;14:427-38.

[128] Cohen AJ, Roe FJ. Evaluation of the aetiological role of dietary salt exposure in gastric and other cancers in humans. *Food Chem Toxicol.* 1997;35:271-93.

[129] Gonzalez CA, Jakszyn P, Pera G, et al. Meat intake and risk of stomach and esophageal adenocarcinoma within the European Prospective Investigation Into Cancer and Nutrition (EPIC). *J Natl Cancer Inst.* 2006;98:345-54.

[130] Larsson SC, Orsini N, Wolk A. Processed meat consumption and stomach cancer risk: a meta-analysis. *J Natl Cancer Inst.* 2006;98:1078-87.

[131] Lissowska J, Gail MH, Pee D, et al. Diet and stomach cancer risk in Warsaw, Poland. *Nutr Cancer.* 2004;48:149-59.

[132] Phukan RK, Narain K, Zomawia E, Hazarika NC, Mahanta J. Dietary habits and stomach cancer in Mizoram, India. *J Gastroenterol.* 2006;41:418-24.

[133] Kim HJ, Chang WK, Kim MK, Lee SS, Choi BY. Dietary factors and gastric cancer in Korea: a case-control study. *Int J Cancer.* 2002;97:531-5.

[134] De Stefani E, Ronco A, Brennan P, Boffetta P. Meat consumption and risk of stomach cancer in Uruguay: a case-control study. *Nutr Cancer.* 2001;40:103-7.

[135] Lee JK, Park BJ, Yoo KY, Ahn YO. Dietary factors and stomach cancer: a case-control study in Korea. *Int J Epidemiol.* 1995;24:33-41.

[136] World Cancer Research Fund - American Institute of Cancer reasearch; *Food, Nutrition and the Prevention of Cancer: A Global Perspective.* Menasha, USA: BANTA Book Group; 1997.

[137] Riboli E, Norat T. Epidemiologic evidence of the protective effect of fruit and vegetables on cancer risk. *Am J Clin Nutr.* 2003;78:559S-569S.

[138] Gonzalez CA, Pera G, Agudo A, et al. Fruit and vegetable intake and the risk of stomach and oesophagus adenocarcinoma in the European Prospective Investigation into Cancer and Nutrition (EPIC-EURGAST). *Int J Cancer.* 2006;118:2559-66.

[139] Campbell PT, Sloan M, Kreiger N. Dietary patterns and risk of incident gastric adenocarcinoma. *Am J Epidemiol.* 2008;167:295-304.

[140] Tricker AR, Preussmann R. Carcinogenic N-nitrosamines in the diet: occurrence, formation, mechanisms and carcinogenic potential. *Mutat Res.* 1991;259:277-89.

[141] Hotchkiss JH. Preformed N-nitroso compounds in foods and beverages. *Cancer Surv.* 1989;8:295-321.

[142] Siddiqi MA, Tricker AR, Kumar R, Fazili Z, Preussmann R. Dietary sources of N-nitrosamines in a high-risk area for oesophageal cancer--Kashmir, India. *IARC Sci Publ.* 1991;210-3.

[143] Mirvish SS. Role of N-nitroso compounds (NOC) and N-nitrosation in etiology of gastric, esophageal, nasopharyngeal and bladder cancer and contribution to cancer of known exposures to NOC. *Cancer Lett.* 1995;93:17-48.

[144] McColl KE. When saliva meets acid: chemical warfare at the oesophagogastric junction. *Gut.* 2005;54:1-3.

[145] Mitacek EJ, Brunnemann KD, Suttajit M, et al. Geographic distribution of liver and stomach cancers in Thailand in relation to estimated dietary intake of nitrate, nitrite, and nitrosodimethylamine. *Nutr Cancer.* 2008;60:196-203.

[146] You WC, Chang YS, Yang ZT, et al. Etiological research on gastric cancer and its precursor lesions in Shandong, China. *IARC Sci Publ.* 1991;33-8.

[147] Sobala GM, Pignatelli B, Schorah CJ, et al. Levels of nitrite, nitrate, N-nitroso compounds, ascorbic acid and total bile acids in gastric juice of patients with and without precancerous conditions of the stomach. *Carcinogenesis.* 1991;12:193-8.

[148] Kim HJ, Lee SS, Choi BY, Kim MK. Nitrate intake relative to antioxidant vitamin intake affects gastric cancer risk: a case-control study in Korea. *Nutr Cancer.* 2007;59:185-91.

[149] Hartman PE. Review: putative mutagens and carcinogens in foods. I. Nitrate/nitrite ingestion and gastric cancer mortality. *Environ Mutagen.* 1983;5:111-21.

[150] Jakszyn P, Bingham S, Pera G, et al. Endogenous versus exogenous exposure to N-nitroso compounds and gastric cancer risk in the European Prospective Investigation into Cancer and Nutrition (EPIC-EURGAST) study. *Carcinogenesis.* 2006;27:1497-501.

[151] Schorah CJ, Sobala GM, Sanderson M, Collis N, Primrose JN. Gastric juice ascorbic acid: effects of disease and implications for gastric carcinogenesis. *Am J Clin Nutr.* 1991;53:287S-293S.

[152] Correa P, Fontham ET, Bravo JC, et al. Chemoprevention of gastric dysplasia: randomized trial of antioxidant supplements and anti-helicobacter pylori therapy. *J Natl Cancer Inst.* 2000;92:1881-8.

[153] Blot WJ, Li JY, Taylor PR, et al. Nutrition intervention trials in Linxian, China: supplementation with specific vitamin/mineral combinations, cancer incidence, and disease-specific mortality in the general population. *J Natl Cancer Inst.* 1993;85:1483-92.

[154] Zhu S, Mason J, Shi Y, et al. The effect of folic acid on the development of stomach and other gastrointestinal cancers. *Chin Med J (Engl).* 2003;116:15-9.

[155] Hennekens CH, Buring JE, Manson JE, et al. Lack of effect of long-term supplementation with beta carotene on the incidence of malignant neoplasms and cardiovascular disease. *N Engl J Med.* 1996;334:1145-9.

[156] Malila N, Taylor PR, Virtanen MJ, et al. Effects of alpha-tocopherol and beta-carotene supplementation on gastric cancer incidence in male smokers (ATBC Study, Finland). *Cancer Causes Control.* 2002;13:617-23.

[157] Virtamo J, Pietinen P, Huttunen JK, et al. Incidence of cancer and mortality following alpha-tocopherol and beta-carotene supplementation: a postintervention follow-up. *JAMA.* 2003;290:476-85.

[158] Plummer M, Vivas J, Lopez G, et al. Chemoprevention of precancerous gastric lesions with antioxidant vitamin supplementation: a randomized trial in a high-risk population. *J Natl Cancer Inst.* 2007;99:137-46.

[159] Nagel G, Linseisen J, Boshuizen HC, et al. Socioeconomic position and the risk of gastric and oesophageal cancer in the European Prospective Investigation into Cancer and Nutrition (EPIC-EURGAST). *Int J Epidemiol.* 2007;36:66-76.

[160] van Loon AJ, Goldbohm RA, van den Brandt PA. Socioeconomic status and stomach cancer incidence in men: results from The Netherlands Cohort Study. *J Epidemiol Community Health.* 1998;52:166-71.

[161] Naess O, Strand BH, Smith GD. Childhood and adulthood socioeconomic position across 20 causes of death: a prospective cohort study of 800,000 Norwegian men and women. *J Epidemiol Community Health.* 2007;61:1004-9.

[162] Amiri M, Kunst AE, Janssen F, Mackenbach JP. Trends in stomach cancer mortality in relation to living conditions in childhood. A study among cohorts born between 1860 and 1939 in seven European countries. *Eur J Cancer.* 2006;42:3212-8.

[163] Menvielle G, Luce D, Geoffroy-Perez B, Chastang JF, Leclerc A. Social inequalities and cancer mortality in France, 1975-1990. *Cancer Causes Control* . 2005;16:501-13.

[164] Lawlor DA, Sterne JA, Tynelius P, Davey Smith G, Rasmussen F. Association of childhood socioeconomic position with cause-specific mortality in a prospective record linkage study of 1,839,384 individuals. *Am J Epidemiol.* 2006;164:907-15.

[165] Weiderpass E, Pukkala E. Time trends in socioeconomic differences in incidence rates of cancers of gastro-intestinal tract in Finland. *BMC Gastroenterol.* 2006;6:41.

[166] Kolonel LN, Nomura AM, Hirohata T, Hankin JH, Hinds MW. Association of diet and place of birth with stomach cancer incidence in Hawaii Japanese and Caucasians. *Am J Clin Nutr.* 1981;34:2478-85.

[167] Shimizu H, Mack TM, Ross RK, Henderson BE. Cancer of the gastrointestinal tract among Japanese and white immigrants in Los Angeles County. *J Natl Cancer Inst.* 1987;78:223-8.

[168] Lee J, Demissie K, Lu SE, Rhoads GG. Cancer incidence among Korean-American immigrants in the United States and native Koreans in South Korea. *Cancer Control.* 2007;14:78-85.

[169] Boysen T, Friborg J, Andersen A, Poulsen GN, Wohlfahrt J, Melbye M. The Inuit cancer pattern--the influence of migration. *Int J Cancer.* 2008;122:2568-72.

[170] Stirbu I, Kunst AE, Vlems FA, et al. Cancer mortality rates among first and second generation migrants in the Netherlands: Convergence toward the rates of the native Dutch population. *Int J Cancer.* 2006;119:2665-72.

[171] Kyobutungi C, Ronellenfitsch U, Razum O, Becher H. Mortality from cancer among ethnic German immigrants from the Former Soviet Union, in Germany. *Eur J Cancer.* 2006;42:2577-84.

[172] Weiderpass E, Vainio H, Kauppinen T, Vasama-Neuvonen K, Partanen T, Pukkala E. Occupational exposures and gastrointestinal cancers among Finnish women. *J Occup Environ Med.* 2003;45:305-15.

[173] Steenland K, Boffetta P. Lead and cancer in humans: where are we now? *Am J Ind Med.* 2000;38:295-9.

[174] Rousseau MC, Parent ME, Nadon L, Latreille B, Siemiatycki J. Occupational exposure to lead compounds and risk of cancer among men: a population-based case-control study. *Am J Epidemiol.* 2007;166:1005-14.

[175] Wong O, Harris F. Cancer mortality study of employees at lead battery plants and lead smelters, 1947-1995. *Am J Ind Med.* 2000;38:255-70.

[176] Cocco P, Ward MH, Dosemeci M. Occupational risk factors for cancer of the gastric cardia. Analysis of death certificates from 24 US states. *J Occup Environ Med.* 1998;40:855-61.

[177] Parent ME, Siemiatycki J, Menzies R, Fritschi L, Colle E. Bacille Calmette-Guerin vaccination and incidence of IDDM in Montreal, Canada. *Diabetes Care.* 1997;20:767-72.

[178] Wingren G, Axelson O. Mortality in the Swedish glassworks industry. *Scand J Work Environ Health.* 1987;13:412-6.

[179] Spinelli JJ, Demers PA, Le ND, et al. Cancer risk in aluminum reduction plant workers (Canada). *Cancer Causes Control.* 2006;17:939-48.

[180] Tsuda T, Mino Y, Babazono A, Shigemi J, Otsu T, Yamamoto E. A case-control study of the relationships among silica exposure, gastric cancer, and esophageal cancer. *Am J Ind Med.* 2001;39:52-7.

[181] Cocco P, Fadda D, Billai B, D'Atri M, Melis M, Blair A. Cancer mortality among men occupationally exposed to dichlorodiphenyltrichloroethane. *Cancer Res.* 2005;65:9588-94.

[182] Krstev S, Dosemeci M, Lissowska J, Chow WH, Zatonski W, Ward MH. Occupation and risk of stomach cancer in Poland. *Occup Environ Med.* 2005;62:318-24.

[183] Travier N, Gridley G, De Roos AJ, Plato N, Moradi T, Boffetta P. Cancer incidence of dry cleaning, laundry and ironing workers in Sweden. *Scand J Work Environ Health.* 2002;28:341-8.

[184] Lynge E, Andersen A, Rylander L, et al. Cancer in persons working in dry cleaning in the Nordic countries. *Environ Health Perspect.* 2006;114:213-9.

[185] Sjodahl K, Jansson C, Bergdahl IA, Adami J, Boffetta P, Lagergren J. Airborne exposures and risk of gastric cancer: a prospective cohort study. *Int J Cancer.* 2007;120:2013-8.

[186] Romundstad P, Andersen A, Haldorsen T. Cancer incidence among workers in the Norwegian silicon carbide industry. *Am J Epidemiol.* 2001;153:978-86.

[187] Li L, Sun TD, Zhang X, et al. Cohort studies on cancer mortality among workers exposed only to chrysotile asbestos: a meta-analysis. *Biomed Environ Sci .* 2004;17:459-68.

[188] Kjaerheim K, Ulvestad B, Martinsen JI, Andersen A. Cancer of the gastrointestinal tract and exposure to asbestos in drinking water among lighthouse keepers (Norway). *Cancer Causes Control.* 2005;16:593-8.

[189] Reid A, Ambrosini G, de Klerk N, Fritschi L, Musk B. Aerodigestive and gastrointestinal tract cancers and exposure to crocidolite (blue asbestos): incidence and mortality among former crocidolite workers. *Int J Cancer.* 2004;111:757-61.

[190] Straughan JK, Sorahan T. Cohort mortality and cancer incidence survey of recent entrants (1982-91) to the United Kingdom rubber industry: preliminary findings. *Occup Environ Med.* 2000;57:574-6.

[191] Straif K, Weiland SK, Bungers M, et al. Exposure to high concentrations of nitrosamines and cancer mortality among a cohort of rubber workers. *Occup Environ Med.* 2000;57:180-7.

[192] Straif K, Keil U, Taeger D, et al. Exposure to nitrosamines, carbon black, asbestos, and talc and mortality from stomach, lung, and laryngeal cancer in a cohort of rubber workers. *Am J Epidemiol.* 2000;152:297-306.

[193] Stucker I, Meguellati D, Boffetta P, Cenee S, Margelin D, Hemon D. Cohort mortality study among French asphalt workers. *Am J Ind Med.* 2003;43:58-68.

[194] Randem BG, Burstyn I, Langard S, et al. Cancer incidence of Nordic asphalt workers. *Scand J Work Environ Health.* 2004;30:350-5.

[195] Sorahan T. Mortality of workers at a plant manufacturing nickel alloys, 1958-2000. *Occup Med (Lond).* 2004;54:28-34.

[196] Waalkes MP. Cadmium carcinogenesis. *Mutat Res.* 2003;533:107-20.

[197] Wernli KJ, Fitzgibbons ED, Ray RM, et al. Occupational risk factors for esophageal and stomach cancers among female textile workers in Shanghai, China. *Am J Epidemiol.* 2006;163:717-25.

[198] Coggon D, Harris EC, Poole J, Palmer KT. Mortality of workers exposed to ethylene oxide: extended follow up of a British cohort. *Occup Environ Med.* 2004;61:358-62.

[199] Prince MM, Ruder AM, Hein MJ, et al. Mortality and exposure response among 14,458 electrical capacitor manufacturing workers exposed to polychlorinated biphenyls (PCBs). *Environ Health Perspect.* 2006;114:1508-14.

[200] Engel LS, Vaughan TL, Gammon MD, et al. Occupation and risk of esophageal and gastric cardia adenocarcinoma. *Am J Ind Med.* 2002;42:11-22.

[201] Sathiakumar N, Delzell E. An updated mortality study of workers at a dye and resin manufacturing plant. *J Occup Environ Med.* 2000;42:762-71.

[202] Band PR, Le ND, Fang R, et al. Cohort cancer incidence among pulp and paper mill workers in British Columbia. *Scand J Work Environ Health.* 2001;27:113-9.

[203] Mallin K, McCann K, D'Aloisio A, et al. Cohort mortality study of capacitor manufacturing workers, 1944-2000. *J Occup Environ Med.* 2004;46:565-76.

[204] Ji J, Hemminki K. Socio-economic and occupational risk factors for gastric cancer: a cohort study in Sweden. *Eur J Cancer Prev.* 2006;15:391-7.

[205] Mills PK, Yang RC. Agricultural exposures and gastric cancer risk in Hispanic farm workers in California. *Environ Res.* 2007;104:282-9.

In: Gastric Cancer: Diagnosis, Early Prevention, and Treatment   ISBN 978-1-61668-313-9
Editor: V. D. Pasechnikov, pp. 43-117   © 2010 Nova Science Publishers, Inc.

Chapter II

GASTRIC CANCER ETIOLOGY AND PATHOGENESIS

Victor Pasechnikov[1], Sergey Chukov[2], Massimo Rugge[3,4]
[1]Department of Therapy, State Medical Academy of Stavropol, Russian Federation
[2]Department of Pathology, State Medical Academy of Stavropol, Russian Federation
[3]Department of Diagnostic Sciences & Special Therapies - Pathology Unit, University of Padova, Italy
[4]Department of Medicine, Veterans Affairs Medical Center and Baylor College of Medicine Houston, Texas USA

ABSTRACT

This Chapter contains the review of the existing and modern representations concerning the Etiology and Pathogenesis of Gastric Cancer. The authors survey the role of the Environmental Factors and Life Style, the role of Helicobacter pylori and some other infectious agents, e.g., Epstein-Barr virus, in the development of gastric carcinoma. The Chapter includes the modern data about the meaning of the genetic susceptibility in the individual risk of Gastric Cancer development. The Recent Advances in Molecular Carcinogenesis of the Gastric Carcinoma, and The Role of Stem Cells in Gastric Cancer Development are also discussed ih the Chapter.

Although the genetic and environmental contributions to gastric carcinogenesis are not yet entirely clear, approximately 10% of gastric cancer shows familial clustering [1]. In other words, a small percentage of gastric cancers (1-3%) arise as a result of clearly identified inherited gastric cancer predisposition syndromes [2-5]. The existence of a familial form of gastric cancer has been known about since the 1800s, when multiple cases of gastric cancer were noted in the Bonaparte family [6].The family cancer syndromes - Hereditary Nonpolyposis Colorectal Cancer (HNPCC) and Peutz-Jeghers syndrome (PJS) are known to be associated with an increased risk of gastric cancer [7]. Recently, a germline mutation in the

CDH1 gene on chromosome l6q has been associated with a very rare autosomal dominant form of gastric cancer called hereditary diffuse gastric cancer (HDGG) [8-10].

Observational studies are useful to determine whether heredity plays a role in gastric cancer and molecular epidemiological studies can be used to identify factors involved in cancer development, progression and metastasis [11]. Studies aimed at determining the role of heredity in stomach cancer include family pedigree reports, twin studies, family aggregation studies and blood typing studies. As discussed by Nomura [12], it has been shown that gastric cancer can be present in families over two to three generations and family members of a stomach cancer case have two to three times the risk than does the general population of developing gastric cancer. Studies involving family members are methodologically limited, however, because they do not distinguish genetic from environmental factors, as family members tend to share a common environment [12]. The results of blood typing studies indicate that blood group A is associated with gastric cancer more frequently than are the other blood groups. The association is stronger in males and for diffuse type gastric cancer as compared with intestinal type gastric cancer [12, 13].

Gastric cancers can be classified in terms of their anatomical site and histopathological subtype. The two major histopathological subtypes are the intestinal type and the diffuse or linitis plastica type. The diffuse types are commoner in endemic areas, tend to have a poorer prognosis and their aetiopathology is less well understood. A subset of these diffuse type gastric cancers are hereditary and recently linkage analysis has implicated E-cadherin (CDH1) mutations in an estimated 25% of them [8]. As mentioned above, this subset of gastric cancer has been termed hereditary diffuse gastric cancer (HDGC).

It is perhaps not surprising that E-cadherin has been implicated in HDGC since in 1994 Becker et al. identified somatic E-cadherin mutations in specimens of diffuse gastric cancer [14]. Since then CDH1 mutations have been found in 40-83% sporadic diffuse cancers but not in intestinal-type gastric cancers [15-17]. The diffuse phenotype probably occurs as a result of aberrant cell-cell adhesion secondary to abnormal E-cadherin expression. A causal role for E-cadherin has been demonstrated in the transition from adenoma to carcinoma in a mouse model of pancreatic tumour progression [18] and silencing of E-cadherin has been described in human carcinomas [19]. So far, there has only been one report of an E-cadherin germline mutation in an apparently sporadic gastric cancer [9].

As a result of the identification of the genetic mutation responsible for HDGC there are far reaching clinical sequelae. First, there is the question of identifying asymptomatic individuals from affected families and providing genetic testing to see if they harbour a CDH1 mutation. Second, once an affected individual is identified there is the opportunity to try to prevent invasive gastric cancer from developing. The current options are regular endoscopic surveillance or else the seemingly radical option of a prophylactic gastrectomy.

As noted already, the histopathology of HDGC is uniformly of the diffuse linitis plastica type of cancer although a minority of tumours may also have a glandular/ intestinal component [20]. To determine whether the HDGCs have any distinctive pathological features among all diffuse carcinomas will require a controlled and blinded analysis of a larger number of such specimens.

The age of onset is typically much younger than sporadic gastric cancers. There is an average age of 38 years compared with sporadic cancer which tends to occur in 60-70 year olds. The youngest cases of HDGC reported have been in persons under 18 years of age.

In order to be considered for a diagnosis of HDGC the following criteria have to be met [21]: (1) two or more documented cases of diffuse gastric cancer in first or second degree relatives, with at least one diagnosed before the age of 50 or (2) three or more cases of documented DGC in 1st/2nd degree relatives, independently of age of onset.

These criteria were set to be over inclusive in order to collect gastric cancer families and to identify other predisposing gene(s). Hence, in a study of Finnish and Japanese gastric cancer families, in which not all of the cases had a diffuse histopathological subtype, no CDH1 mutations were found [22, 23]. Despite the negative Finnish and Japanese data, HDGC families harbouring CDH1 mutations have been identified from varied ethnic backgrounds (Caucasian, Japanese, Korean, African-American), [8,14,24,25]. Therefore, HDGC does not seem to be restricted to one ethnic group but the inclusion/exclusion criteria are likely to be critical in order to identify affected individuals.

Research on these families has also shown that penetrance of the gene is high, with an estimated range of 70-80%; therefore if you carry the abnormal E-cadherin gene you have a 70-80% lifetime risk of developing gastric cancer [26]. This high penetrance is similar to medullary thyroid cancers in MEN2 syndromes and breast cancer in BRCA1 carriers.

The longest follow-up data of patients with HDGC comes from Maori kindred which were first described in 1964. Indeed, it was from this kindred that Guilford et al. first identified the germline mutations of CDH1 in 1998 [8]. In this kindred over 25 family members have died from gastric cancer, with an increased frequency of colo-rectal cancer in these patients. The age of death from gastric cancer ranges from 14 years and the majority of affected persons die when they are under 40 years of age. Hence, data from these Maori families and from other series suggest that individuals with CDH1 mutations may be predisposed to the development of other cancers (lobular breast, colorectal and prostate) [9, 10, 26]. However, it was felt that the inclusion of other associated cancers into the definition of HDGC was too premature [21].

The working definition for HDGC appears to be fulfilling its aims since recent work has shown that whereas 36.4% of families fulfilling the criteria for HDGC harboured CDH1 mutations, no mutations were found in those kindred not fulfilling the criteria [27].

Before discussing the clinical implications of CDH1 mutations with regards to genetic testing and therapeutic strategies, it is important to appreciate the molecular genetics of these tumours since clearly future methods to obviate the need for gastric surgery are preferable.

The analysis of all the reported genetic abnormalities in CDH1 found in HDGC reveals that the majority are inactivating mutations (splice-site, frameshift and nonsense) rather then missense. Furthermore, the CDH1 germline mutations are evenly distributed along the E-cadherin gene, in contrast to the clustering in exons 7-9 observed in sporadic diffuse gastric cancer [28]. These germline mutations affect one allele, leaving a wild-type E-cadherin allele.

CDH1 is a tumour suppressor gene and hence loss or inactivation of the remaining normal allele would be expected to be a required initiating event in susceptible individuals with a germline mutation. The 'second hit' is normally deletion of the whole gene or else silencing of the gene by promoter methylation. Aberrant CDH1 promoter methylation has been demonstrated in three out of six HDGC with negative E-cadherin expression [29]. Reduction of E-cadherin expression by hypermethylation of the CDH1 promoter region is common in a number of non-inherited tumours such as breast, prostate, hepatocellular and thyroid [30, 31, 19] as well as in sporadic diffuse gastric cancer [32]. Interestingly, a demethylating agent, 5-azacytidine, restored E-cadherin expression in a gastric cancer cell line (SNU-1) that tested positive for promoter CDH1 methylation [33]. Hence, it is tempting to consider the potential value of prophylactic treatment of these mutation carriers with demethylating agents such as 5-azadeoxycytidine.

In contrast, some individuals with germline E-cadherin mutations have E-cadherin protein detectable immunohistochemically. Hence it has been suggested that the germline mutations identified have a dominant negative effect similar to forms of N-cadherin in embryonic cell adhesion [34]. Alternatively, it has also been suggested that a 50% reduction in E-cadherin function may be sufficient to promote tumourigenesis.

E-cadherin is a 120 kDa calcium-dependent adhesion molecule that is a member of the cadherin family of proteins, a class of cell surface proteins that establish intercellular connections through homophilic interactions and maintain epithelial tissue polarity and structural integrity. The E-cadherin gene coding sequence gives rise to a 27 amino acid signal peptide (exons 1-2), a 154 amino acid precursor peptide (exons 2-4) and a 728 amino acid mature protein [28]. This mature protein consists of 3 major domains, a large extracellular domain (exons 4-13) and smaller transmembrane domains (exons 13-14) and cytoplasmic domains (exons 14-16). The extracellular portion mediates homophilic interactions, whereas its intracellular part provides a link to the actin cytoskeleton through an association with the catenins. One of these, P-catenin, is not only involved in cell adhesion but also in signal transduction.

The mechanism by which these E-cadherin mutations actually lead to cancer is probably complex. It is likely that disrupted cell-cell adhesion could play a role in the initiation of cell proliferation by allowing escape from growth control signals. Furthermore, the cytoplasmic domain of E-cadherin may modulate the Wnt signalling pathway by inhibiting the availability of free cytoplasmic P catenin, in a manner complimentary to the product of the colorectal tumour suppressor APC.

Underexpression of E-cadherin protein is a prognostic marker of poor clinical outcome in many tumour types [35]. Specifically, there is overwhelming evidence that loss of E-cadherin function is associated with invasiveness, lymph node metastasis, distant metastasis and other poor prognostic factors [36-38]. Furthermore, restored E-cadherin expression in tumour models can suppress invasiveness of epithelial tumour cells [39,40]. Recently, Perl et al. used a transgenic mouse model of pancreatic beta cell tumourigenesis to demonstrate that abrogation of E-cadherin mediated cell adhesion induces tumour invasion and metastasis [18]. However, since loss of membranous staining appears to be a late event in tumourigenesis this would be unlikely to be clinically useful for identifying early gastric cancers.

Genetic testing for HDGC is currently available only through research protocols. Due to the current ambiguity and lack of evidence-based practice concerning cancer risk rates and screening guidelines in HDGC, genetic testing at this time is only being offered to at- risk individuals if a mutation has been identified previously in an affected blood relative. Because knowledge and understanding of this genetic mutation is relatively new and may undergo further developments in the near future, it is recommended that all individuals who wish to receive germline testing for the E-cadherin mutation be enrolled in research protocol as well as a cooperative registry [20]. It also is recommended that any positive test result furnished by a research lab be confirmed at a separate laboratory that has been approved for clinical gene testing [20].

Upper endoscopy is believed to be an effective screening technique for gastric cancer associated with HNPCC and PJS, but the most effective screening modalities for HDGC are not yet currently known. As mentioned, the early malignant lesions associated with diffuse gastric cancer usually are not visible on gross examination [20], so the usefulness of upper endoscopy is questionable. In fact, there are case reports of individuals who underwent numerous negative endoscopies, but were found to have diffuse gastric cancer on open biopsy or at the time of "prophylactic" gastrectomy [41].

Because it has proven difficult to identify any early lesion associated with diffuse gastric cancer, the option of prophylactic gastrectomy should be discussed with individuals who carry an identified CDH1 mutation [20]. There have been no clinical trials to support the use of this treatment in known carriers, but based on the published case reports, it appears to be a prudent option [20, 42, 41]. Total gastrectomy is associated with substantial long-term morbidity, including dumping syndrome, weight loss, and diarrhea, a fact that must be fully explained to individuals considering surgical prophylaxis [20]. The option of prophylactic gastrectomy should not be recommended for individuals without a documented CDH1 mutation [20]. Known mutation carriers, who choose not to undergo gastrectomy, and at-risk individuals without a known mutation, should receive upper endoscopy screening every 6 to 12 months, preferably with the most current technological advances, including endoscopic ultrasound and chromoendoscopy, which uses staining dyes [20].

The primary management of an individual or family with an E-cadherin gene mutation must be provided by health professionals with experience in cancer genetic counseling and risk management. Because these recommendations are based on current knowledge and not clinical trials at this time, the management of CDH1 mutation carriers and families, as well as management of at risk families, should be carried out in the context of a research protocol [20]. As in pancreatic cancer, participation in trials of gastric screening will assist in the development of new screening tests and the refinement of screening recommendations.

ENVIRONMENTAL FACTORS AND LIFE STYLE

There are geographic and ethnic differences in gastric cancer incidence in the world and in its trends for each population with time. The incidence patterns observed among immigrants change according to where they live. These factors indicate the close association of gastric cancer with modifiable factors such as diet. Substantial evidence from ecological, case-control, and cohort studies strongly suggest that the risk of cancer increases with a high intake of various traditional salt-preserved foods as well as salt per se and that this risk could be decreased with a high intake of fruit and vegetables [43,44]. A recent report of a joint World Health Organization (WHO)/Food and Agriculture Organization (FAO) Expert Consultation concluded that salt-preserved food and salt "probably" increase the risk of gastric cancer, whereas fruit and vegetables "probably" decrease the risk [45]. Other established non-dietary factors include cigarette smoking [46] and infection with the bacterium Helicobacter pylori (H. pylori) [47]. In addition, there is some evidence that the intake of green tea and vitamin C is associated with the risk of gastric cancer.

Occupational factors have been regarded as playing a smaller part in the aetiology of gastric cancer than dietary and other environmental exposures, although they may interact with various non-occupational factors at key stages in the development of gastric cancer [48]. According to epidemiological studies, occupational exposures reported to increase the risk of stomach cancer include dusts, nitrogen oxides, N-nitroso compounds, and ionizing radiation [48]. Excess risks have been found for several occupational groups, including miners and quarrymen, farmers, fishermen, masonry and concrete workers, machine operators, nurses, food industry workers, cooks, launderers and dry cleaners [49-53].

A number of medical conditions have been suggested to increase risk of stomach cancer. These include pernicious anaemia, peptic ulcer disease, and also prior experience of gastric surgery [54]. However, the use of non-steroidal anti-inflammatory drugs (NSAIDS) has been suggested to reduce risk of stomach cancer. In a meta-analysis of nine studies (eight case—control and one cohort) with a total of 2831 gastric cancer cases, NSAID use was associated with a reduced risk of gastric cancer, with a summary odds ratio of 0.78 (95% Cl = 0.69 to 0.87) [55].

Whilst measures of obesity are generally positively related to risk of cancer, for stomach cancer there is a lack of consistency in the epidemiological literature. Variation in the impact of obesity on stomach cancer risk could be attributed to problems in obtaining unbiased reports of pre-disease weight, to differential risk according to tumour location and to publication bias. Within case—control studies, measures of obesity are generally lower in stomach cancer cases than in control populations [56-60], but this may be due to bias in reporting in individuals who have experienced pre-diagnostic weight loss or a reflection of confounding by other factors, such as smoking, rather than indicating a benefit of excess adiposity. Large prospective cohort studies that reported risk of stomach cancer without differentiation according to tumour site also tend to show either negative or no association with body mass index (kg/m2) or other indices of obesity [61-67]. However, some more recent prospective studies that have been able to report risk according to site of tumour origin have tended to suggest that risk of cancer occurring in the cardia or proximal region of the stomach may be somewhat elevated in obese individuals [62,68,70], but reduced for cancers occurring in the non-cardia or distal region of the stomach [71-73].

Although overweight and obesity have traditionally not been linked to gastric cancer risk, recent prospective evidence suggests that the risk of GCC is positively associated with BMI [72]. In a British cohort study, BMI was associated with risk of GCC, in a dose-dependent manner, but not with risk of GNCC. The association with obesity (BMI>30 kg/m2) was stronger for EAC (RR=1.93) than for GCC (RR=1.46); both associations seemed independent of gastro-esophageal reflux and were found in men and women [72].

Compared to the literature base for a number of other gastrointestinal cancers, there are relatively few studies that have examined the relationship between physical activity and stomach cancer. One prospective cohort study of Japanese residents of Hawaii found an elevated risk of stomach cancer associated with the highest levels of both recreational and occupational physical activity when compared with mostly sedentary activity levels [74]. However, neither resting heart rate nor activity during a 24 h period were related to stomach cancer risk. Within the UK, neither the Whitehall Study of London civil servants [75] or the British Regional Heart Study [76] found any relationship with self-reported recreational physical activity levels. While currently there is insufficient evidence to indicate whether this lack of association will also be found in studies that are able to examine risk according to gastric tumour location, one recent population-based case—control study found no significant association for cancer of the gastric cardia with occupational activity even after comprehensive adjustment for socio-economic variables [77].

Evidence that salt intake is inversely associated with risk of stomach cancer has accumulated over many decades. Salt intake has been assessed in numerous ways, including salt preference, consumption of salted foods, use of table salt, salt added during cooking and more accurately urinary sodium excretion. There are of course many problems regarding the evaluation of studies of this particular exposure. In particular, the measurement of salt intakes poses particular problems since dietary survey methodology may not accurately capture salt added at the table and during cooking. However, 24 h urinary sodium excretion, which is generally regarded as a better reflection of salt intake, is also not devoid of measurement bias and error [78]. Furthermore, since the mechanism of action of salt on gastric cancer risk is thought to be via irritation of the stomach lining [79] and ultimately the development of atrophic gastritis, and this is also thought to occur with H. pylori infection, the effects of salt intake may be readily confounded by lack of adjustment for infection. Additionally, the consumption of salted foods commonly correlates with the intake of secondary amines and fresh vegetables as well as the method of preservation and storage of foods such as refrigeration and curing. There is consequently further potential for significant confounding of this exposure with other diet-related exposures.

Most case-control studies have shown a positive association between intake of salt or salted food and gastric cancer. The few cohort studies that reported results on salt or salted food and stomach cancer risk found no clear associations [80]. In one recent Japanese cohort study no significant association with intake of pickled foods and traditional soups and gastric cancer risk was found [81] while in another cohort study a significant positive association between salt intake and risk of gastric cancer was seen in men, but not in women [82]. In the NLCS, the results suggested that intake of dietary salt and several types of cured meat were weakly positively associated with gastric cancer risk [83]. Thus, the link between salt and gastric cancer is not consistently observed. It is possible that the increased risks could be attributed to other compounds of the foods (possible carcinogens) developed during the preservation process, and not to salt content of the foods [84]. As in the NLCS, use of table salt was not associated with stomach cancer risk in the only other cohort study that reported on this association [85]. Also, gastric cancer rates in the USA are low, even though salt intake is not.

In experimental studies in rats, ingestion of salt is known to cause gastritis and, on co-administration, to enhance the carcinogenic effects of known gastric carcinogens such as N-methyl-N'-nitro-N-nitrosoguanidine (MNNG) [86,87]. A high salt concentration in the stomach destroys the mucosal barrier and leads to inflammation and damage such as diffuse erosion and degeneration. Furthermore, the induced proliferative change may act to promote the effect of food-derived carcinogens. It is therefore biologically plausible that high salt intake increases the risk of gastric cancer in humans.

There are substantial geographic differences in the incidence of and mortality associated with gastric cancer worldwide, as well as nationwide in Japan. Using data from the INTERSALT study, in which randomly selected 24-h urine samples from 39 populations were sampled from 24 countries (n = 5756), Joossens and colleagues analyzed median sodium levels in samples from subjects aged 20-49 years in relation to the national gastric cancer mortality rates [88]. For the 24 countries, the Pearson correlation of gastric cancer mortality with sodium was 0.70 in men and 0.74 in women (both $P < 0.001$). In an ecological study of 65 rural counties in China, the consumption of salt-preserved vegetables was correlated with gastric cancer mortality (r = 0.26 in men, 0.36 in women) [89].

Approximately threefold differences in age-standardized mortality rates have been identified in Japan, with higher rates in Akita and Yamagata prefectures, lower rates in Kyushu district prefectures such as Kagoshima and Miyazaki, and an especially low rate in Okinawa (Vital Statistics: Ministry of Health, Labor and Welfare, Japan). Our ecological study of five selected areas in Japan showed an almost linear correlation between the cumulative mortality rate for gastric cancer in subjects up to 75 years of age and the urinary salt excretion level in 24-h urine samples [90, 91].

Both age-adjusted mortality and incidence rates have been decreasing for several decades in Japan. In the United States [92] and Europe [93], gastric cancer used to be one of the most common cancers; however, mortality rates have fallen dramatically over the last 50 years in all Western countries without any specific intervention taken, and gastric cancer is now rare. This worldwide decline in incidence is likely attributable to the spread of refrigeration, the use of which would inversely correlate with salting and other salt-based methods of preservation such as curing and smoking, and with the overall volume of salt in the diet [43].

Studies in migrants offer clues about the relative importance of genetic and environmental factors in the etiology of cancer and are particularly useful when large differences exist between the original and host countries in incidence and lifestyle. Age-adjusted (world population) incidence rates of gastric cancer among Japanese residents in Hawaii (USA) were significantly lower than in Japan among both men and women, whereas rates in Sao Paulo, Brazil, were relatively similar to those in Japan [94]. These differences in incidence among three Japanese populations suggest that lifestyle changes, mainly dietary, are associated with a decreased risk of gastric cancer depending on the degree of westernization and the individual incidence rate in the respective host country (United States or Brazil) [95,96].

The substantial decrease in the incidence of gastric cancer among Japanese immigrants in the United States and the minimal decrease among Japanese immigrants in Brazil can be explained on the basis of the manner in which they continue to maintain Japanese dietary habits, which are typically high in salt.

Many but not all case-control studies have found a positive association between gastric cancer and the intake of highly salted foods such as salted fish, cured meat, and salted vegetables or the use of table salt [44]. Several studies have quantitatively estimated total salt intake and found a strong positive association with the risk of gastric cancer, and several others evaluated its association with the intake of salted food such as salted fish and vegetables. In an evaluation performed by the World Cancer Research Fund (WCRF) and the American Institute for Cancer Research (AICR) in 1997 [43], 16 case-control studies reported an association between salt or salted food and the risk of gastric cancer. Eight of these estimated overall dietary salt or sodium intake; four showed strong statistically significant increases in risk [odds ratio (OR) = 2.1-5.0 for the highest intake level], whereas the remaining four showed no substantial association. Six of sixteen studies specifically exam-ined the use of table salt, with three reporting statistically significant increased risks (OR = 1.6-6.2 for highest intakes) and two nonsignificant ORs. Several recent case-control studies have also revealed an association between salted food and the risk of gastric cancer [84, 98, 100, 101].

Prospective data are scarce, and only two studies were evaluated in the 1997 report by the WCRF and AICR [43]. One reported no association with the intake of table salt or soy sauce, although the second found an association between salted fish intake and an increased risk of gastric cancer in white American men, largely of Scandinavian and German descent [relative risk (RR) = 1.9 for the highest intake level].

Four more recent studies have also reported this association. Ngoan and colleagues examined 13000 Japanese men and women and identified 116 gastric cancer deaths during a 10-year follow-up. Higher consumption of pickled foods and traditional soups were associated with increased risk, although without statistical significance [81].

The Netherlands Cohort Study examined 120852 men and women and identified 282 gastric cancer cases at a 6.3-year follow-up [83]. Salt intake was measured by calculating the mean daily sodium intake (dietary salt) from 150 food items and by specific questions related to the consumption of salt. The intake of dietary salt and several types of cured meat showed a weak positive association with the risk of gastric cancer.

The Hisayama study examined 2476 men and women and identified 93 gastric cancer cases during a 14-year follow-up [104]. Dietary salt intake from a 70-item food frequency questionnaire was significantly associated with the risk of gastric cancer after considering H. pylori infection.

Our population-based prospective study examined a total of 18684 men and 20381 women aged 40-59 years and documented 358 men and 128 women with histologically confirmed gastric cancer during the 12 years of follow-up [82]. After adjustment for potential confounding factors, the category salt intake by quintile was dose-dependently associated with the risk of gastric cancer in men (for trend, $P < 0.001$), whereas no clear trend was seen in women ($P = 0.48$). The weak association between salt intake and gastric cancer in women may have been due to the relatively low validity of the estimated salt intake: the Spearman rank correlation with a 2-day urinary excretion level was only 0.12 for women but 0.38 for men. Although the association was less clear for miso soup, pickled vegetables, and dried fish, the frequency categories of highly salted food (e.g., salted fish roe and salted fish preserves) were strongly associated with gastric cancer risk in both sexes.

These findings imply that either the intake of highly salted food increases the risk of gastric cancer or that it is merely a good marker of a preference for salted food or salt intake in general. An alternative explanation for the strong association between highly salted food and gastric cancer might involve the presence of chemical carcinogens such as N-nitroso compounds, which are formed by the reacting nitrate or nitrite during the process of preservation and during digestion in the stomach. A recent meta-analysis based on six prospective and nine case-control studies showed that the consumption of processed meat was associated with an increased risk of gastric cancer [106]. Of note, processed meat often contains chemical carcinogens such as the N-nitroso compounds as well as high amounts of salt.

More than 37 case-control studies have been published on gastric cancer and fruit intake. A recent IARC report [107] concluded from the case-control studies that the mean OR was 0.63 (95% CI, 0.58–0.69), range 0.31–1.39, comparing subjects from high fruit intake categories with subjects from low intake categories. A total of 11 cohort studies have been reported; the mean RR of these studies was 0.85 (95% CI, 0.77–0.95), range 0.55–1.92, comparing high to low intakes. Regarding vegetables, IARC arrived for the 20 available case-control studies at a mean OR of 0.66 (95% CI, 0.61–.71), range 0.30– 1.70. The five cohort studies on vegetables and stomach cancer showed a mean RR of 0.94 (95% CI, 0.84–1.06), range 0.70–1.25, comparing high to low intakes. For both fruits and vegetables, the IARC analyses showed significant heterogeneity between the ORs from case-control studies, but not from cohort studies [107]. Two case-control and two cohort studies have reported on GCC specifically; no differences in the associations between GCC and GNCC. Prospective studies have shown weaker inverse associations than case-control studies, and evidence is available that the apparent inverse association seen in case-control studies might be due to recall bias because of lower intake following prediagnostic symptoms [108].

Due to differences in type and amount of phytochemicals (isothiocyanates, polyphenols, phytoestrogens, flavonoids etc.) it may be that certain types of vegetable have a more potent impact on risk of stomach cancer than others. In particular, there has been a considerable epidemiological research focus on the effects of vegetables from the Allium family (onions, garlic, leeks). A recent meta-analysis on the effects of garlic intake found a risk estimate of 0.53 (95% Cl: 0.31, 0.92) associated with high levels of consumption [109], indicating a protective effect. However, the authors caution that since there was significant heterogeneity among studies the validity of this summary estimate is questionable. Interestingly, an aqueous extract of garlic cloves standardised for its thiosulphinate concentration and tested for its antimicrobial activity on H. pylori has been shown to exhibit a potent antimicrobial action even at low concentrations [110]. In a cross-sectional survey of 214 adults who participated in a gastroscopic screening survey in Cangshan County in China (an area with low cancer risk) consumption of garlic showed non-significant protective effects and an inverse association with H. pylori infection [111].

Fruit and vegetables are rich sources of carotenoids, vitamin C, folate, and phytochemicals, which may have a protective role in the carcinogenesis process. It is likely that modulation of xenobiotic-metabolizing enzymes, in particular phase II enzymes, contributes to this putative preventive mechanism. The mechanisms of antioxidant activity may be also possible.

In 1997, an expert panel assembled by the WCRF and AICR concluded that diets high in fruit and vegetables "convincingly" protect against gastric cancer [43]. This evaluation was based mainly on reports of case-control studies. Since then, however, several cohort studies have reported conflicting results. The joint WHO/FAO Expert Consultation in 2003 concluded that fruit and vegetables "probably," but not "convincingly," decrease the risk of gastric cancer [45].

A subsequent report by the International Agency for Research on Cancer (IARC) determined that higher intake of fruit "probably" and higher intake of vegetables "possibly" reduce the risk of gastric cancer [107]. For fruit, the association has been evaluated in 10 cohort studies, most of which reported an inverse association with a summary value of 0.85 (95% CI = 0.77-0.95). Inverse associations were more striking in the 28 evaluable case-control studies, with summary ORs of 0.63 (95% CI = 0.58-0.69). For vegetables, the association has been evaluated in five cohort studies, most of which reported RRs below 1.0. However, none of these RR values were statistically significant, and the summary value was 0.94 (95% CI = 0.84-1.06). In contrast, most of the 20 evaluable case-control studies provided statistically significant ORs below 1.0 and a summary value of 0.66 (95% CI = 0.61-0.71). The reason case-control studies were more likely to show an inverse association is not clear, although one explanation might be the recall bias inherent to case-control studies. Furthermore, people with preclinical symptoms of gastric cancer or stomach disorders may change their dietary habits months or years before diagnosis.

A meta-analysis of cohort studies published up to 2004 reported nonsignificant summary estimates (RR for the highest versus the lowest consumption category) of 0.89 (95% CI =

0.78-1.02) for fruit (13 studies) and 0.98 (95% CI = 0.86-1.13) for vegetables (8 studies) [112]. However, the inverse associations became clearer when the studies were limited to those with incidence data (seven studies for fruit: RR = 0.82, 95% CI = 0.73-0.93; five studies for vegetables: RR = 0.88, 95% CI = 0.69-1.13) and with follow-up periods of 10 years or longer (three studies for fruit: RR = 0.66, 95% CI = 0.52-0.83; two studies for vegetables: RR = 0.71, 95% CI = 0.53-0.94).

Subsequent to the evaluation by the IARC [107] and the meta-analysis of Lunet et al. [112], several cohort studies have reported the association with fruit and vegetables. In a study in Sweden (139 gastric cancer cases among 70000 men and women) [113], subjects who consumed 2.5 servings of vegetables or more per day had a hazard ratio of 0.56 (95% CI = 0.34-0.93) compared with those who consumed less than 1.0 serving per day. The respective hazard ratio for fruit consumption was 0.86 (95% CI = 0.52-1.43). In the European Prospective Investigation into Cancer and Nutrition (330 gastric cancer cases among 520000 men and women) [114], a protective role for vegetable intake was observed for the intestinal type of gastric cancer. Citrus fruit consumption may play a role in protection against gastric cardia cancer.

In the cohort study of Tsugane S. and Sasazuki S. [115] with 400 gastric cancer cases among 40000 men and women, the RR associated with intake 1 day or more per week compared with less than 1 day per week was 0.64 (95% CI = 0.45-0.92) for yellow vegetables, 0.48 (95% CI = 0.25-0.89) for white vegetables, and 0.70 (95% CI = 0.49-1.00) for fruit. RRs associated with the quintile of total vegetable consumption were 1.00, 0.86, 0.75, 0.90, and 0.75 (for trend, P = 0.17). This association became clearer for the differentiated type of gastric cancer, at 1.00, 0.96, 0.78, 0.88, and 0.53 (for trend, P = 0.03). These findings suggest that vegetable and fruit intake, even in relatively low amounts, is associated with a lower risk of gastric cancer.

In summary, consumption of fruit and vegetables, particularly fruit, is probably protective against gastric cancer. Nevertheless, it remains unknown which constituents in fruit and vegetables play a significant role in gastric cancer prevention.

The relationship between vitamin C intakes, vitamin C status and risk of gastric cancer is further complicated by the relationship of this nutrient to H. pylori infection. Infection with H. pylori is known to substantially reduce the bioavailability of vitamin C and, when combined with the reduced vitamin C intake in H. pylori-positive people, this markedly reduces plasma vitamin C concentrations [116]. This lower circulating level of vitamin C may be in itself a potential causative factor in the development of gastric cancer. Successful eradication of H. pylori in a small patient sample has been shown to improve secretion of vitamin C into gastric juice. The speculation that this approach might increase protection against gastric cancer is supported by the results of a randomised controlled trial conducted in Columbia, in which treatment of patients at high risk of gastric cancer with a combination of vitamin C, beta-carotene and H. pylori eradication successfully promoted the regression of pre-malignant lesions [117].

Fruit and vegetables are rich sources of vitamin C. Vitamin C acts as an antioxidant and can quench reactive oxygen species produced in the gastric environment [118]; it is also known to inhibit production of carcinogenic N-nitroso compound in the stomach [119]. A possible relation between H. pylori infection and ascorbic acid is under investigation, as some research has indicated that high-dose vitamin C is effective in inhibiting H. pylori infection [120,121].

The WCRF/AICR report [43] concluded that high dietary vitamin C intake probably decreases the risk of gastric cancer. This conclusion is based on 1 of 2 cohort studies and 12 of 13 case-control studies showing inverse associations between dietary vitamin C intake and the risk of gastric cancer. In addition, one prospective study showed that baseline plasma vitamin C levels among subjects who died from gastric cancer (n = 20) was 20% lower than those who remained cancer-free (n = 2421) during more than 12 years of follow-up [122].

Since then a limited number of prospective studies have directly tested the association between dietary intake or blood level of vitamin C and the risk of gastric cancer. Dietary intake from comprehensive food frequency questionnaires was inversely associated with the risk of noncardia gastric cancer (n = 179) during a median follow-up of 12 years in Finnish male smokers [123] and with the risk of gastric cancer (n = 282) over 6.3 years in a Dutch cohort [124], with an inverse association, albeit diminished, in the latter study after excluding cases diagnosed within 2 years of baseline.

A nested case-control study in the European Prospective Investigation into Cancer and Nutrition (EPIC) compared the levels of dietary and prediagnostic plasma vitamin C between 215 gastric cancer cases and 416 matched controls [125]. No association with gastric cancer risk was observed for dietary vitamin C, whereas an inverse association was seen in the highest versus lowest quartile of plasma vitamin C (OR = 0.55, 95% CI = 0.31-0.97; for trend, P = 0.04). This inverse association was more pronounced in subjects consuming high levels of red and processed meat, a factor that may increase endogenous N-nitroso compound production. In a nested case-control study in a cohort of 20000 Chinese men (191 cases and 570 matched controls), increased serum levels of vitamin C were significantly associated with a reduced risk of gastric cancer among never-smoker and non-heavy-alcohol drinking men (for trend, P = 0.02) [126].

The use of vitamin C supplements was inversely and nonsignificantly associated with the risk of gastric cancer mortality (n = 1725; RR = 0.83, 95% CI = 0.68-1.01) among a million U.S. adults followed for 16 years (Cancer Prevention Study II) [127]. However, the decrease in risk was observed among users of shorter duration only, not among those of longer duration.

A nutritional intervention trial in Linxian, China, showed that supplementation with beta-carotene, alpha-tocopherol, and selenium reduced the risk of gastric cancer mortality by approximately 20% after 5.25 years [128]. Other micronutrients, including vitamin C (120 mg), however, were associated with no reduction. In contrast, a chemoprevention trial of gastric dysplasia in Colombia in which vitamin C supplementation at 2g/day for 6 years was tested as one of three treatment regimens showed that vitamin C as well as 30 mg beta-carotene and anti-H. pylori therapy increased the regression rate of gastric precancerous lesions [117].

In our population-based, double-blind, randomized controlled trial to examine the effect of 5 years of vitamin C supplementation, a statistically significant difference was seen between the high-dose group (500 mg/day) and the low-dose group (50 mg/day) (P = 0.046) in the change in the pepsinogen I/pepsinogen II ratio, a marker of mucosal atrophic change in the stomach. This finding suggests that vitamin C supplementation may protect against the progression of gastric mucosal atrophy [130].

In summary, when the relatively consistent epidemiological evidence and biological plausibility are considered, dietary or supplemental vitamin C intake probably decreases the risk of gastric cancer.

Adverse effects of a number of dietary exposures (particularly cured or salted meat and fish), are thought to be linked to the N-nitroso model of gastric carcinogenesis. N-nitroso compounds are potent carcinogens formed in vivo by the nitrosation of amides or amines in the stomach by nitrites, a process that is inhibited by vitamin C in gastric juice. In the stomach, nitrites are mainly derived from food and water sources, with the proportions varying according to dietary pattern and water source. For example, in one UK-based survey, approximately 90% of the nitrate intake was derived from vegetables. Cured meats provided about 65% of the nitrite intake [131]. The contribution from drinking water was estimated to add a further 13.5 mg, about 12% of total intake. However, in the USA, about 80% of nitrite intake is vegetable in origin and about 10% is derived from drinking water. Despite continuing concern that the formation of nitrosamines from dietary pre-cursors may be causally related to gastrointestinal cancer, the epidemiological literature has failed to support this link with any degree of conviction [43].

Nitrate can be converted into nitrite and in a nitrosation reaction to N-nitroso compounds (e.g. nitrosamines); these are carcinogenic in animal experiments. However, the extrapolation of these results—often obtained with high intakes—to humans and human intake levels is uncertain. In case-control and cohort studies, little evidence has been found regarding nitrate or nitrite intake from food or drinking water and gastric cancer risk [132,133]. It seems fair to conclude that nitrate does not increase gastric cancer risk, and it is not advisable to reduce vegetable intake because of nitrate, given the possible beneficial effects of high vegetable intake on gastric cancer risk. There are very few epidemiological studies on dietary nitrosamines and stomach cancer. Nitrosamines occurred in the past in smoked and salted fish, cured meats and beer, and appeared to increase the risk of gastric cancer in a French study [132], but not in a Finnish study [134]. Due to other methods of food preservation (e.g. refrigeration, addition of vitamin C and E to cured meats, which block the nitrosation reaction) levels of nitrosamines in foods have substantially decreased.

The recent IARC Monograph on Tobacco Smoke and Involuntary Smoking concluded that the results from both cohort and case—control studies are consistent with a causal role of tobacco smoking in the development of stomach cancer [46]. In a recent publication from a large European prospective Study (EPIC), an estimated 17.6% (95% Cl = 10.5—29.5%) of gastric cancer cases were attributable to smoking [135]. This is somewhat higher than the worldwide estimated 11% attributable risk derived from a 1997 meta-analysis of smoking and stomach cancer. This meta-analysis suggested a risk of stomach cancer among smokers compared to non-smokers of the order of 1.5—1.6, with a somewhat higher summary estimate in males than in females [136].

A possible increase in risk of gastric cancer associated with alcohol intake has been suggested from a meta-analysis of 16 cohort and case—control studies of gastric cancer. Bagnardi et al. [137], reported a pooled relative risk of 1.3 for a high intake of alcohol (100 g/day) but on the basis of the significant heterogeneity observed between studies the authors concluded that it was not possible to infer causality from these data. Evidence is still insufficient to establish whether cancer of the cardia or proximal region of the stomach is related to alcohol intake to any different extent than the rest of the stomach. However, one prospective study [71] and four case—control studies that reported a quantitative assessment of alcoholic drinks found no association with cancer of the gastric cardia [139-142]. What is clear is that in direct contrast to the cardiovascular system, there is less evidence that moderate consumption of alcoholic beverages has beneficial health effects on the stomach.

In a recent meta-analysis, based on 14 case-control studies and two cohort studies, a positive association was found between drinking alcoholic beverages and gastric cancer risk [143]. Regarding GCC specifically, the results are mixed.

Green tea contains polyphenols, more commonly known as catechins. Antioxidant activities and the ability to inhibit the nitrosation of polyphenols have been isolated from green tea in both in vitro and in vivo studies [144-146]. In addition, recent research has proposed many other possible mechanisms for the cancer-inhibitory effects of green tea, including modulation of signal transduction pathways, leading to the inhibition of cell proliferation and transformation, induction of apoptosis and cell cycle arrest, and inhibition of tumor invasion and angiogenesis [147-149].

The WCRF/AICR report [43] included five case-control studies investigating the relation between green tea intake and gastric cancer risk. Among these studies, four suggested a protective effect. Although a Japanese study showed a significant decrease in risk only among those consuming 10 cups or more per day, a Chinese study identified a clear dose relation. In contrast, a case-control study in Japan observed no material associations for green tea. Based on these findings, the WCRF/AICR report concluded that high consumption of green tea "possibly" decreases the risk of gastric cancer. More recent case-control studies have also shown a reduction in the risk with green tea intake, most with statistical significance [150-153].

In contrast to laboratory studies and most case-control studies, however, all but one recent cohort study have shown no protective effect of green tea for gastric cancer [154-157]. In a population-based prospective study conducted in Miyagi Prefecture in northern Japan, the RRs associated with drinking one or two, three or four, and five or more cups of green tea per day, as compared with less than one cup per day, were 1.3 (95% CI = 0.8-1.9), 1.2 (95% CI = 0.8-1.8), and 1.5 (95% CI = 1.0-2.1), respectively, in men (for trend, P = 0.03), and 0.8 (95% CI = 0.5-1.5), 0.7 (95% CI = 0.4-1.3), and 0.8 (95% CI = 0.5-1.3), respectively, in women (for trend, P = 0.46) [154]. In a nationwide multicenter prospective study, no inverse association was found between green tea consumption and gastric cancer death, with the risks associated with drinking 1 or 2, 3 or 4, 5-9, and > 10 cups of green tea per day, relative to those of drinking less than 1 cup per day, of 1.6 (95% CI = 0.9-2.9), 1.1 (95% CI = 0.6-1.9), 1.0 (95% CI = 0.5-2.0), and 1.0 (95% CI = 0.5-2.0), respectively, in men (for trend, P = 0.669), and 1.1 (95% CI = 0.5-2.5), 1.0 (95% CI = 0.5-2.5), 0.8 (95% CI = 0.4-1.6), and 0.8 (95% CI = 0.3-2.1), respectively, in women (for trend, P = 0.448) [155]. Furthermore, green tea consumption was virtually unrelated to the incidence of any cancer, including gastric cancer, in a follow-up study of atomic bomb survivors in Hiroshima and Nagasaki [156].

In a cohort study, among 73 000 subjects with 890 gastric cancers, although no association between green tea consumption and gastric cancer was observed among men, decreased risk was suggested in women, with RRs and 95% CI for one or two, three or four, and five or more cups per day compared to less than one cup per day of 0.85 (95% CI = 0.53-1.38), 1.04 (95% CI = 0.68-1.58), and 0.67 (95% CI = 0.43-1.04), respectively (for trend, P = 0.08) [157]. This association was further strengthened when cancer was restricted to the distal portion, with a RR of 0.51 (95% CI = 0.30-0.86) for consumption of five or more cups of green tea (for trend, P = 0.01). These results are consistent with those of previous prospective studies in that decreased risk was more apparent in women. In summary, consumption of green tea is possibly associated with decreased risk of gastric cancer, especially in Japanese women, most of whom are nonsmokers. Further prospective studies with detailed information are needed to clarify the role of green tea on gastric carcinogenesis.

Although catechin levels in black tea are only about 30% of those in green tea, the inhibitory activity of black tea against tumorigenesis has been shown to be comparable to that of green tea in several animal models [158]. Most of three prospective studies and 12 case-control studies showed no association with the risk of gastric cancer. Thus, the WCRF/AICR found that high consumption of black tea "probably" has no association with the risk of gastric cancer [43]. Only one prospective study in Japan has been conducted since then, and it showed a nonsignificant increase in the risk of gastric cancer among women who drink black tea more than several times per week [159]. It is possible that lifestyle, which was not investigated in this study, was associated with the increased risk of gastric cancer. Thus, the evidence is less clear for black tea than for green tea.

Caffeine, kahweol, and cafestol in coffee may contribute to a protective effect against cancer [160]. Based on the evaluation of two prospective and eight case-control studies, which showed no statistically significant association between coffee consumption and gastric cancer, the WCRF/AICR concluded that high consumption of coffee "probably" has no relation with the risk of gastric cancer [43]. In a more recent systematic review and meta-analysis of 23 studies (7 cohort studies and 16 case-control studies) [160], coffee intake showed no effect on gastric cancer when all studies were combined (OR = 0.97, 95% CI = 0.86-1.09), with a combined risk estimate of 1.02 (95% CI = 0.76-1.37) for cohort studies, 0.90 (95% CI = 0.70-1.15) for population-based case-control studies, and 0.97 (95% CI = 0.83-1.13) for hospital-based case-control studies. Notwithstanding that risk estimates differed significantly according to country of origin, with North American studies presenting a significantly higher risk, this meta-analysis showed no overall effect of coffee consumption on gastric cancer risk. In summary, there is no apparent evidence that black tea or coffee consumption has any effect on the risk of gastric cancer.

H.PYLORI INFECTION

The role of Helicobacter pylori and its association with gastric cancer has been acknowledged [180]. Our understanding about the causal relationship between H. pylori with gastric cancer has changed dramatically in recent years and become perspicuous. Through epidemiological studies, animal models and progresses in analyzing molecular mechanisms of carcinogenesis, the role of H. pylori has been elaborated. The results document that the development of gastric cancer is a multi-factorial process. H. pylori generates its many effects by interacting with the host and the environment. Together bacterial, host and environment factors interact as dangerous liaisons in triggering off a cascade of events resulting in host-pathogen disequilibrium. This interaction seems to be most important in the initial stages of tumor development. Identification of these mechanisms at various stages of neoplasia is important in preventing the progress of the disease. Recent advances in cell kinetics including findings on stem cell origin of gastric cancer have paved the way for further research.

Even though the etiology is thought to be multifactorial, inflammation seems to be the most important trigger. The major areas of colonization in the stomach are the antrum and the corpus. Histologically, these areas show chronic active gastritis characterized by polymorphonuclear leukocytes infiltrating the lamina propria, the glands, and the surface epithelium, sometimes even spilling over into the lumen forming micro abscesses. Lymphoid aggregates or follicles are seen in the lamina propria. Longer duration of the disease results in gastric atrophy (loss of glands) or intestinal metaplasia (replacement of epithelium with intestinal type of epithelium). The risk of gastric cancer is higher as the grade of atrophy and intestinal metaplasia increases [181]. In general, chronic inflammation seems a precancerous common factor. There are several links which serve as evidence to this domino effect of H. pylori.

The prevalence of H. pylori has been shown to be directly proportional to the incidence of gastric carcinoma. It is therefore low in western and northern Europe and high in Asia and Eastern Europe [182]. The EURO-CAST study has evaluated 17 populations and found that H. pylori-infected populations had a 6-fold increase in gastric cancer compared with noninfected populations [183]. This association was also shown in other prospective studies in which the odds ratio varied from 0.9 to 6.0 [184], Based on three large, well-controlled trials the International Agency for Research on Cancer (IARC) designated H. pylori as a definitive carcinogen (group I) [1, 47,185,186]. Cohort studies have shown that a decline in gastritis is associated with a similar waning in gastric cancer rates. Eradication of H. pylori caused a decrease in the progression of gastritis with an increased rate of regression of preneoplastic lesions (atrophy, intestinal metaplasia), a delay in the development of gastric cancer, and finally, prevention of gastric cancer in subjects without pre-existing lesions [187-189]. Uemura et al. [190] studied patients with early gastric cancer treated by endoscopic mucosal resection, and eradication of H. pylori in them decreased the incidence of recurrent cancer. Correa and co-workers [117, 191] studied the benefit of eradication of H. pylori as well as antioxidant treatment in a randomized control trial and observed regression of gastric atrophy as well as intestinal metaplasia after a 6-year follow-up.

These and ongoing studies point to a causal relationship of H. pylori involvement in the development of adenocarcinoma. It remains, however, to be proven whether the statement is true for all subsets of patients. Further epidemiological studies will have to focus on different populations with larger prolonged data collection.

H. pylori infection has been studied in gnotobiotic piglets, beagle dogs, Japanese monkeys and mice [181]. The Mongolian gerbil (MG) has, however, been the best studied animal model as it shows close resemblance to the colonization and infection of H. pylori in humans [192, 193]. Sugiyama et al. [194] could show an increased incidence of N-methyl-N-nitroso-urea induced gastric cancer in this model. Watanabe et al. [195] found that 37% of the animals infected with H. pylori developed 62 weeks after inoculation well-differentiated carcinomas corresponding to the intestinal type of gastric cancer in humans. Either alone or along with a chemical carcinogen, studies have shown the potentiating effect of H. pylori infection in carcinogenesis in these models. In other transgenic models such as the hypergastrinaemic (INS-GAS) mice that usually develop gastric cancer, H. pylori accelerated the time taken to neoplasia [196]. Further studies point to the importance of a pyloric lesion (spasmolytic polypeptide expressing metaplasia [SPEM] expressing the Trefoil factor family 2) as a precursor to gastric cancer in H.felis infected C57BL/6 mice [197]. Transgenic mice infected with Helicobacter have shown a gastric mutagenic effect and an inactivation of p53 tumor suppresser gene [198]. Cai et al. [199] documented that treatment with antibiotics in murine models with dysplasia prevented progression onto cancer in 70%. Even though Koch' s postulates have been fulfilled in these models, there remain differences in carcinogenesis in mouse models as compared to humans.

Cytotoxin-Associated Antigen A (CagA) is one of the principle virulence factors of H. pylori. The cagA gene is partially responsible for eliciting signaling mechanisms leading to oncogenesis. The cagA gene product, CagA is delivered into gastric epithelial cells by the type IV secretory system, a functional microinjection device of the bacterium (Figure 1). Within the gastric epithelial cells, CagA undergoes a series of biochemical modifications which include tyrosine phosphorylation. Upon phosphorylation it activates a cytoplasmic Src Homology 2 Domain - containing protein tyrosine phosphatase (FTP) called SHP2 and the complex forms a humming bird morphology of the cell [200]. This complex acts as an oncoprotein transmitting signals for cell growth, migration and adhesionBased on the sequence variation of the SHP2-binding site, two subtypes of CagA have been described - East Asian CagA and West Asian CagA, the former showing stronger SHP2 binding and therefore greater cellular growth and motility [201]. Nearly all East Asian strains bear cagA compared to as many as half in the west showing some diversity of cagA pathogenicity in different regions. The CagA-SHP2 complex can be detected in patients having chronic atrophic gastritis but not in intestinal metaplasia or cancer suggesting its role in pre-gastric cancer.

In vitro studies show that other genes within the cag island (examples: cagE, cagG, cagH, cagI, cagL, cagM) are also required for release of inflammatory cytokines such as IL-8 [202]. Inactivation of these genes result in decreased activation of NF-KB and mitogen-activated protein kinase (MAPK) signal transduction cascades regulating pro-inflammatory signals [203]. Current concepts suggest that NF-KB acts as key intermediary player in promoting the cellular changes leading to the uncontrolled growth of cancer cells; cag+ strains act as a 'switching on' mechanism of this protein [204].

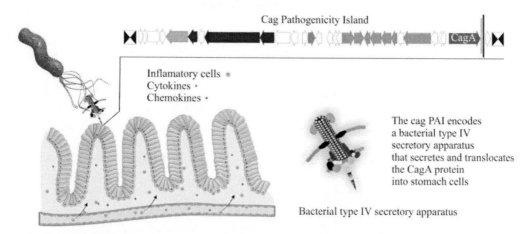

Figure 1. Cag Pathogenicity Island and Bacterial Type IV Secretory Apparatus.

Vacuolating Toxin (VacA) is another virulence factor of H. pylori and the vacA gene maps to separate loci from the cagA on the H. pylori chromosome. It functions as an anion channel. All strains of H. pylori carry the vacA gene unlike the cag island and encodes for the VacA toxin. In mice, VacA induces gastric erosions. In addition to this, it is thought to inhibit the T lymphocyte activation through induction of a G1/S cell cycle arrest, impedance of transcription of IL-2 and downregulation of IL-2a through the targeting the nuclear factor of activated T cells (NFAT) signaling pathways [205]. The exact role of vacA in oncogenesis is not yet known. However, strains possessing si/ml allele are associated with increased risk of gastric cancer [206],

Adhesion factors such as BabA, which binds to fucosylated Lewis b (Leb) blood group antigen forming an apparatus for bacterial proteins to enter epithelial cells, have been implied in gastric cancer though this has not been verified in animal models [207, 208]. The enzyme unease of H. pylori helps in buffering the acidic environment for its survival and this is controlled by a pH-gated urea channel, UreI [209]. The urease complex also upregulates inducible nitric oxide synthase (iNOS) and thereby releases nitric oxide causing inflammation [210]. The risk of developing more serious gastric lesions increases in parallel to the number of virulence factor genes accumulated in a given H. pylori strain. Zambon et al. [211] noted that H. pylori strains carrying babA2, cagA, and the vacA genotype s1m1 were associated with the highest risk of developing intestinal metaplasia, whereas this condition was rarely (<10%) associated with strains having a cagA-, babA2-, vacA s2m2 genotype. We infer from these observations a synergistic action of the factors.

The H. pylori adhesion SabA binds with sialyl-Lewis antigen promoting persistent inflammation and further dysplasia [212]. Recently, epithelial decay accelerating factor (DAF), which is a regulator of complement-mediated lysis, has been identified as a receptor for H.pylori [213, 251].

At the other side, Host Factors may play the determinative role in the consequences of the interaction between H.pylori and the host.

The protective role of the host immune system and the role of inflammation in the protection of the host have been studied widely. The initial innate immune response to Helicobacter colonization seems to be determined by Toll-like receptors (TLRs) in gastric epithelium. These receptors participate in innate immune recognition of pathogen-associated molecular patterns. Various components of the bacterium activate members of the TLR family [214]. CagA may activate the TLR-2 type of receptors. In the mouse model the progression to atrophy and cancer is dependent on a Th1 (pro-inflammatory) immune response. Therefore, susceptible strains (c57 BL6) mount a strong Th1 response while resistant strains such as the Balb/C respond with Th2 response, which protects the gastric mucosa from colonization [215]. TLR signaling is required for Th1 adaptive immunity. It is this difference between cytokine responses in different populations which are important co-factors for promoting neoplasia in some populations as compared to others [216].

Genetic susceptibility of the host is an important determinant for carcinogenesis. Increased risk of gastric cancers has been reported in IL-1β-511T carriers, IL-1-RN 2/2 genotype and tumor necrosis factor (TNF) α-308A carriers [217, 218]. IL-1 β acts as a powerful acid inhibitor and individuals with polymorphism of this gene are at a risk of developing hypochlorhydria, gastric atrophy with a 2- to 3-fold increased risk for gastric cancer. The risk seems to increase with the presence of multiple alleles coding for pro-inflammatory cytokines [219]. It is interesting to see that synergistic effect of both bacterial and host factors produce more severe clinical outcome in H. pylori infection. Therefore individuals who were cag A+, vacA+ and had IL-1β genotype had histologically a more severe disease [220].

H. pylori seems to downregulate E-cadherin, a molecule involved in cell adhesion and proliferation control [221]. The defect in cell adhesion contributes to early neoplasia; somatic mutations of this gene are found in at least half of the patients with diffuse type gastric cancers [8, 14]. Chan et al. [222] studied in gastric mucosa the relationship of E-cadherin methylation and H. pylori infection and noted that this association was increased in all stages of gastric cancer.

Alterations in the balance between apoptosis and proliferation pathways are prime to the progression of metaplasia onto cancer. Increased apoptosis secondary to H. pylori infection leads to gastric atrophy while inhibition of apoptosis results in cell proliferation and transformation into cancer. H. pylori can induce directly or indirectly (through cytokines IL-lβ, TNFα and IFNγ) Fas Ag- and ligand-mediated apoptosis [223]. This occurs early in the course of the infection and as it persists, cells become resistant to Fas-mediated apoptosis [224, 225]. The Fas pathway may then be used for proliferation and increased cell turnover. Helicobacter can also bind to MHC-II in cultured cells and inhibit Fas Ag-mediated apoptosis [226]. Different genetic susceptibility such as the MHC DQ*0102 allele can induce different expressions of the MHC II with an increased risk for the development of gastric adenocarcinoma [227].

Other pathways of apoptosis include cytokine triggered nitric oxide action on the mitochondrial systems, or VacA-induced Cytochrome c release [221]. H. pylori also upregulates Smads5 proteins belonging to the group of R-Smads which are stimulated by bone morphogenetic protein (BMP) mediating apoptosis [228].

The activating protein 1 (AP-1) plays an important role in the cell kinetics of proliferation in epithelial cells. The AP-1 complex consists of heterodimers and homodimers of proto-oncogenes c-Fos, c-Jun and ATF. These are activated by co-action of growth factors, cytokines and cellular stress signals. The activities of the oncoproteins are exerted by kinase cascades-MAPK. H. pylori activates the MAP kinase cascade resulting in stimulation one of its pathways - extracellular signal-regulated kinase 1/2 (ERK) leading to phosphorlyation of the transcription factor Elk-1 and increase in c-fos expression as well as c-Jun transcription [229].

Finally, H. pylori can trigger cell motility in the target cell which is important for invasive cell proliferation. These changes are similar to that of the hepatocyte growth factor (HGF). CagA activates the HGF/scatter factor receptor c-Met in host cells, thereby promoting a mutagenic response in the cells, which may be necessary for tumor progression [230].

As a response to H. pylori infection, the gastric mucosa expresses epidermal growth factor (EGF) for mucosal repair. This is through activation of the EGF receptor (EGFR), metalloprotease and MEK1 which results in the upregulation of the heparin binding-EGF gene transcription and amphiregulin expression. These effects in turn increase the mucosal levels of EGF and EGFR transcripts [231, 232, 233]. Increased gastrin levels induced by H. pylori is a cell proliferative factor which acts via CCK-2 receptor. Infection in hypergastrinemic transgenic mice (INS-GNS) progresses onto atrophy, dysplasia, and invasive gastric cancer [234]. Reg protein is produced by enterochromaffin-like cells (ECL cells) and act as growth factor necessary for epithelial cell proliferation. The production of this protein is in part stimulated by high gastrin levels or by increased cytokine production, both induced by H. pylori [235].

Cyclo-oxygenase-2 (COX-2) expression has been demonstrated in cell cultures co-cultured with H. pylori [236]. Higher levels are also seen in the gastric mucosa of infected subjects [237, 238]. COX-2 expression is more pronounced in pre- and malignant lesions associated with H. pylori [239, 240]. COX-2 increases the level of Bcl-2 protein, which is involved in controlling apoptosis. An over-expression of COX-2 therefore leads to the development of resistance towards apoptosis, with dysregulation of cell death and cell growth in epithelial cells. This inhibition of apoptosis is associated with the initial phase of carcinogenesis [241]. H. pylori also induces the release of PGE2 (another product of the AA pathway) in gastric mucosa resulting in similar effects [242].

Reactive Oxygen (ROS) and Nitrogen Species (RNS) cause DNA damage of the host cell and lead to altered cell turnover [243]. H. pylori decreases the antioxidant properties of gastric mucosa as it decreases vitamin C levels - a naturally occurring antioxidant [244, 245]. In vivo studies show that H. pylori causes oxidative damage in gastric epithelial cells, whereas eradication of H. pylori causes an attenuation of oxidative stress [246, 247]. Glutathione-S-transferases (GSTs) are a superfamily of enzymes helping in protecting the DNA. Genetic polymorphisms and null mutations of GSST1 and GSTM1 cause increased risk of developing H. pylori-related gastric cancer [248]. Further strengthening evidence has been shown in interventional trials using antioxidants which act as chemopreventive agents in reducing histological changes secondary to H. pylori in a similar way as vitamin C sup-plementation may protect against gastric atrophy and further neoplastic growth [130, 191].

Recent research in mice suggests that H. pylori-induced inflammation caused migration of bone marrow stem cells to the stomach where they progress under certain circumstances onto gastric cancer. Stem cells have the features of 'plasticity', i.e. ability to differentiate into multiple cell lineages and 'transdifferentiation' or differentiation of cells from one organ-specific lineage to that of another organ. Houghton and colleagues [249, 250] studied this on a mouse model replacing the bone marrow-derived (BMD) cells through irradiation with transgenic cells which would express detectable markers. After infection with H.felis the authors began to detect BMD cells migrating into the gastric epithelium. After 20 weeks they had differentiated into cells with characteristics of gastric epithelial cells. The cells rapidly proliferated and by 52 weeks the mice developed early stages of gastric cancer and the tumors stained positively for markers indicating their bone marrow cell line origin. These fascinating studies are just in their early stages and further work is awaited to confirm the observations.

The ongoing studies on the role of H. pylori in the development of gastric cancer give us a way for identifying early treatment strategies before the 'point of no return'. Eradication of infection seems to decrease the risk of developing gastric carcinomas and these strategies will have to be further worked on [252, 253].

H.pylori and the Intestinal Type of Gastric Cancer

According to Correa, intestinal type GC may be considered a multistep process starting from chronic gastritis and progressing through chronic atrophic gastritis, IM and dysplasia [255]. This sequence is usually triggered by H. pylori infection and affected by a variety of genetic and environmental factors that may act synergistically [256].

Chronic Atrophic Gastritis

Long-standing H. pylori-induced gastric inflammation often leads to atrophic gastritis which is considered the first important step in the histogenesis of GC [255]. In a large population study on 2455 subjects in Japan, Asaka reported gastric atrophy in 80% of H. pylori-infected patients compared with 10% of H. pylori-negative patients [257]. According to previous European studies, the overall prevalence of gastric atrophy, in asymptomatic adults, ranges from 22 to -37%, with a GC incidence ranging from 7 to -13%, in patients with chronic atrophic gastritis, after a follow-up of more than 11 years [258, 259] Recently, observing 5375 subjects for a 10-year follow-up period, 117 GCs were identified. The risk of GC was greatest among the subjects with moderate atrophy at baseline (HR: 2.22; 95% CI: 1.08-4.58) and 4-6 years of follow-up (HR: 4.6-5.0) [260]

Gastric atrophy, particularly when it affects a large part of the gastric body, is associated with acid hyposecretion and impaired pepsinogen levels [261] The low acidity of the gastric juice will, moreover, allow colonization with other bacteria, that, in turn, may promote the formation of carcinogenic factors, i.e. N-nitroso formation, inducing cellular DNA methylation [256,262]. This finding is particularly important since in chronic atrophic gastritis, the increased proliferation of mucosal epithelium, results in the presence of relatively immature cells in the glands [263]. Ornithine decarboxylase (ODC), the first and rate-limiting enzyme in the biosynthesis of polyamines, is required for normal and neoplastic growth [264, 265]. ODC is up-regulated by H. pylori and strongly expressed in atrophic and IM areas [266, 267]. Therefore, the expression of ODC may be considered an important marker of premalignancy in the stomach [266].

Intestinal Metaplasia

Chronic atrophic gastritis is often associated with IM, both lesions being closely related to H. pylori infection [255, 268, 269]. Indeed, the prevalence of IM was significantly higher in H. pylori-positive (43%) than in H. pylori-negative subjects (6.2%) [257]. In Japan, using a GC index, IM was the only criterion associated with the development of intestinal type GC [270]. Intestinal metaplasia has been classified according to Jass and Filipe as complete or type I, or incomplete which comprises types II and III [271]. The expression of mucin core proteins (MUC) differs in the different types of IM. Whilst all types showed de novo expression of MUC2, the expression of MUC1, MUC5AC and MUC6 was decreased in the complete type of IM and preserved in the incomplete type [272, 273].

Based on retrospective data, the risk of GC is related to the type of IM [274, 275]. In a 10-year follow-up study from Slovenia, patients with IM showed an overall 10-fold increased risk of GC compared with those without IM [274]. In another study, the risk of GC was fourfold higher in patients with IM type III than in those with type I [276]. In a cohort study of 4655 healthy asymptomatic subjects observed for a mean period of 7.7 years, the risk of GC increased in a stepwise fashion from H. pylori-positive chronic gastritis group (HR: 7.13; 95% CI: 0.95-53.33) to H. pylori-positive chronic atrophic gastritis group (HR: 14.85; 95% CI: 1.96-107.7) and finally to severe chronic atrophic gastritis with extensive IM (HR: 61.85; 95% CI: 5.6-682.64) [277]. The association between the risk of GC development and IM subtypes is, however, not universally accepted. Cassaro et al. have recently shown that IM involving the lesser curvature, from the cardia to the pylorus, or the entire stomach, was associated with a higher risk of GC than focal or antral predominant IM [278]. Thus, the distribution of IM rather than IM subtype may provide a higher predictive value of cancer risk. Molecular alterations could be involved in the progression of IM to GC [279-284]. The pattern of gene expression determining the cell phenotype is under the control of a complex hierarchy of transcription factors of which homeodomain proteins are important members.

CDX1 and CDX2, homeobox genes are intestinal transcription factors regulating the proliferation and differentiation of intestinal epithelial cells. CDX1 and CDX2 proteins are expressed predominantly in the small intestine and colon but not in the normal adult stomach [285]. In a recent study from Japan, CDX2 expression was found in patients with chronic gastritis closely associated with IM [286].

Telomerases, generally activated in GC, were reported to be elevated in 18% (eight of 43) of patients with IM [284]. Microsatellite instability (MSI) can be detected in IM obtained both from cancer and non-cancer patients thus suggesting that MSI may be an early event in the multistep progression of GC [280, 287, 288]. Accumulation or mutations of the p53 protein have been demonstrated in IM, particularly in type III, and in IM areas adjacent to GC [282, 289, 290, 291]. Overexpression of COX-2 and cyclin D2 and decreased p27 expression, all involved in cell cycle regulation, were detected in H. pylori-associated IM [239, 241, 283]. Interestingly, type III IM, carrying a higher risk for GC, is that harboring more numerous genetic changes than type I or II IM [287, 289, 292].

However, IM can also be categorized by the preservation of pyloric cells or the appearance of goblet cells, resembling the gastric and intestinal phenotype respectively [513]. Essentially, however, IM shows absorptive intestinal type cells with a brush border, goblet cells containing mucin and Paneth cells, harbouring eosinophilic granules in their cytoplasm and found typically at the base of the glands and also neuroendocrine cells. Mixtures of gastric and intestinal phenotypes occur at the cellular as well as the glandular level. Thus, IM subtypes should not be considered as independent entities but rather as a part of a dynamic process with a gradual change from gastric to intestinal character associated with stem cell differentiation patterns that can initially produce both gastric and intestinal type cells and ultimately move to a wholly metaplastic gland [514]. Multipotent progenitor cells are thought to be located in the proliferative cell zone in the isthmus of gastric glands, giving rise to all the various differentiated gastric cell types [510]. Gutierrez-Gonzalez et al. have shown that gastric glands are clonal, contain multiple stem cells and divide by fission. These data also suggest that an individual progenitor cell has populated the entire population of that gland – so called monoclonal conversion [510]. Mixed IM, where pyloric cells and goblet cells are present in the same gland has been postulated to be a novel form of IM [515]: the authors propose that mixed glands are in the process of converting from gastric to intestinal type via monoclonal conversion and the presence of mixed IM is therefore simply a step in this process of monoclonal conversion.

Furthermore, along with IM, an additional type of metaplasia in the stomach is growing in importance – so called SPEM lineage, named because of its characteristic expression of trefoil factor family 2 (TFF2; spasmolytic polypeptide). This change is associated with loss of parietal cells (oxyntic atrophy) [516] and develops characteristically in the fundus of the stomach in mice infected with H. felis [197] and also in humans [517]. SPEM appears to have some common characteristics with the well-recognized pseudopyloric metaplasia (PPM) of the intestine and biliary tract and the global gut ulcer-associated cell lineage [518, 519]. Given the epidemiological association of Helicobacter species infection with gastric cancer, SPEM has a strong association with both chronic Helicobacter pylori infection and gastric adenocarcinoma and may represent another pathway to gastric neoplasia [520,521]. Defective epidermal growth factor receptor (EGFR) signalling accelerates SPEM development [522], possibly though loss of the parietal cells, which secrete at least three EGFR ligands. Although all of the actions of EGFR ligands are mediated through a common EGFR protein, individual ligands may produce different physiological responses [516] and regulate gastric differentiation in different ways; while the loss of amphiregulin (AR) causes acceleration of SPEM development and its progression after acute oxyntic atrophy, the loss transforming growth factor (TGF-α) produces foveolar hyperplasia [516]. This gives an epithelial field which is in inherently genetically unstable [523], with an increased risk of progression into carcinoma, suggesting a relationship between the metaplastic population with malignancy. Classically, the development of IM has been associated with downregulation of p27, telomerases, mutation of p53 protein, upregulation of c-myc, loss of heterozygosity, microsatellite instability, cyclin D2 [524], Helicobacter pylori infection, APC mutations and cyclooxygenase (COX-2) expression [525]. Recent investigations have led to re-evaluation of the true origin of IM. For the moment, this pathogenesis has been elucidated as a combination of bacterial, environmental factors and cytokines that modulate inflammatory responses and exert synergistic effects, but there are few studies on the important role of the molecular factors in this development. The homeobox genes Cdx1 and Cdx2 are one of the most important genes involved in the development, maintenance and proliferation of intestinal phenotype in the gut, but they are only expressed in the upper digestive epithelium (oesophagus and stomach) when Helicobacter pylori infection and chronic gastritis occurs, leading to the development of intestinal epithelium in the gastric mucosa. However, each gene plays a different role in the development of IM: while Cdx1 permits the transdifferentiation of the gastric mucosa to an intestinal phenotype, the maintenance of intestinal differentiation appears to require the presence that Cdx2. In Cdx2 transgenic mice, normal gastric mucosa was completely replaced by IM, confirming the central role of Cdx2 in the induction of IM [526,527], but other important genes are over-expressed in IM, such as Pdx1, Oct1 and TFF3, although Sox2, Shh are downregulated and Runx3 is deactivated by epigenetic silencing. Nevertheless, the control of gene expression in the development of IM is complex, depending on several families of signalling molecules such as Wnt, RA, FGF, Hhh and MAPK/ERK that may serve as future molecular markers of metaplastic epithelium. Moreover multiple, specific somatic mutations in metaplastic epithelium have been suggested as potential biomarkers. The most promising mark ers to date are the presence of aneuploidy, growth factor expression, loss of heterozygosity of p53, p16 and cyclin Dl overexpression. Given the acceptance of IM as a precursor of dysplasia and cancer in many gastric tumours, more extensive studies on the molecular origin of IM is necessary if we are to prevent cancer development in individuals with such lesions.

The loss of parietal cells, oxyntic atrophy, is the most reliable correlate with gastric cancer in human beings [528]. Nozaki et al [528] suggest that the loss of parietal cells in gastrin-deficient mice leads to the rapid appearance of metaplastic cells at the bases of fundic glands expressing both mature chief cell markers and TFF2. In addition, the authors observed an upregulation of genes involved in G1/S-phase transition leading to re-entry of a population of cells into the cell cycle. The metaplastic process also was associated with the up-regulation of a number of putative soluble regulators not usually present in the normal stomach mucosa. In particular, HE4 was up-regulated in gastric metaplasia in both mice and human beings and its expression was maintained in gastric adenocarcinomas. Thus, examination of the induction of gastric metaplasia in mice has revealed a number of critical regulators relevant to the preneoplastic process in human beings. Although most views of the stomach mucosa have centered on lineage production from the normal progenitor zone in the neck of gastric fundic glands [529], the present investigations focus attention on a potential compartment at the bases of fundic glands induced after parietal cell loss [531]. Three explanations could account for this observation [528]. First, a cryptic progenitor cell population may exist at the base of fundic glands, distinct from the normal progenitor region in the neck, which would be suppressed by mucosal differentiation factors released by parietal cells. At least in gastrin-deficient mice, this explanation seems less likely because of the rapidity of metaplastic changes and the low amount of proliferation. Second, SPEM may develop from transdifferentiation of chief cells. Previous studies have shown that acute oxyntic atrophy leads to the observation of proliferating cells expressing intrinsic factor, a marker of differentiated chief cells in mice [531]. Although intrinsic factor is expressed in rare prezymogenic cells, the transcription factor Mist1 is expressed only in mature chief cells [530]. The observation here of Mist1-immunoreactive cells also expressing TFF2 supports chief cell transdifferentiation as the origin of SPEM. The transdifferentiation of zymogenic cells to mucous metaplasia may be a general mechanism underlying preneoplastic transition in the upper gastrointestinal tract. Means et al [532] have shown that over expression of transforming growth factor α leads to the transdifferentiation of pancreatic zymogen cells into mucous-secreting metaplastic cells. Acinar cell transdifferentiation contributes to preneoplastic lesion in the pancreas [533]. Similarly, loss of parietal cells may elicit the transdifferentiation of gastric zymogen-secreting chief cells. Thus, although previous views have suggested that gastric metaplasia originates from normal mucosal progenitor cells, the results obtained by Nozaki et al [528] indicate that the loss of parietal cells from the gastric fundic mucosa induces alterations in the transcriptional profile of chief cells leading to changes in the cellular secretory phenotype and transdifferentiation into a mucous cell metaplasia.

Dysplasia

The next step in the cascade of morphological changes in gastric carcinogenesis is dysplasia that usually develops in the IM setting [255]. This process includes a continuum of progressively dedifferentiated phenotypes which may result in a new cell. According to the definition of the World Health Organization, dysplasia is now called non-invasive gastric neoplasia, indicating a preinvasive neoplastic change in the gastric glands [293]. In dysplasia, cellular morphology is characterized by uncontrolled growth and the potential to migrate and implant in other areas. The higher the grade of dysplasia, the greater the risk of developing invasive GC [294]. Helicobacter pylori is clearly associated with the progressive development of metaplastic changes [295]. From a molecular viewpoint, dysplastic cells are endowed with an increased amount of DNA, partly due to the increased number of proliferating cells. A mixture of polyploidy and aneuploidy cells, in high grade dysplasia, has been demonstrated [296, 297]. Several markers, such as APC/MCC loss of heterozygosity, carcinoembryonic antigen, p21ras, tumour suppressor gene p53 and the apoptosis inhibitor bcl-2 gene, which are overexpressed in GC, have also been detected in dysplastic areas [282, 289, 290, 298, 299]. According to our current understanding, dysplastic cells resemble malignant cells, and, in fact, may sometimes already be malignant. The majority of carcinoma found in follow-up studies and which were discovered within 1 year of the diagnosis of dysplasia may indicate that the carcinoma was already present at the time of diagnosis of dysplasia [256].

Helicobacter Pylori and Diffuse Type Gastric Cancer

Diffuse GC, often associated with familial distribution, is more prevalent in younger women and blood group A patients [300]. The cancer develops in the stomach following chronic inflammation without passing through the intermediate steps of atrophic gastritis or IM. The severity of the mucosal inflammation and host characteristic may directly induce mutagenetic events ultimately leading to cancer [301, 302]. Many molecular alterations have been detected in diffuse type GC that differ substantially from those found in the intestinal type, i.e. MSI-H phenotype, implicated in the repair of spontaneous and toxic DNA damage; SC-1 antigen, an apoptotic receptor; E-cadherin mutation and the growth factors c-met and k-sam [25, 288, 303, 304, 305, 306]. The onset of these molecular alterations is strongly associated with H. pylori infection. Indeed, a recent meta-analysis showed a close correlation between diffuse type GC and H. pylori infection, similar to those found between intestinal type and H. pylori (OR: 2.58, 95% CI: 1.47-4.53; OR: 2.49, 95% CI: 1.41-4.43, respectively) [307]. Therefore, even if intestinal and diffuse type GCs are characterized by a different genetic pathway, they depend prevalently upon the same triggering factor. It is likely that H. pylori-associated inflammatory reaction may trigger a cascade of events (atrophy, IM and dysplasia) progressing to intestinal type GC or directly induce diffuse type GC. Once the cascade of events is activated, it may also progress independently of the bacterium. A prospective, randomized, placebo-controlled, population study, has recently been carried out in a high-risk area of China [252]. Healthy carriers of H. pylori infection (1630 subjects) were observed from 1994 until 2002. A comparable incidence of GC development was found in the subjects receiving H. pylori eradication treatment and those receiving placebo. However, in a subgroup of H. pylori carriers not presenting precancerous lesions, eradication of H. pylori significantly decreased the development of GC. Therefore, eradication of H. pylori might immediately reduce the risk of diffuse cancer whereas cancers of the intestinal type may be less effectively prevented if patients are treated later in the evolution of their carcinogenic process.

EPSTEIN–BARR VIRUS-ASSOCIATED GASTRIC CARCINOMA

Epstein-Barr virus (EBV)-associated gastric carcinoma (EBVaGC) is the most common among various lethal malignancies associated with EBV [69]. Epstein-Barr virus, a gammaherpes virus, is the first virus that was identified in a human neoplastic cell [97]. More than 90% of the world population is infected with EBV before adolescence, and it has been shown that some limited populations develop EBV-associated malignancy in an endemic manner, such as Burkitt lymphoma in equatorial Africa [99] and nasopharyngeal carcinoma (NPC) in Southern China [102]. However, recent advances in molecular techniques have demonstrated an unexpectedly wide variety of neoplasms associated with EBV [103, 105], among which EBVaGC is the most common, with a worldwide distribution [129,138,161,162]. In Japan, for example, 5000 patients are estimated to develop gastric carcinoma annually in association with EBV [138].

EBVaGC consists of two types of carcinomas, most of lymphoepithelioma (LE)-like gastric carcinoma [163] and 10% or less of ordinary gastric carcinoma [138]. Although the relative frequency of both types depends on the strictness of the histological criteria, LE-like carcinoma appears to constitute one-fifth of EBVaGC. The pathological features of both types have been well described, such as male predominance, location primarily in the proximal stomach, and moderately or poorly differentiated type of histology. However, the developmental process of EBVaGC has yet to be clearly demonstrated. In nonneoplastic gastric mucosa, rarity or complete absence of epithelial cells showing positive signal by EBER (EBV-encoded small RNA) with in situ hybridization (ISH) suggests that EBV infection is relatively rare in gastric epithelia [69]. On the other hand, Yanai et al. [164] and Jing et al. [165], using a commercially available DNA ISH kit, recently insisted that EBV infection was occasionally observed in epithelial cells of intestinal metaplasia. However, the signals in the epithelial cells presented in the studies were too strong for the DNA probe ISH without any enhancing procedure, as the copy number of EBV in EBVaGC is generally considered to reach only a few hundred at most [69], the lower limit for detection. Because the methods in both studies lacked sufficient control studies [166], their finding should be interpreted with caution and needs reexamination. Thus, EBV seems to play a direct role in the development of this carcinoma [69, 162], or at least the carcinoma cells are tagged with clonal EBV, which makes EBVaGC a distinct entity among gastric carcinomas.

EBVaGCs occur much more frequently as multiple carcinoma than expected if it develops independently [138, 167], suggesting that the nonneoplastic mucosa of the proximal stomach bearing EBVaGC has been conditioned to develop EBVaGC (field cancerization). To help reconcile these findings with the recently hypothesized EBV infection in the intestinal metaplasia, we attempt here to evaluate the detailed pathology of non-neoplastic mucosa of EBVaGC, and to analyze the EBV infection by ISH of EBV DNA using RNA probes and by polymerase chain reaction (PCR) detection of EBV DNA, which was applied to the microdissected gastric mucosa with or without intestinal metaplasia.

In 1990, Burke et al. [168] first demonstrated the relationship between EBV and gastric carcinoma, by identifying EBV-DNA by polymerase chain reaction (PCR) in a lymphoepithelioma-like carcinoma of the stomach that has been termed "gastric carcinoma with lymphoid stroma", which shows a favorable prognosis compared with that of other poorly differentiated adenocarcinomas [169]. Based on the results of a highly sensitive in-situ hybridization (ISH) method targeting EBV-encoded small RNA (EBER) [170], most lymphoepithelioma-like gastric carcinomas are now considered to be associated with EBV [163, 167, 171, 172]. In the stomach, the association with EBV is not limited to lymphoepithelioma-like carcinoma, but is also observed in some gastric carcinomas with ordinary histology.

There are three possible mechanisms by which EBV may be related to cancer initiation in the stomach [69]. (A) EBV may be the sole factor that initiates EBVaGC. If mucosal damage delays the flow of epithelial cells, then EBV-infected cells can grow within the gland. (B) EBV may cooperate with other promoting factors. EBV-infected cells may be prone to subsequent genetic alterations, which initiate carcinomatous growth. (C) Alternatively, proliferating cells, which have already started neoplastic growth but remain a small fraction within the mucosa, may be more likely to be infected by EBV. This mechanism is based on the assumption that EBV-infected cells have some advantage for monoclonal growth over other, uninfected, cancer cells. Using PCR-KFLP and micro-satellite markers, Chong JM, et al., observed that deletion of 5q and/ or 17p and microsatellite instability were extremely rare in EBVaGC, in contrast to their high frequency in EBV-negative carcinoma, particularly its intestinal type [173]. This indicates that the genetic pathways of EBVaGC and EBV-negative carcinoma may be different. An immunohistochemical study reported that EBVaGC was independent of bcl-2 expression and p53 accumulation [174].

Few studies have investigated the cellular characteristics of EBVaGC in detail. Both the frequency of apoptosis and the proportion of proliferative cells were significantly lower in EBV-associated lymphoepi-thelioma-like carcinoma than in conventional EBV-negative gastric carcinomas [175]. However, whether the determinant of these phenomena was the presence of EBV or the particular histologic type of gastric carcinoma was not clear. Mucin histochemistry has revealed gastric type mucin to be predominant in most EBVaGC [176]. Some isoforms of CD44, an adhesion molecule of the cell surface, have been associated with the metastatic potential of carcinomas, such as colon and breast carcinomas. When CD44 variants 3-5 and 6 were immunohistochemically determined in gastric carcinoma, a multivariate analysis showed that EBV association and lymph node metastasis contributed independently to CD44 variant-expression [177]. Thus, the mechanism and significance of CD44 variant expression are different in gastric carcinoma with and without EBV. It is possible that EBV infection may influence CD44 expression by interacting with cytokine genes, such as those for tumor necrosis factor (TNF)α, interferon (INF)γ and interleukin 10, which are known to modulate CD44 expression. Infiltration of lymphocytes, most of which are CDS-positive in EBVaGC [176], may be induced by such a mechanism [178], rather than as a reaction to carcinoma cells.

The number of reports on the detection of EBV in gastric cancer cases is rapidly increasing. However, the mechanism of EBV-induced gastric carcinogenesis remains to be elucidated. It appears that in gastric carcinoma, EBV infection precedes malignant transformation in a significant fraction of cases, but neither bcl-2 expression (an inhibitor of apoptosis) nor p53 accumulation was found to be consistently associated with the presence of the virus [174]. Ojima et al. [179] studied 412 patients with gastric adenocarcinoma and detected EBV-specific RNA in tumor cell nuclei of 83 patients (20.1 %), of which 60 were histologically subclassified as gastric carcinoma with lymphoid stroma. Overexpression of p53 was demonstrated in only seven (8.4%) of 83 EBV-positive gastric carcinomas, but in 31 (34.4%) of 90 randomly selected EBV-negative gastric carcinomas. The authors of this study believed that EBV-associated gastric carcinomas may arise through a different mechanism from other types of gastric carcinomas without EBV infection [179].

GENETIC POLYMORPHISMS AND GASTRIC CANCER SUSCEPTIBILITY

In recent years, genetic susceptibility has been extensively studied as one of the most important possible explanations for interindividual variation in GC risk [468,486]. Multiple studies have demonstrated proinflammatory genetic polymorphisms as risk factors for both precancerous lesions and GC through determining the extent and severity of gastric mucosal inflammation [191,487]. Besides chronic inflammation, other mechanisms including mucosal protection, carcinogen metabolism, antioxidant protection, cell cycle regulation, tumour invasion and metastasis are likely to contribute to GC development. Gene variants related to these mechanisms were also widely assessed as potential risk markers for GC [468,486].

Single nucleotide polymorphisms (SNPs) have potential as markers for identifying genes responsible for common diseases and for personalized medicine.

With the completion of the human genome project and appreciation of the implications of disease-associated SNP for tailoring medicines, attention is now rapidly shifting towards the study of individual genetic variation in determining clinical diseases [488]. SNP is the most abundant source of genetic variation in the human genome, and likely accounts for heritable inter-individual differences in the phenotypes for complex genetic and environmentally determined diseases [489].

The fact that cytokines such as γ-interferon (INF-γ), interleukin-lβ (IL-1β), IL-1 receptor antagonist (IL-1RN), and tumor necrosis factor-α (TNF-α) are considerably upregulated during H. pylori infection and that some H. pylori -infected persons develop clinical disease, has stimulated the drive to search for polymorphisms of these and related genes [490]. Polymorphic regions of cytokine genes could alter gene transcription, thereby influencing inflammatory processes in response to H. pylori infection [491]. IL-1β and IL-1RN are the cytokine genes studied most extensively for gene polymorphisms. IL-1β gene is an important pro-inflammatory cytokine and a powerful inhibitor of gastric acid secretion [492]. Two SNP sites exist in the promoter region at positions -511 and -31, representing C-T and T-C transitions, respectively. These SNP have been shown to be associated with clinical outcomes of H. pylori infection, including gastric ulcer or cancer. Further, within the IL-1RN gene, a variable number of tandem repeats (VNTR) of an 86 bp length in intron 2 have been reported [492]. Besides their significant disease associations, these SNP of either IL-l β or IL-1RN appear to impose functional abnormalities. In particular, they promote hypochlorhydria, which favors further colonization of H. pylori, leading to a more severe gastritis and gastric atrophy, after which adenocarcinoma may develop [493].

El-Omar et al. showed the IL-1 β polymorphism is a risk factor for gastric cancer [218,219]. Furuta et al. also showed that pro-inflammatory IL-l β polymorphisms, IL-1B-511 T, are associated with hypochlorhydria and atrophic gastritis in Japanese people [494]. Later, El-Omar reported not only IL-1 gene polymorphism, but also other cytokine polymorphisms, such as IL-10 and TNF-α, increased the risk of non-cardia gastric adenocarcinoma [217]. Garza-Gonzalez et al. showed that IL-1B-31 is associated with increased risk of distal gastric cancer [495].

Two large meta-analyses concerning the association between IL-1 gene polymorphisms and gastric cancer were published [496,497]. Both reached the same conclusion, that IL-1B-511 T was associated with an increased risk of gastric cancer. In addition, IL-1RN*2 was also associated with an increased risk of gastric cancer among Caucasians [497]. In contrast, in studies of Chinese people, IL-lβ gene polymorphisms were not associated with gastric cancer risk [498]. Another report from Spain also showed no association between variable cytokine gene polymorphisms (IL-l β, IL-1RN, IL-12p40, LTA, IL-10, IL-4 and TGF- β1) and gastric cancer [499]. Shin et al. showed that IL-1B-511, IL-1RN and IL-2 gene polymorphisms were not the determining factor that discriminated gastric ulcer, gastric cancer and duodenal ulcer [500]. Therefore, although IL-lβ and IL-1RN gene polymorphism is generally proven as risk factor in Caucasians, there was no relationship between these cytokine gene polymorphisms and gastric cancer in Korean studies.

A systematic review of Gao L . et al. [485] showed that genetic polymorphisms in tumour invasion could be candidate biomarkers of GC risk. The review summarized the associations between tumour invasion-related genetic polymorphisms and GC susceptibility. Fourteen polymorphisms, significantly related to GC risk in at least one published study, were identified. Meta-analysis was performed for CDH1-160C>A, the most widely studied polymorphism. While results were often inconsistent, the analysis suggested the inconsistencies to be explained in part by differences between study populations. Furthermore, because of the multistage character of GC, genetic factors may play a role at specific stages only and they may interfere with nongenetic risk factors, such as smoking and high intake of salted foods, which strongly vary between populations.

RECENT ADVANCES IN MOLECULAR CARCINOGENESIS IN GASTRIC CARCINOMA

Over the past several years, there have been many new developments in our understanding of the molecular biology of gastric carcinoma. Integrated research in molecular pathology over the past 15 years has uncovered the molecular mechanism of invasion and metastasis in gastric cancer [308-312]. Many studies have clearly demonstrated that multiple genetic alterations are responsible for the development and progression of gastric cancer [313-316]. It is now evident that different genetic pathways lead to diffuse- and intestinal-type gastric cancer. Alterations in specific genes that play important roles in diverse cellular functions, such as cell adhesion, signal transduction, cell differentiation, development, metastasis, DNA repair, and glycosylation changes, have been identified, although much less is known about the mixed types or rare variants of gastric carcinoma [313-316, 317-320]. Molecular biology is equally important for developing diagnostic and prognostic molecular markers. Therefore, the challenge is to detect stage-specific genetic abnormalities that may result in early diagnosis and even aid in selecting therapy.

At present, a number of molecular abnormalities participating in proliferation, invasion, and metastasis have been identified, including microsatellite instability (MSI), inactivation of tumor suppressor genes, activation of oncogenes and reactivation of telomerase, abnormalities in growth factors and their receptors, cell-cycle regulators, cell-adhesion molecules, matrix-degrading enzymes, and other factors (Figure 2).

MSI is defined as the presence of replication errors in simple repetitive microsatellite sequences due to DNA mismatch repair deficiency [321]. It is classified as high-frequency (MSI-H), low-frequency (MSI-L), or stable (MSS) [322]. MSI has been recognized as one of the earliest changes in carcinogenesis and results in genomic instability [323]. MSI is present in a subset of gastric cancers [324], ranging from 13% to 44% of gastric tumors [316]; in particular, MSI-H occurs in 10% to 16% of gastric cancers [316]. Furthermore, hypermethylation of CpG islands in the promoter region of the hMLH1 gene is associated with decreased hMLH1 protein expression and often occurs in gastric cancer cases with MSI-H, indicating that epigenetic inactivation of this gene in association with promoter methylation may underlie MSI [325]. MSI in gastric cancer cases is also associated with antral tumor location, intestinal-type differentiation, and a better prognosis [313, 316]. Such cancer cases exhibit a different genetic background from those without MSI, i.e., they exhibit mutations of transforming growth factor (TGF) receptor II and do not have p53 mutations [326]. MSI-H-positive gastric cancers are clinicopathologically distinct; thus, it may be valuable to identify subgroups of gastric cancers [327]. The MSI technique is promising for the early detection of cancer: rather than searching for a specific gene, it may be used as a screening tool [328]. Additional genes with simple, tandem repeat sequences within their coding regions that have been found to be specifically altered in gastric cancers displaying MSI include BAX, hMSHS, hMSH6, E2F-4, TGF-β receptor II, and insulin-like growth factor receptor II, which are known to be involved in the regulation of cell-cycle progression and apoptotic signaling [315, 316].

Inactivation of tumor suppressor genes due to mutations and/or loss of heterozygosity (LOH) is also a frequent event in gastric carcinogenesis. For example, inactivation of p53 and p16 has been reported in both diffuse- and intestinal-type gastric cancers, whereas adenomatous polyposis coli (APC) gene mutations seem to occur more frequently in intestinal-type gastric cancers [290, 329]. Other candidate tumor suppressor genes that have exhibited genomic alterations in gastric cancers include fragile histidine triad (FHIT) and deleted in colon cancer (DCC).

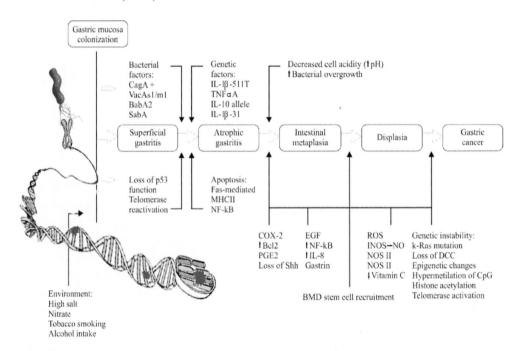

Figure 2. Multistep model for the casual relationship of H.pylori and gastric cancer. EGF – Epidermal growth factor; iNOS – inducible nitric oxide synthase; NOS –nitric oxide synthase; ROS – reactive oxygen species; BMD – bone marrow derived; MHC II – major histocompatibility complex Class II; DCC – deleted in colon cancer; NF-kB – nuclear factor kappa B; Shh – Sonic Hedgehog gene. (Adapted from Shajan P., Beglinger C. [534]).

Mutation or LOH of the p53 gene has been reported in up to 80% of gastric cancer cases independent of the histological subtype, and predominately in cases of metastatic disease [329 - 333]. However, p53 mutations have also been identified in early dysplastic and meta-plastic lesions (about 10%) [329, 334, 335], and some studies have reported that p53 alterations have a crucial role in early intestinal-type gastric carcinogenesis, likely acting at the transition step between metaplasia and dysplasia, and that the alterations are mainly associated with tumor progression in diffuse-type cancer [329]. However, because of the use of different techniques, including immunohistochemistry, polymerase chain reaction single-strand conformation polymorphism, and sequencing, the results are not consistent [336].

Up to 60% of intestinal-type gastric tumors and approximately 25% of adenomas have mutation and/or LOH of the tumor suppressor gene APC [337-341]. These alterations are rare in diffuse-type carcinomas but may be associated with signet-ring cell carcinomas [342]. However, a recent study indicated that somatic mutation of the APC gene plays an important role in the pathogenesis of gastric adenoma and dysplasia, but has a limited role in the progression of it to adenocarcinoma [343]. In addition, the APC protein is important for the degradation of β-catenin [344, 345]. Specifically, it binds to β-catenin, whose free concentration within the cell is tightly regulated and kept at a low level. After interaction with the transcription factor lymphoid enhancer factor-1 (LEF-1), β-catenin translocates into the nucleus, where it regulates gene expression [346]. β-Catenin mutations have also been detected in intestinal-type gastric tumors, but are absent from diffuse-type tumors [347, 348]. In intestinal-type gastric cancers, the accumulation of β-catenin protein may result from impaired degradation of the β-catenin protein due to alterations of the β-catenin and APC genes [313].

In previous studies, P16INK4 somatic mutations with LOH were noted in several cases of esophageal cancer, but not in those of gastric carcinoma [349, 350]. A significant portion (>40%) of gastric cancers exhibited CpG island methylation of the promoter region of p16 [351, 352]. Many of these cases exhibiting hypermethylation of promoter regions displayed the MSI-H phenotype and multiple sites of methylation, including the hMLH1 promoter region [353, 354], suggesting that CpG island hypermethylation occurs early in multistep gastric carcinogenesis.

Aberrant methylation of promoters may lead to the transcriptional silencing of various genes (e.g., E-cadherin, p16, p15, MGMT, and hMLH1) in gastric cancer [309, 354, 355]. It has been reported that approximately 40% of gastric cancers are CpG island methylator phenotype (CIMP) tumors, which frequently exhibit methylation of the p16 and hMLH1 genes [356]. The genetic and molecular changes in these cancers are different from those in CIMP-negative cancers, suggesting an alternative pathway of gastric cancer pathogenesis. Because these changes can also be found in normal mucosa, they are probably early events in gastric carcinogenesis [356].

FHIT is a putative tumor suppressor gene that was isolated from the common fragile site FRA3B at 3p14.2 and found to have abnormal transcripts, with deleted exons in five of nine gastric cancer cases [357]. In other studies, genomic alterations and abnormal expression of FHIT were demonstrated in the majority of gastric carcinoma cases [358, 359], suggesting that FHIT can play an important role in gastric carcinogenesis [359]. A recent study showed that abnormalities of FHIT, which are presumably associated with the unstable nature of FRA3B within the gene, are involved in the carcinogenesis of gastric cancer and that lack of mismatch repair possibly promotes its alteration in a subset of gastric cancer cases [360].

The candidate tumor suppressor gene DCC is located on chromosome 18q. LOH is frequently observed at the DCC locus in well-differentiated but not poorly differentiated gastric cancer [303, 361-363]. Yoshida et al. [362] observed decreased DCC mRNA expression in 52 gastric cancers and reported that this decreased expression was closely associated with liver metastasis. A more recent study also reported that altered expression of DCC was detectable in gastric carcinomas, albeit more commonly at advanced stages of tumor progression [364]. Yet another gene, trefoil factor family 1 (TFF1), resides on chromosome 21q22, a region that has been noted to be deleted in gastric cancers in LOH studies [365]. TFF1 is synthesized and secreted by normal stomach mucosa and gastrointestinal cells of injured tissue. The link between mouse TFF1 inactivation and the fully penetrant antropyloric tumor phenotype prompted the classification of TFF1 as a gastric tumor suppressor gene [366]. There is increasing evidence that TFF1 is a stabilizer of the mucous gel overlying the gastrointestinal mucosa, which provides a physical barrier against various noxious agents [365]. Altered expression, deletion, and/or mutations of the TFF1 gene have been frequently observed in human gastric carcinomas [366]. Also, loss of expression of TFF1 was observed in about 44% of gastric carcinoma cases [365, 367], while loss of the trefoil peptide was described in approximately 50% of gastric carcinoma cases [365, 368]. Recently, researchers found evidence of a dual antiproliferative and antiapoptotic role of the TFF1 gene [366].

The group of activated oncogenes consists primarily of various growth factors and growth factor receptors. For example, in previous studies, the c-met protoonco-gene, which encodes a tyrosine kinase receptor for the hepatocyte growth factor, was overexpressed in 50% of both diffuse- and intestinal-type gastric cancers, indicating poor prognosis on multivariate analysis [311, 341, 369-371]. Tumors having overexpression of c-met have tended to display increased invasiveness and be poorly differentiated (including scirrhous tumors). Also, c-met is amplified and/or overexpressed but not mutated in several tumors, suggesting that over-expression of normal c-met, rather than structural alteration, is responsible for activation of the tyrosine kinase receptor [372, 373]. Furthermore, rearrangement of the tpr and c-met genes has been reported in gastric cancer and identified in a small subset of gastric cancers [374].

The c-erB2 (HER-2/neu) gene, another protooncogene, is a transmembrane tyrosine kinase receptor. HER-2/neu protein overexpression or gene amplification is associated with approximately one-fourth of all gastrointestinal tract malignancies [375]. HER-2/neu overexpression also appears to be linked with advanced rather than early disease with limited invasion. The majority of studies of this protein have reported a significant prognostic value of HER-2/neu status, and overexpression of HER-2/neu has been implicated as a potential marker of poor prognosis in gastric cancers [373, 376-378]. Other studies, however, have not found any prognostic value of HER-2/neu expression in these cancers [379]. Other oncogenes, such as cyclin E, c-erbB3, K-sam, Ras, and c-myc, have also been found to be amplified and overexpressed in gastric carcinomas [380, 381, 382]. In particular, K-sam, which belongs to the fibroblast growth factor receptor family, is frequently overexpressed in diffuse-type gastric cancers, due to amplification of it [336, 383]. Additionally, more enhanced expression of the Ras gene was found in intestinal-type gastric cancers than in diffuse-type cancers [384] and in advanced rather than in early gastric cancer [385, 386]. Expression of c-myc has also been found to correlate with the disease stage, depth of invasion [387], and peritoneal dissemination [388].

The maintenance of telomeres by telomerase activation induces cellular immortalization and participates in carcinogenesis [389]. Strong telomerase activity associated with human telomerase reverse transcriptase (hTERT) expression is present in a majority of gastric carcinomas, regardless of tumor staging [311, 390, 391]. Protection of telomeres 1 (POT1), a telomere end-binding protein, is proposed not only to cap telomeres but also to recruit telomerase to the ends of chromosomes [392]. POT1 expression levels are significantly higher in gastric cancer of advanced stage, and POT1 downregulation is frequently observed in gastric cancers of early stage, suggesting that POT1 may be a marker of high-grade malignancy [392].

Gastric cancer cells express a variety of growth factors and their receptors to make autocrine and paracrine loops [308, 309, 311]. These factors induce not only cell growth but also extracellular matrix degradation and angiogenesis for tumor invasion and proliferation. The simultaneous expression of epidermal growth factor (EGF)/ transforming growth factor (TGF)-alpha and EGF receptor correlates with deep invasion, advanced stage, and poor prognosis. The amplification of the c-met encoding receptor for hepatocyte growth factor is frequently associated with poor prognosis of gastric cancer, especially of scirrhous type. The amplification and overexpression of the K-sam and HER-2/c-erbB2 genes may be prognostic factors for well-differentiated type and poorly differentiated or scirrhous type, respectively [309, 322]. Angiogenesis is a prerequisite for tumor growth and metastasis that depends on the production of angiogenic factors by host and tumor cells. Neovascularization enhances the growth of primary tumors and provides an avenue for hematogenous metastasis. Gastric cancer cells produce various angiogenic factors, including vascular endothelial growth factor (VEGF), interleukin (IL)-8, basic fibroblast growth factor (bFGF), and platelet-derived endothelial cell growth factor (PD-ECGF) [393-395]. Because increasing vascu-larity correlates with lymph-node metastasis, hepatic metastasis, and poor prognosis, all of these may be candidate prognostic factors of gastric cancer. In fact, the prognosis in patients with tumors displaying high IL-8 and VEGF expression levels is significantly poorer than that in patients whose tumors with low expression levels [396].

Cell-cycle checkpoints are regulatory pathways that control cell-cycle transitions, DNA replication, and chromosome segregation. Abnormalities in cell-cycle regulators are involved in stomach carcinogenesis through genomic instability and unbridled cell proliferation [309, 311, 397]. The cyclin E gene is amplified in 15%-20% of gastric cancers, and the overexpression of cyclin E correlates with the aggressiveness of the cancer. Reduction in the expression of p27Kip1, a cyclin-dependent kinase (CDK) inhibitor, is frequently associated with advanced gastric cancers, and the reduced expression of p27Kip1 also significantly correlates with deep invasion and lymph-node metastasis. It has been shown that reduced p27 expression is a negative prognostic factor for patients with a cyclin E-positive-tumor [398]. Aberrant expression (reduced or overexpression) of the p16 gene is frequently found in gastric cancers, but does not correlate with patients' prognosis [399]. An important regulator at the Gl/S checkpoint is retinoblastoma (RB) protein. RB expression is lower in lymph-node metastasis than in the corresponding primary tumors [390]. Univariate and multivariate survival analyses have revealed that reduced expression of RB is associated with worse overall survival. The product of the tumor suppressor gene, p53, is multifunctional and participates in cell-cycle regulation partly through p21 induction. Although nearly 200 articles concerning p53 abnormality in gastric cancer in relation to patients' prognoses have been published, the prognostic impact remains controversial. Recent reports indicate that abnormal expression of p53 significantly affects cumulative survival and that p53 status may also influence response to chemotherapy [400, 401]. The overexpression of checkpoint kinase 1 (Chk1) and Chk2, DNA damage-activated kinases involved at the G2/M checkpoint, is associated with p53 mutations, but has no prognostic impact. The overexpression of CDC25B is found in 70% of gastric cancers, and is associated with invasion and metastasis.

In addition to the activation of oncogenes and inactivation of tumor suppressor genes, alteration of adhesion molecules seems to be critical for the development of gastric cancer.

Cell-adhesion molecules may function as tumor suppressors. For instance, E-cadherin is a binding partner of β-catenin and plays a crucial role in establishing intercellular adhesion and the structural integrity of epithelial tissues [402, 403]. E-cadherin belongs to the cadherin superfamily and is involved in maintenance of the epithelial phenotype. Reduction or loss of E-cadherin expression has been found often in gastric cancers, probably because of hypermethylation of the E-cadherin promoter [314, 404]. Multivariate analyses have revealed that reduced E-cadherin expression is an independent prognostic factor [405]. Dysadherin, a cancer-associated cell-membrane glycoprotein, downregulates E-cadherin expression and promotes metastasis [405]. Patients with both dysadherin positivity and reduced E-cadherin have the worst prognosis, although dysadherin is not an independent prognostic factor [405]. Soluble fragment of E-cadherin is known to be increased in the sera of cancer patients [406]. Serum soluble E-cadherin is a valid prognostic marker for gastric cancer, and a high concentration predicts palliative/conservative treatment and extensive tumor invasion [406]. CD44 is an important cell-adhesion molecule, and its variants, generated by alternative splicing, modulate cell-to-cell interaction, movement, and finally metastatic potential. There is a significant survival advantage in patients with low expression of CD44 sharing variant exon 6 (CD44v6) compared with those with high expression [407]. Furthermore, The serum level of soluble CD44v6 is a prognostic indicator in patients with poorly differentiated type gastric cancer [408]. The expression of CD44v9 is associated not only with tumor invasion, metastasis, and advanced stage but also with the tumor-recurrence mortality of gastric cancer [311, 409].

A balance of activities between matrix-degrading enzymes and their inhibitors is important in determining tumor invasion and metastasis. Among various MMPs, The expression of MMP-7, also known as matrilysin, is correlated with vessel invasion and both lymphatic and hematogenous metastases [410], while the prognosis of patients with MMP-1-positive tumors is significantly worse than that of patients with MMP-1-negative tumors [411]. Membrane-type 1 (MT-1) MMP is an activator of MMP-2. MT1-MMP expression is an independent factor influencing both tumor invasion and metastasis. Although MT1-MMP is not an independent prognostic factor, patients with tumors having a high tumor/normal (T/N) ratio of MT1-MMP show a significantly poorer prognosis than those with a low ratio [412]. Tissue inhibitors of MMP (TIMPs) inhibit tumor invasion through the inactivation of MMPs. In a multivariate analysis, the T/N ratio of TIMP-1 was shown to be an independent factor influencing tumor invasion and the second most important factor in determining the prognosis of the patients [413].

Nitric oxide (NO) is a potent biological molecule that mediates a diverse array of activities, including vasodilatation, neurotransmission, iron metabolism, and immune defense [414, 415]. Recent studies have suggested that tumor-associated NO, which is, presumably, produced by tumor and/or host cells (e.g., macrophages) that infiltrate and surround tumors, has pleiotropic effects on carcinogenesis, tumor growth, and metastasis [416-421]. The outcome apparently depends on the genetic and epigenetic makeup of tumor cells as well as the source and level of NO production, which itself is dictated by the isoforms of NO synthases (NOSs), i.e., NOS I, NOS II, and NOS III [421]. It is generally believed that a low level of NO production, mostly from elevated expression of NOS I and NOS III (constitutive NOS), most likely benefits tumor growth through increasing tumor blood perfusion and angiogenesis [416, 421]. However, expression of NOS II (inducible NOS) can have the opposite effects, mainly because of the high NO production and long-lasting half-life of the NOS II enzyme.

NOS II expression and NO production within tumor cells can directly or indirectly influence the fate of the cells themselves [416-421]. For example, overproduction of endogenous NO is autocytotoxic through the induction of apoptosis [421] and suppresses tumor growth and metastasis [421, 422]. Expression of NOS II in tumor stromal cells, e.g., infiltration macrophages and vascular endothelial cells, has also been implicated in tumor progression and may be the major source of tumor-associated NO [414, 415, 421, 423]. Activated macrophages and endothelial cells may produce NO at cytotoxic levels in vitro [414, 421, 423] and prevent tumor growth and metastasis, presumably by killing tumor cells passing through vascular lumens [421].

Conversely, the role of NOS II in tumor growth is complex and not fully understood. There is a body of evidence indicating that NOS II may promote tumor growth and metastasis. Specifically, tumor-associated NOS II activity correlates with more advanced human tumors of the breast [424] and central nervous system [425]. In fact, NOS II expression directly correlates with the metastatic potential of UV-2237 murine fibrosarcoma cells [414]. In addition, macrophage-derived NO may promote tumor growth and metastasis through multiple mechanisms, such as regulation of immune response, cell survival, blood flow, and vessel formation [414, 415, 426]. Consistently, enforced low levels of NOS II expression have been shown to positively influence tumor progression by protecting tumor cells from apoptosis [427] and altering tumor blood supply through changing vascular tone and/or formation [416,428]. NO also stimulates vascular endothelial cell proliferation and migration directly or indirectly by inducing the expression of VEGF [429, 430].

However, the expression and potential role of NOS II and NOS III in the pathogenesis of human gastric cancer are mostly unknown. Recent studies showed elevated NOS II and NOS III expression in human gastric cancer specimens, which has been interpreted as inhibiting or promoting tumor progression [431-437]. Clearly, the definitive roles of NO in gastric cancer development and progression remain to be determined.

Cyclooxygenase (COX)-2

COX-2, one of the two key enzymes in the conversion of arachidonic acid to prostanoids, is the target of inhibition by nonsteroidal anti-inflammatory drugs. Increased expression of COX-2 has been associated with inflammatory processes and carcinogenesis [431, 438] and has been detected in several common human malignancies, predominantly of the gastrointestinal tract, including colorectal, esophageal, and gastric carcinomas [439]. COX-2 overexpression is common in intestinal-type gastric carcinoma and dysplastic precursor lesions, suggesting a relatively early role for COX-2 expression in gastric carcinogenesis [440, 441]. Additionally, COX-2 overexpression is inversely associated with MSI in gastric cancer [442]. COX-2 overexpression in epithelial cells inhibits apoptosis and increases the invasiveness of malignant cells, favoring tumorigenesis and metastasis [443]. Transcriptional repression of COX-2 has been shown to be caused by hypermethylation of the COX-2 CpG island in gastric carcinoma cell lines [444]. In addition, promoter methylation regulates H. pylori-stimulated COX-2 expression in gastric epithelial cells [445]. Loss of COX-2 methylation may facilitate COX-2 expression and promote gastric carcinogenesis associated with H. pylori infection [446]. In one study, after successful eradication of H. pylori, expression of COX-2 was reduced but not eliminated in the epithelium [447]. Other candidate genes that have been identified to play an important role in cell-cell adhesion and metastasis include CD44 [448], nm23 [449], matrix metalloproteinase-2 [328], and plasminogen activator type 1 (PAI-1) [450]. Moreover, the expression and regulation of mucin and glycoconjugate also play important roles in the pathological processes of H. pylori infection and gastric carcinogenesis [451]. Interestingly, several recent studies have shown that the aberrant expression of transcription factors contributes to gastric cancer development and progression. These factors included CDX1, CDX2 [452], Etsl [453, 454], NF-KB [455], and Sp1 [456]. For example, Sp1 Overexpression has been shown to predict poor clinical outcome of gastric cancer [456].

Among the various epigenetic alterations that lead to modified gene expression, the most important are believed to be DNA methylation and chromatin remodeling by histone modification [312]. Some aberrant epigenetics modifications are associated with tumor progression of gastric cancer, and could be candidate prognostic factors.

Histone Acetylation

Inactivation of chromatin by histone deacetylation is involved in the transcriptional repression of several tumor suppressor genes, including p21WAF1/CIP1. Hypo-acetylation of histones H3 and H4 in the p21WAF1/Cip1 promoter region is observed in more than 50% of gastric cancer tissues by chromatin immunoprecipitation [457]. By using anti-acetylated histone antibody, the global acetylation status of histone can be analyzed immunohistochemically in tissue specimens of gastric cancer [312]. The level of acetylated histone H4 expression is reduced in 70% of gastric cancers in comparison with non-neoplastic mucosa, indicating global hypo-acetylation in gastric cancer. Reduced expression of acetylated histone H4 correlated well with advanced tumor stage, deep tumor invasion, and lymph-node metastasis. Thus, low levels of global histone acetylation may serve as a marker of high-grade malignancy. In fact, trichostatin A, a histone deacetylase inhibitor, induces growth arrest and apoptosis and suppresses the invasion of gastric cancer cells [312, 458].

Accumulation of DNA methylation in multiple genes

The hypermethylation of CpG islands is associated with the silencing of various tumor suppressor genes and participates in tumorigenesis. These genes include p16MTS1/INK4A, CDH1 (E-cadherin), hMLH1, RAR-beta, RUNX3, MGMT, TSP1, HLTF, RIZ1, and SOCS-1 [311, 459-465]. Among these, DNA methylation of CDH1, RAR-beta, and SOCS-1 is significantly associated with tumor invasion and metastasis. Gastric cancers frequently have the CpG island methylator phenotype (CIMP), which may be an important pathway involved in stomach carcinogenesis [466]. However, no significant association has been found between CIMP and tumor progression. Yasui W, et al. [467] analyzed DNA methylation in 12 tumor-related genes (hMLH1, MGMT, p16, CDH1, RAR-beta, HLTF, RIZ1, TM, FLNs, LOX, HRASLS, HAND1) in gastric cancers and found that the average number of methylated genes per tumor was about five. The authors [467] then divided cancers into two groups; cancers with five or more methylated genes (high-methylation group) and those with four or fewer methylated genes. The high-methylation group was found more frequently in stage III and stage IV cancers than in stages I and II. Thus, the number of methylated genes may serve as a molecular marker of tumor progression, although the prognostic implication remains to be elucidated.

Genetic polymorphism is an important determinant of endogenous causes of cancer. An overview of genetic susceptibility and gastric cancer risk has been described by Gonzalez et al. [468]. Representative genetic polymorphisms modifying gastric cancer risk include IL-Ibeta, IL-1 receptor antagonist, and N-acetyltransferase. The relation between genetic polymorphisms of tumor-related genes and gastric cancer was studied in case-control and case-case studies, in about 500 subjects [469-472]. A single-nucleotide polymorphism (SNP; A > G, Ile > Val) was present in the transmembrane domain of the HER-2/c-erbB2 gene, while there were SNPs in the promoter regions of the EOF (61 A/G), E-cadherin (-160 C/A), MMP-1 (-1607 1G/2G), and MMP-9 (-1562 C/T) genes. All the promoter SNPs described above are known to influence the respective gene expression. According to the results of case-control studies [469-472], SNPs of the HER-2, EOF, and E-cadherin genes significantly affected gastric cancer risk, while the genotypes of the MMP-1 and MMP-9 genes did not differ between the gastric cancer cases and the controls. Among the gastric cancer patients, the genotypes of the HER-2, E-cadherin, and MMP-9 genes were associated with tumor invasion, metastasis, or stage grouping. As for the MMP-1 gene, a significant association was detected only with histological differentiation. Therefore, SNPs of the HER-2, E-cadherin, and MMP-9 genes could serve as a predictor of risk for a malignant phenotype [467]. The prognostic significance must be clarified. Controversial observations have been reported in regard to the association between E-cadherin SNP and gastric cancer [473-474].

Sonic Hedgehog and Gastric Carcinogenesis

The role of Hedgehog (Hh) signaling in the development of gastric cancer has become evident from studies of both various gastrointestinal cancer cell lines and analysis of patient gastric samples [475,476]. Sonic hedgehog (Shh) is an essential regulator of patterning processes throughout development, and CDX proteins act as the master regulators for intestinal development and differentiation. Shh and CDX2 seem to be interdependently linked with cellular differentiation through different signal cascades [477]. A Shiotani et al. [478] have recently shown that the loss of Shh and aberrant expression of CDX2 in H. pylori – associated atrophic gastritis can be modified by H. pylori eradication prior to incomplete intestinal metaplasia. On the other hand, abnormal signaling of the hedgehog pathway has been reported in gastric cancer, especially diffuse-type cancer and advanced gastric cancer, and Shh acts as a proliferation factor in both the normal mucosa and malignant lesions. CDX2 expressed in the early stage of gastric carcinogenesis is associated with the intestinal phenotypic region and thus with a better outcome. However, it remains unclear how Shh and CDX2 are involved with intestinal transformation and further carcinogenesis.

It was clearly demonstrated that elevated Hh signaling activity, supported by increased Ptch receptor expression, occurred in gastric carcinoma [476]. The overactivity of the Hh pathway during carcinoma was explained by overexpression of the Hh ligand that was blocked by both cyclopamine (hedgehog signaling antagonist) and a Hh blocking antibody [476]. Conversely, when patients with evidence of precancerous lesions such as atrophy and intestinal metaplasia are studied, there is a strong loss of Shh protein expression [475]. Interestingly, a recent study showed that during pseudopyloric metaplasia, a lesion induced by

Helicobacter infection, resulted in the reactivation of Shh [479]. It may be that such conflicting data indicates that Hh signaling is active in the later stages of gastric carcinogenesis in response to inflammatory cytokines [480]. There may also be differences in the expression of Shh and tumor subtype. Testing Hh pathway activation in a cohort of patients with gastric cancer would address the role of Hh ligand production and expression in tumors. This also underscores the need for genetically modified mice to study the role of Hh signaling in tumorigenesis.

THE ROLE OF STEM CELLS IN GASTRIC CANCER DEVELOPMENT

Stem cells, regardless of their source, are defined as cells with the following properties: self-renewal, primitive or nondifferentiated phenotype, and the ability to give rise to specialized cells. There are many recognized types of stem cells with varying degrees of differentiation potential. The most primitive is the embryonic stem cell, derived from early preimplantation embryos. These cells give rise to all of the cell types of the body, and as such are the most versatile stem cells recognized, carrying the greatest differentiation potential. Adult stem cells, also capable of self renewal, are derived from tissues of the adult animal and are responsible for tissue maintenance and repair [501]. In recent years, the theory of stem cell lineage restriction has been challenged with emerging evidence from multiple laboratories that adult stem cells possess a greater degree of plasticity than previously imagined. For example, neural stem cells have been shown to differentiate into several cells of the hematopoietic lineages [502], and epithelial cells within the GI tract, muscle, lung, and skin [503]. Cells originating in the bone marrow have been isolated from virtually every organ of the body as differentiated cells and seem to not only take on the phenotypic characteristics of peripheral cells, but also to function appropriately in their new location [504, 505].

Cancer is increasingly recognized as a stem cell disease [501]. Bone marrow – derived stem cells (BMDCs) possess the plasticity for transdifferentiation, reside in peripheral organs in increasing numbers as a result of inflammation and damage, and depend heavily on environmental cues and cell–cell signaling for differentiation decisions and growth regulation. It seems logical then, to entertain the notion that BMDCs might contribute to cancer either directly or indirectly in situations such as chronic tissue damage and inflammation [501]. Several studies describe the Helicobacter– infected mouse model for evaluating the effects of chronic inflammation on bone marrow cell migration and engraftment in the stomach. In this model, inflammation is maximal at about 8 weeks of infection, and then continues at a more modest level for the life of the mouse. Between 8 and 20 weeks of infection, there is loss of the oxyntic glands, and a restructuring of the gastric architecture to include metaplastic cell lineages, reflecting the effects of an abnormal tissue milieu on rapidly proliferating cells [199]. After several months, mucosal atrophy, parietal cell loss, and mucus cell metaplasia are prominent. Interestingly, engraftment of BMDCs first becomes evident at about 20 weeks of infection, and corresponds with the appearance of these metaplastic cell lineages. With time, the number of bone marrow–derived glands increases dramatically, suggesting a threshold for recruitment needs to be reached [249]. Based on these studies, it seems that longstanding inflammation and inflammatory-mediated damage to the epithelium are required for BMDC engraftment within the gastric epithelium, an environment strongly linked to the development of cancer in many settings. On the basis of the data that the chronic inflammatory environment is sufficient for BMDC engraftment within the gastric mucosa, Houghton J.M., and Wang T. C. [501] reasoned that bone marrow–derived stem cells, as the ultimate uncommitted adult stem cell, might represent the ideal candidate for transformation if placed in a favorable environment (Figure 3). The C57BL/6 model of H. felis–induced gastric cancer is optimal for studying the role of stem cells in inflammatory-mediated cancers because C57BL/6 mice do not develop gastric cancer under control conditions, and reliably develop cancer with infection. With Helicobacter infection, the gastric mucosa progresses through a series of changes including metaplasia and dysplasia [508], culminating in GI intraepithelial neoplasia [507] by 12–15 months of infection [506, 508]. This reiterates human disease, where gastric cancer in the absence of Helicobacter infection is unusual, and longstanding infection carries a significant (up to 1%–3%) risk of gastric cancer [186]. Progressive parietal and chief cell loss is a hallmark of chronic Helicobacter infection. Of the few parietal or chief cells that were isolated from the infected mice [249], none were bone marrow derived, strongly suggesting that marrow cells do not differentiate toward the parietal or chief cell phenotype under the experimental conditions used. At 30 weeks of infection, antralized glands and metaplastic cells at the squamocolumnar junction were replaced by marrow-derived cells. The severity of intraepithelial dysplasia increased over time, and by 1 year of infection, most mice developed invasive neoplastic glands. All of the intraepithelial neoplasia in mice infected for 12–16 months arose from donor marrow cells, strongly suggesting an inherent vulnerability of this population of cells to transformation. In addition to epithelial cells within the tumor, BMDCs also comprise a subset of cells within the tumor stroma and within seemingly uninvolved epithelium and subepithelial spaces adjacent to the tumors. There have been recovered adipocytes, fibroblasts, endothelial cells, and myofibroblasts derived from bone marrow precursors in areas adjacent to dysplasia and neoplasia [249, 509].

Thus, the accumulated evidence suggests that chronic inflammation promotes many types of cancers, and that this occurs in part through the mobilization of BMDCs. Therefore, it is likely that the interaction between bone marrow–derived epithelial cells and bone marrow–derived stromal and nonepithelial cells is central to tumor development. In addition, BMDCs have contributed to the metastatic niche. In recent reports, bone marrow–derived vascular endothelial growth factor receptor -1 positive hematopoietic progenitor cells were shown to home to tumor-specific premetastatic sites before the arrival of tumor cells [506]. Thus, BMDCs seem to be contributing to both tumor cells and the tumor niche, and have roles in both cancer initiation and cancer progression.

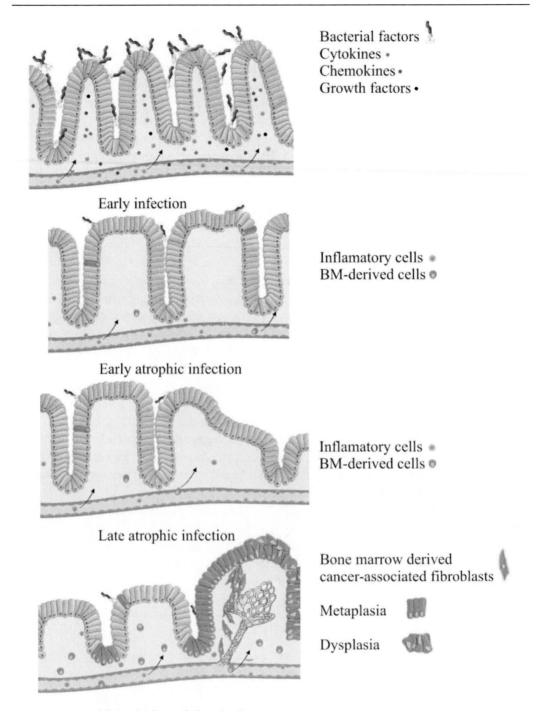

Bacterial factors
Cytokines ·
Chemokines ·
Growth factors ·

Early infection

Inflamatory cells ·
BM-derived cells ◌

Early atrophic infection

Inflamatory cells ·
BM-derived cells ◌

Late atrophic infection

Bone marrow derived
cancer-associated fibroblasts

Metaplasia

Dysplasia

Metaplasia and dysplasia

Figure 3. The role of BMDC in gastric carcinogenesis. H.pylori – induced chronic inflammation results in mucosal atrophy with rare engrafts of BMDC. Chemokines recruit BMDC into stem cell niche. The stem cells proliferate and repopulate the entire gastric units. Later, BMDC acquire mutations and transform into cancer cells, contributing to cancer-accosiated fibroblasts and incorporating into newly formed blood vessels. (Adapted from Houghton J.M., Wang T. C. [501]).

THE CANCER STEM CELLS (CSCs) HYPOTHESIS

Somatic stem cells are present in all highly regenerating tissues such as skin, intestinal epithelium and the hematopoietic system, and are critically important for their maintenance during homeostasis and repair after injury. Smaller pools of somatic stem cells are present in tissues with less regenerative potential, such as the brain or the heart. On a single-cell basis, long-lived stem cells have the capacity to produce both stem cells of the same type by self-renewal and more-differentiated lineage-restricted progenitors. Although these progenitors show only limited self-renewal capacity, they divide rapidly and give rise to a large number of functionally mature cells, which replace those cells constantly lost during normal tissue turnover [481–483]. This hierarchical design of regenerative tissues allows lifelong production of mature cells without exhausting the stem-cell pool. Net cellular expansion occurs primarily at the progenitor cell level and not in the predominantly dormant stem cells. Trumpp A., and Wiestler O. D. have published the review on the concept of cancer stem cells (CSCs) [484]. According to this concept, many human neoplasms are likely to contain an often minor population of cancer cells within the tumor mass called CSCs, which are the only cells required for both initiation and maintenance of the disease. CSCs have unlimited self-renewal activity, and also can give rise to a large number of more differentiated cells, which generate the bulk of the tumor. CSCs can either originate from normal stem cells or from more-differentiated progenitors. Long-lived CSCs seem to be resistant to radiation and classical chemotherapy and thus serve as an often small but highly malignant reservoir of cells. Due to their potential for migration and seeding in specific tissue niches, these CSCs might also drive disease recurrence and metastatic growth even after a significant latency period. The mechanisms that allow CSCs to escape current therapies remains to be elucidated, but are likely to be caused by several inherent features of CSCs, which include relative quiescence/dormancy, expression of multidrug resistance transporters, localization in a protective and hypoxic niche and highly effective DNA repair mechanisms.

McDonald et al. [510] have published the results of their investigation of mitochondrial DNA (mtDNA) mutations as a marker of clonal expansion in human stomach. The authors conclude that human gastric units contain multiple multipotential stem cells, one of which, once mutated, can colonize the entire unit, resulting in a new clonal unit by monoclonal conversion. The simplest model for stem cell architecture suggested by these data is that the multiple stem cells are housed in a niche in the isthmus/neck of the gastric unit, above where several glands enter and that these cells give rise to all lineages in the gland and in the foveolus. Obviously, the situation is complicated by the presence of up to 7 glands associated with each unit, and a further model might be that each gland may have its own multipotential stem cell. However, whatever model is appropriate, it will have to incorporate the observation that the same stem cell(s) also give rise to lineages in the foveolus. The authors propose that monoclonal conversion is a mechanism for the colonization of crypts seen in intestinal metaplasia, where gastric stem cells commit to the intestinal phenotype. Additionally, it was shown that mixed gastric/intestinal units in this process of clonal conversion can be observed. Tatematsu et al [511] considered this to be a new form of IM (mixed intestinal metaplasia), in which gastric units contained both goblet cells and pyloric mucous cells. McDonald et al. [510], based on their data, suggest that rather than a new form of metaplasia, these units actually were undergoing monoclonal conversion to become entirely metaplastic. Moreover,

IM crypts are derived clonally and contain multiple multipotential stem cells. McDonald et al. [510] have provided definitive evidence that mutations spread through the human stomach by gland fission, a process first suggested by Hattori and Fjuita [512]. Here a bud forms from the stem cell zone in the neck of the gland, and budding continues until a new gland and foveolus is formed. This is analogous to crypt fission in the colon where crypts bifurcate from the base upward. Crypt or gland fission takes place close to or at the site of the stem cell zone, although the initiating factors for fission to occur still are unknown. Thus, McDonald et al. [510] have concluded that fission of mutated units is a mechanism of field cancerization in the human gastric mucosa and elsewhere in the gastrointestinal mucosa.

REFERENCES

[1] Parsonnet J, Friedman GD, Vandersteen DP, Chang Y, Vogelman JH, Orentreich N, Sibley RK. Helicobacter pylori infection and the risk of gastric carcinoma. *N Engl J Med* 1991; 325: 1127–1131.

[2] Vasen HF, Wijnen JT, Menko FH, Kleibeuker JH, Taal BG, Griffioen G, Nagengast FM, Meijers-Heijboer EH, Bertario L, Varesco L, Bisgaard ML, Mohr J, Fodde R, Khan PM. Cancer risk in families with hereditary nonpolyposis colorectal cancer diagnosed by mutation analysis. *Gastroenterology* 1996;110:1020-1027.

[3] Keller G, Rudelius M, Vogelsang H, Grimm V, Wilhelm MG, Mueller J, Siewert JR, Hofler H: Microsatellite instability and loss of heterozygosity in gastric carcinoma in comparison to family history. *Am J Pathol* 1998;152:1281-1289.

[4] Varley JM, McGown G, Thorncroft M, Tricker KJ, Teare MD, Santibanez-Koref MF, Martin J, Birch JM, Evans DG: An extended Li-Fraumeni kindred with gastric carcinoma and a codon 175 mutation in TP53. *J Med Genet* 1995; 32:942-945.

[5] La Vecchia C, Negri E, Franceschi S, Gentile A: Family history and the risk of stomach and colorectal cancer. *Cancer* 1992; 70:50-55.

[6] Sokoloff B: Predisposition to cancer in the Bonaparte family. *Am J Surg* 1938;40:673-678.

[7] ASHG/ACMG. Points to consider: ethical, legal and psychosocial implications of genetic testing in children and adolescents. *Am J Hum Genet*, 1995;57-1233-1241.

[8] Guilford P, Hopkins J, Harraway J, McLeod M, McLeod N, Harawira P, Taite H, Scoular R, Miller A, Reeve AE: E-cadherin germline mutations in familial gastric cancer. *Nature* 1998; 392:402-405.

[9] Guilford PJ, Hopkins JB, Grady WM, Markowitz SD, Willis J, Lynch H, Rajput A, Wiesner GL, Lindor NM, Burgart LJ, Toro TT, Lee D, Limacher JM, Shaw DW, Findlay MP, Reeve AE: E-cadherin germline mutations define an inherited cancer syndrome dominated by diffuse gastric cancer. *Hum Mutat* 1999; 14:249-255.

[10] Richards FM, McKee SA, Rajpar MH, Cole TR, Evans DG, Jankowski JA, McKeown C, Sanders DS, Maher ER. Germline E-cadherin gene (CDH1) mutations predispose to familial gastric cancer and colorectal cancer. *Hum Mol Genet*. 1999;8:607-610..

[11] Stadtlander C.T.K.-H. and Waterbor J.W. Molecular epidemiology, pathogenesis and prevention of gastric cancer. *Carcinogenesis*. 1999;20(12):2195-2208.

[12]   Nomura A. Stomach. In: Schottenfeld,D. and FraumeniJ.F. (eds) Cancer Epidemiology and Prevention. W.B. Saunders, Philadelphia, PA, 1982: pp. 624-637.

[13]   Kramer B.S. and Johnson K.A. Other gastrointestinal cancers: stomach, liver. In: Greenwald, P, Kramer,B.S. and Weed, D.L. (eds) Cancer Prevention and Control. Marcel Dekker, New York, NY, 1995: pp. 673-694.

[14]   Becker KF, Atkinson MJ, Reich U, Becker I, Nekarda H, Siewert JR, Hofler H: E-cadherin gene mutations provide clues to diffuse type gastric carcinomas. *Cancer Res* 1994;54:3845- 3852.

[15]   Becker KF, Hofler H: Frequent somatic allelic inactivation of the E-cadherin gene in gastric carcinomas. *J Natl Cancer Inst* 1995;87:1082-1084.

[16]   Machado JC, Soares P, Carneiro F, Rocha A, Beck S, Blin N, Berx G: Sobrinho-Simoes M: E-cadherin gene mutations provide a genetic basis for the phenotypic divergence of mixed gastric carcinomas. *Lab Invest* 1999;79:459- 465.

[17]   Oda T, Kanai Y, Oyama T, Yoshiura K, Shimoyama Y, Birchmeier W, Sugimura T, Hirohashi S: E-cadherin gene mutations in human gastric carcinoma cell lines. *Proc Natl Acad Sci USA* 1994;91:1858-1862.

[18]   Perl AK, Wilgenbus P, Dahl U, Semb H, Christofori G: A causal role for E-cadherin in the transition from adenoma to carcinoma. *Nature* 1998;392:190-193.

[19]   Yoshiura K, Kanai Y, Ochiai A, Shimoyama Y, Sugimura T, Hirohashi S: Silencing of the E-cadherin invasion-suppressor gene by CpG methylation in human carcinomas. *Proc Natl Acad Sci USA* 1995;92:7416-7419.

[20]   Caldas C, Carneiro F, Lynch HT, Yokota J, Wiesner GL, Powell SM, Lewis FR, Huntsman DG, Pharoah PD, Jankowski JA, MacLeod P, Vogelsang H, Keller G, Park KG, Richards FM, Maher ER, Gayther SA, Oliveira C, Grehan N, Wight D, Seruca R, Roviello F, Ponder BA, Jackson CE: Familial gastric cancer: over view and guidelines for management. *J Med Genet* 1999;36:873-880.

[21]   IGCLC: First Worskshop of the International Gastric Cancer Linkage Consortium (IGCLC). Cambridge, University of Cambridge, 1999.

[22]   Iida S, Akiyama Y, Ichikawa W, Yamashita T, Nomizu T, Nihei Z, Sugihara K, Yuasa Y: Infrequent germ-line mutation of the E-cadherin gene in Japanese familial gastric cancer kindreds. *Clin Cancer Res* 1999;5:1445-1447.

[23]   Avizienyte E, Launonen V, Salovaara R, Kiviluoto T, Aaltonen LA: E-cadherin is not frequently mutated in hereditary gastric cancer. *J Med Genet* 2001;38:49-52.

[24]   Yoon KA, Ku JL, Yang HK, Kim WH, Park SY, Park JG: Germline mutations of E-cadher in gene in Korean familial gastric cancer patients. *J Hum Genet* 1999;44:177-180.

[25]   Gayther SA, Gorringe KL, Ramus SJ, Hunts man D, Roviello F, Grehan N, Machado JC, Pinto E, Seruca R, Hailing K, MacLeod P, Powell SM, Jackson CE, Ponder BA, Caldas C: Identification of germ-line E-cadherin mutations in gastric cancer families of European origin. *Cancer Res* 1998;58:4086-4089.

[26]   Pharoah PD, Guilford P, Caldas C: Incidence of gastric cancer and breast cancer in CDH1 (E-cadherin) mutation carriers from hereditary diffuse gastric cancer families. *Gastroenterology* 2001;121:1348-1353.

[27]   Oliveira C, Bordin MC, Grehan N, Huntsman DG, Gianpaolo S, Machado JC, Kiviluoto TA, Aaltonen L, Jackson CE, Seruca R, Caldas C: Screening E-Cadherin in

gastric cancer families reveals germ-line mutations only in hereditary diffuse gastric cancer kindred. *Hum Mut* 2002 May;19(5):510-7.

[28]   Berx G, Becker KF, Hofler H, van Roy F: Mutations of the human E-cadherin (CDH1) gene. *Hum Mutat* 1998;12:226-237.

[29]   Grady WM, Willis J, Guilford PJ, Dunbier AK, Toro TT, Lynch H, Wiesner G, Ferguson K, Eng C, Park JG, Kim SJ, Markowitz S: Methylation of the CDH 1 promoter as the sec ond genetic hit in hereditary diffuse gastric cancer. *Nat Genet* 2000;26:16-17.

[30]   Graff JR, Herman JG, Lapidus RG, Chopra H, Xu R, Jarrard DF, Isaacs WB, Pitha PM, Davidson NE, Baylin SB: E-cadherin expression is silenced by DNA hypermethylation in human breast and prostate carcinomas. *Cancer Res* 1995;55:5195-5199.

[31]   Graff JR, Greenberg VE, Herman JG, Westra WH, Boghaert ER, Ain KB, Saji M, Zeiger MA, Zimmer SG, Baylin SB: Distinct patterns of E-cadherin CpG island methylation in papillary, follicular, Hurthle's cell, poorly differentiated human thyroid carcinoma. *Cancer Res* 1998;58: 2063-2066.

[32]   Machado JC, Oliveira C, Carvalho R, Soares P, Berx G, Caldas C, Seruca R, Carneiro F, Sobrinho-Simoes M: E-cadherin gene (CDH1) promoter methylation as the second hit in sporadic diffuse gastric carcinoma. *Oncogene* 2001;20:1525-1528.

[33]   Fang J, Xiao S: Alteration of DNA methylation in gastrointestinal carcinogenesis. *J Gastroenterol Hepatol* 2001;16:960-968.

[34]   Kintner C: Regulation of embryonic cell adhesion by the cadherin cytoplasmic domain. *Cell* 1992;69:225-236.

[35]   Bracke ME, Roy FM, Mareel MM: The E-cadherin/catenin complex in invasion and metastasis. *Curr Top Microbiol Imm* 1996;213:123-161.

[36]   Nigam AK, Savage FJ, Boulos PB, Stamp GW, Liu D, Pignatelli M: Loss of cell-cell and cell- matrix adhesion molecules in colorectal cancer. *Br J Cancer* 1993;68:507-514.

[37]   Kinsella AR, Lepts GC, Hill CL, Jones M: Reduced E-cadherin expression correlates with in creased invasiveness in colorectal carcinoma cell lines. *Clin Exp Metastasis* 1994; 12:335-342.

[38]   Berx G, Cleton-Jansen AM, Nollet F, de Leeuw WJ, van de Vijver M, Cornelisse C, van Roy F: E-cadherin is a tumour/invasion suppressor gene mutated in human lobular breast cancers. *EMBO J* 1995;14:6107-6115.

[39]   Frixen UH, Behrens J, Sachs M, Eberle G, Voss B, Warda A, Lochner D, Birchmeier W: E-cadherin-mediated cell-cell adhesion prevents invasiveness of human carcinoma cells. *J Cell Biol* 1991;113:173-185.

[40]   Jones EG: Familial gastric cancer. *NZ Med J* 1964;63:287-296.

[41]   Huntsman DG, Carneiro F, Lewis FR, MacLeod PM, Hayashi A, Monaghan KG, Maung R, Seruca R, Jackson CE, Caldas C. Early gastric cancer in young, asymptomatic carriers of germline E-cadherin mutations. *N EngJMed.* 2001 ;344; 1904-1909.

[42]   Stone J, Bevan S, Cunningham D, Hill A, Rahman N, Peto J, Marossy A, Houlston RS. Low frequency of germline E-cadherin mutations in familial and nonfamilial gastric cancer. *Br J Cancer.* 1999;79:1935-1937.

[43] World Cancer Research Fund, American Institute for Cancer Research. Food, nutrition and the prevention of cancer: a global perspective. Washington, DC: American Institute for Cancer Research; 1997.

[44] Kono S, Hirohata T. Nutrition and stomach cancer. *Cancer Causes Control* 1996;7:41-55.

[45] World Health Organization. Diet, nutrition and the prevention of chronic diseases. WHO technical report series 916. Geneva: World Health Organization; 2003

[46] International Agency for Research on Cancer. Tobacco smoking and tobacco smoke. IARC monographs on the evaluation of the carcinogenic risk of chemicals to humans. Vol. 83. Lyon: International Agency for Research on Cancer; 2004.

[47] International Agency for Research on Cancer. Schistosomes, liver flukes, and Helicobacter pylori. IARC monographs on the evaluation of carcinogenic risks to humans. Lyon: International Agency for Research on Cancer;1994; 61: 218–220.

[48] Cocco P, Palli D, Buiatti E, Cipriani F, DeCarli A, Manca P, Ward MH, Blot WJ, Fraumeni JF Jr. Occupational exposures as risk factors for gastric cancer in Italy. *Cancer Causes Control* 1994; 5: 241-248.

[49] Aragones N, Pollan M & Gustavsson P. Stomach cancer and occupation in Sweden: 1971—89. *Occup Environ Med* 2002; 59: 329-337.

[50] Simpson J, Roman E, Law G, Pannett B. Women's occupation and cancer: preliminary analysis of cancer registrations in England and Wales, 1971-1990. *Am J Ind Med* 1999; 36: 172-185.

[51] Kang S-K, Burnett CA, Freund E, Walker J, Lalich N, Sestito J. Gastrointestinal cancer mortality of workers in occupations with high asbestos exposures. *Am J Ind Med* 1997; 31:713-718.

[52] Swanson GM & Burns PB. Cancer incidence among women in the workplace: a study of the association between occupation and industry and I I cancer sites. *J Occup Environ Med* 1995; 37: 282-287.

[53] Chow WH, McLaughlin JK, Malker HS, Weiner JA, Ericsson JL, Stone BJ, Blot WJ. Occupation and stomach cancer in a cohort of Swedish men. *Am J Ind Med* 1994; 26: 51 1-520.

[54] Kelley JR & Duggan JM. Gastric cancer epidemiology and risk factors. *J Clin Epidemiol* 2003; 56: 1-9.

[55] Wang WH, Huang JQ, Zheng GF, Lam SK, Karlberg J, Wong BC. Non-steroidal anti-inflammatory drug use and the risk of gastric cancer: a systematic review and meta-analysis. *J Natl Cancer Inst* 2003; 95: 1784-1791.

[56] Chatenoud L, La Vecchia C, Franceschi S, Tavani A, Jacobs DR Jr, Parpinel MT, Soler M, Negri E.. Refined-cereal intake and risk of selected cancers in Italy. *Am J Clin Nutr* 1999; 70: 1107-1110.

[57] De Stefani E, Correa P, Boffetta P, Deneo-Pellegrini H, Ronco AL, Mendilaharsu M. Dietary patterns and risk of gastric cancer: a case-control study in Uruguay. *Gastric Cancer* 2004; 7: 21 1-220

[58] Huang XE, Tajima K, Hamajima N, Xiang J, Inoue M, Hirose K, Tominaga S, Takezaki T, Kuroishi T, Tokudome S. Comparison of lifestyle and risk factors among Japanese with and without gastric cancer family history. *Int J Cancer* 2000; 86: 421-424.

[59]   Inoue M, Ito LS, Tajima K, Yamamura Y, Kodera Y, Takezaki T, Hamajima N, Hirose K, Kuroishi T, Tominaga S. Height, weight, menstrual and reproductive factors and risk of gastric cancer among Japanese postmenopausal women: analysis by subsite and histologic subtype. *Int J Cancer* 2002; 97: 833-838.

[60]   Munoz N, Plummer M, Vivas J, Moreno V, De Sanjosé S, Lopez G, Oliver W. A case-control study of gastric cancer in Venezuela. *Int J Cancer* 2001:93:417-423.

[61]   Calle EE, Rodriguez C, Walker-Thurmond K, Thun MJ. Overweight, obesity, and mortality from cancer in a prospectively studied cohort of U.S. adults. *N Engl J Med* 2003; 348: 1625-1638.

[62]   Kuriyama S, Tsubono Y, Hozawa A, Shimazu T, Suzuki Y, Koizumi Y, Suzuki Y, Ohmori K, Nishino Y, Tsuji I. Obesity and risk of cancer in Japan. *Int J Cancer* 2005; 113: 148-157.

[63]   Lukanova A, Bjor O, Kaaks R, Lenner P, Lindahl B, Hallmans G, Stattin P. Body mass index and cancer: results from the Northern Sweden Health and Disease Cohort. *Int J Cancer* 2006; 118: 458-466.

[64]   Sauvaget C, Lagarde F, Nagano J, Soda M, Koyama K, Kodama K. Lifestyle factors, radiation and gastric cancer in atomic-bomb survivors. *Cancer Causes Control* 2005; 16: 773-780.

[65]   Tulinius H, Sigfússon N, Sigvaldason H, Bjarnadóttir K, Tryggvadóttir L. Risk factors for malignant diseases: a cohort study on a population of 22,946 Icelanders. *Cancer Epidemiol Biomarkers Prev* 1997; 6: 863-873.

[66]   Wolk A, Gridley G, Svensson M, Nyrén O, McLaughlin JK, Fraumeni JF, Adam HO. A prospective study of obesity and cancer risk (Sweden). *Cancer Causes Control* 2001; 12: 13-21.

[67]   Zhang J, Su XQ, Wu XJ, Liu YH, Wang H, Zong XN, Wang Y, Ji JF. Effect of body mass index on adenocarcinoma of gastric cardia. *World J Gastroenterol* 2003; 9: 2658-2661

[68]   Power C, Hypponen E & Smith GD. Socioeconomic position in childhood and early adult life and risk of mortality: a prospective study of the mothers of the 1958 British birth cohort. *Am J Public Health* 2005; 95: 1396-1402.

[69]   Fukayama M, Hayashi Y, Iwasaki Y, Chong JM, Ooba T, Takizawa T, Koike M, Mizutani S, Miyaki M, Hirai K. Epstein-Barr virus-associated gastric carcinoma and Epstein-Barr virus infection of the stomach. *Lab Invest* 1994;71:73-81.

[70]   Jansson C, Johansson AL, Bergdahl IA, Dickman PW, Plato N, Adami J, Boffetta P, Lagergren J. Occupational exposures and risk of esophageal and gastric cardia cancers among male Swedish construction workers. *Cancer Causes Control* 2005; 16: 755—764.

[71]   Tran GD, Sun XD, Abnet CC, Fan JH, Dawsey SM, Dong ZW, Mark SD, Qiao YL, Taylor PR. Prospective study of risk factors for esophageal and gastric cancers in the Linxian general population trial cohort in China. *Int J Cancer* 2005; I 13: 456—463.

[72]   Lindblad M, Rodriguez LA & Lagergren J. Body mass, tobacco and alcohol and risk of esophageal, gastric cardia, and gastric non-cardia adenocarcinoma among men and women in a nested case-control study. *Cancer Causes Control* 2005; 16: 285-294.

[73]   Tretli S & Robsahm TE. Height, weight and cancer of the oesophagus and stomach: a follow-up study in Norway. *Eur J Cancer Prev* 1999; 8: I 15-122.

[74] Severson RK, Nomura AM, Grove JS, Stemmermann GN. A prospective analysis of physical activity and cancer. *Am J.Epidemiol* 1989; 130: 522-529.

[75] Smith GD, Shipley MJ, Batty GD, Morris JN, Marmot M. Physical activity and cause-specific mortality in the Whitehall study. *Public Health* 2000; 114: 308-315.

[76] Wannamethee SG, Shaper AG & Walker M. Physical activity and risk of cancer in middle-aged men. *Br J Cancer* 2001; 85: 1311-1316.

[77] Vigen C, Bernstein L & Wu AH. Occupational physical activity and risk of adenocarcinomas of the esophagus and stomach. *Int. J Cancer* 2006; 11

[78] Johansson G, Bingham S & Vahter M. A method to compensate for incomplete 24-hour urine collections in nutritional epidemiology studies. *Public Health Nutr* 1999; 2: 587—591.

[79] Charnley G & Tannenbaum SR. Flow cytometric analysis of the effect of sodium chloride on gastric cancer risk in the rat. *Cancer Res* 1985; 45: 5608-5616.

[80] Galanis DJ, Kolonel LN, Lee J & Nomura A. Intakes of selected foods and beverages and the incidence of gastric cancer among the Japanese residents of Hawaii: a prospective study. *Int J Epidemiol* 1998; 27(2): 173–180.

[81] Ngoan LT, Mizoue T, Fujino Y, Tokui N, Yoshimura T. Dietary factors and stomach cancer mortality. *Br J Cancer* 2002; 87(1):37–42.

[82] Tsugane S, Sasazuki S, Kobayashi M & Sasaki S. Salt and salted food intake and subsequent risk of gastric cancer among middle-aged Japanese men and women. *Br J Cancer* 2004; 90(1): 128–134.

[83] van den Brandt PA, Botterweck AA & Goldbohm RA. Salt intake, cured meat consumption, refrigerator use and stomach cancer incidence: a prospective cohort study (Netherlands). *Cancer Causes Control* 2003; 14(5): 427–438.

[84] Ward MH, Lopez-Carrillo L. Dietary factors and the risk of gastric cancer in Mexico City. *Am J Epidemiol* 1999;149: 925-32.

[85] Nomura A, Grove JS, Stemmermann GN & Severson RK. A prospective study of stomach cancer and its relation to diet, cigarettes, and alcohol consumption. *Cancer Res* 1990; 50(3): 627–631.

[86] Tatematsu M, Takahashi M, Fukushima S, Hananouchi M, Shirai T. Effects in rats of salt on experimental gastric cancers induced by N-methyl-N'-nitro-N-nitrosoguanidine or 4-nitroquinoline-1-oxide. *J Natl Cancer Inst* 1975; 55:101-6.

[87] Takahashi M, Hasegawa R. Enhancing effects of dietary salt on both initiation and promotion stages of rat gastric carcinogenesis. Princess Takamatsu Symp 1985;16:169-82.

[88] Joossens JV, Hill MJ, Elliott P, Stamler R, Lesaffre E, Dyer A, Nichols R, Kesteloot H. Dietary salt, nitrate and stomach cancer mortality in 24 countries: European Cancer Prevention (ECP) and the INTER-SALT Cooperative Research Group. *Int J Epidemiol* 1996;25: 494-504.

[89] Kneller RW, Guo WD, Hsing AW, Chen JS, Blot WJ, Li JY, Forman D, Fraumeni JF Jr. Risk factors for stomach cancer in 65 Chinese counties. *Cancer Epidemiol Biomarkers Prev* 1992;1:113-18.

[90] Tsugane S, Gey F, Ichinowatari Y, Miyajima Y, Ishibashi T. Matsushima S, et al. Cross-sectional epidemiologic study for assessing cancer risks at the population level. I. Study design and participation rate. *J Epidemiol* 1992;2:75-81.

[91]   Tsugane S, Gey F, Ichinowatari Y, Miyajima Y, Ishibashi T. Matsushima S, et al. Cross-sectional epidemiologic study for assessing cancer risks at the population level. II. Baseline data and correlation analysis. *J Epidemiol* 1992;2:83-9.

[92]   National Program of Cancer Registries (NPCR) United States Cancer Statistics (USCS) 1999–2005. Cancer Incidence and Mortality Data. http://apps. nccd.cdc.gov/uscs/.

[93]   La Vecchia C, Franceschi S, Levi F. Epidemiological research on cancer with a focus on Europe. *Eur J Cancer Prev* 2003;12:5-14.

[94]   Tsugane S, de Souza JM, Costa ML Jr, Mirra AP, Gotlieb SL. Laurenti R, Watanabe S. Cancer incidence rates among Japanese immigrants in the city of Sao Paulo, Brazil, 1969-78. *Cancer Causes Control* 1990;l:189-93.

[95]   Tsugane S, Hamada GS, Souza JM, Gotlieb SLD, Takashima Y. Todoriki H, et al. Lifestyle and health related factors among randomly selected Japanese residents in the city of Sao Paulo, Brazil, and their comparisons with Japanese in Japan. *J Epidemiol* 1994;4:37-46.

[96]   Tsugane S, Hamada GS, Karita K, Tsubono Y, Laurenti R. Cancer patterns and lifestyle among Japanese immigrants and their descendants in the city of Sao Paulo, Brazil. *Gann Monogr Cancer Res* 1996;44:43-50.

[97]   Shibata D, Weiss LM. Epstein-Barr virus-associated gastric adenocarcinoma. *Am J Pathol* 1992;140:769-74.

[98]   Ye WM, Yi YN, Luo RX, Zhou TS, Lin RT, Chen GD. Diet and gastric cancer: a case-control study in Fujian Province, China. *World J Gastroenterol* 1998;4:516-18.

[99]   McClain KL, Leach CT, Jenson HB, Joshi VV, Pollock BH, Parmley RT, DiCarlo FJ, Chadwick EG, Murphy SB. Association of Epstein-Barr virus with leiomyosarcomas in children with AIDS. *N Engl J Med* 1995;332:12-8.

[100] Kim HJ, Chang WK, Kim MK, Lee SS, Choi BY. Dietary factors and gastric cancer in Korea: a case-control study. *Int J Cancer* 2002;97:531-5.

[101] Lee SA, Kang D, Shim KN, Choe JW, Hong WS, Choi H. Effect of diet and Helicobacter pylori infection to the risk of early gastric cancer. *J Epidemiol* 2003;13:162-8.

[102] Anagnostopoulos I, Hummel M. Epstein-Barr virus in tumours. *Histopathology* 1996;29:297-315.

[103] Raab-Traub N. Epstein-Barr virus and nasopharyngeal carcinoma. *Cancer Biol* 1992;3:297-307.

[104] Shikata K, Kiyohara Y, Kubo M, Yonemoto K, Ninomiya T. Shirota T, Tanizaki Y, Doi Y, Tanaka K, Oishi Y, Matsumoto T, Iida M. A prospective study of dietary salt intake and gastric cancer incidence in a defined Japanese population: the Hisayama study. *Int J Cancer* 2006; 119:196-201.

[105] Osato T. Epstein-Barr virus infection and oncogenesis. In: Osato T, Takada K, Tokunaga M, editors. Epstein-Barr virus and human cancer. Tokyo: Japan Scientific Societies Press; 1998:3-16.

[106] Larsson SC, Orsini N, Wolk A. Processed meat consumption and stomach cancer risk: a meta-analysis. *J Natl Cancer Inst* 2006;98: 1078-87.

[107] IARC, Fruit and vegetables. IARC Handbooks of Cancer Prevention, Vol. 8. Lyon: IARC Press; 2003.

[108] Botterweck AA, van den Brandt PA & Goldbohm RA. A prospective cohort study on vegetable and fruit consumption and stomach cancer risk in The Netherlands. *Am J Epidemiol* 1998; 148(9): 842–853.

[109] Fleischauer AT, Poole C & Arab L. Garlic consumption and cancer prevention: meta-analyses of colorectal and stomach cancers. *Am J Clin Nutr* 2000; 72: 1047-1052.

[110] Sivam GP, Lampe JW, Ulness B, Swanzy SR, Potter JD. Helicobacter pylori — in vitro susceptibility to garlic (Allium sativum) extract. *Nutr Cancer* 1997; 27: 118-121.

[111] You WC, Zhang L, Gail MH Ma JL, Chang YS, Blot WJ, Li JY, Zhao CL, Liu WD, Li HQ, Hu YR, Bravo JC, Correa P, Xu GW, Fraumeni JF Jr. Helicobacter pylori infection, garlic intake and precancerous lesions in a Chinese population at low risk of gastric cancer. *Int J Epidemiol* 1998; 27: 941—944.

[112] Lunet N, Lacerda-Vieira A, Barros H. Fruit and vegetables consumption and gastric cancer: a systematic review and meta-analysis of cohort studies. *Nutr Cancer* 2005;53:1-10.

[113] Larsson SC, Bergkvist L, Wolk A. Fruit and vegetable consumption and incidence of gastric cancer: a prospective study. *Cancer Epidemiol Biomarkers Prev* 2006;15:1998-2001.

[114] Gonzalez CA, Pera G, Agudo A, Bueno-de-Mesquita HB, Ceroti M, Boeing H, et al. Fruit and vegetable intake and the risk of stomach and oesophagus adenocarcinoma in the European Prospective Investigation into Cancer and Nutrition (EPIC-EURGAST). *Int J Cancer*. 2006; 118:2559-66.

[115] Tsugane S. and Sasazuki S. Diet and the risk of gastric cancer: review of epidemiological evidence. *Gastric Cancer* 2007; 10: 75-83.

[116] Woodward M, Tunstall-Pedoe H & McColl K. Helicobacter pylori infection reduces systemic availability of dietary vitamin C. *Eur J Gastroenterol Hepatol* 2001; 13: 233-237.

[117] Correa P, Fontham ET, Bravo JC, Bravo LE, Ruiz B, Zarama G, Realpe JL, Malcom GT, Li D, Johnson WD, Mera R. Chemoprevention of gastric dysplasia: randomized trial of antioxidant supplements and anti-Helicobacter pylori therapy. *J Natl Cancer Inst* 2000;92:1881-8.

[118] Drake IM, Davies MJ, Mapstone NP, Dixon MF, Schorah CJ. White KL, et al. Ascorbic acid may protect against human gastric cancer by scavenging mucosal oxygen radicals. *Carcinogenesis* 1996;17:559-62.

[119] Tannenbaum SR, Wishnok JS, Leaf CD. Inhibition of nitrosamine formation by ascorbic acid. *Am J Clin Nutr* 1991;53:247S-50S.

[120] Zhang HM, Wakisaka N, Maeda O, Yamamoto T. Vitamin C in hibits the growth of a bacterial risk factor for gastric carcinoma: Helicobacter pylori. *Cancer* 1997;80:1897-903.

[121] Jarosz M, Dzieniszewski J, Ufniarz ED, Wartanowicz M. Ziemlanski S, Reed PI. Effects of high dose vitamin C treatment on Helicobacter pylori infection and total vitamin C concentration in gastric juice. *Eur J Cancer Prev* 1998;7:449-54.

[122] Stahelin HB, Gey KF, Eichholzer M, Ludin E, Bernasconi F. Thurneysen J, Brubacher G. Plasma antioxidant vitamins and subsequent cancer mortality in the 12-year follow-up of the prospective Basel study. *Am J Epidemiol* 1991; 133:766-75.

[123] Nouraie M, Pietinen P, Kamangar F, Dawsey SM, Abnet CC. Albanes D, Virtamo J, Taylor PR. Fruits, vegetables, and antioxidants and risk of gastric cancer among male smokers. *Cancer Epidemiol Biomarkers Prev* 2005;14:2087-92.

[124] Botterweck AA, van den Brandt PA, Goldbohm RA. Vitamins, carotenoids, dietary fiber, and the risk of gastric carcinoma: results from a prospective study after 6.3 years of follow-up. *Cancer* 2000;88:737-48.

[125] Jenab M, Riboli E, Ferrari P, Sabate J, Slimani N, Norat T. et al. Plasma and dietary vitamin C levels and risk of gastric cancer in the European Prospective Investigation into Cancer and Nutrition (EPIC-EURGAST). *Carcinogenesis* 2006;27:2250-7.

[126] Yuan JM, Ross RK, Gao YT, Qu YH, Chu XD, Yu MC. Predi- agnostic levels of serum micronutrients in relation to risk of gastric cancer in Shanghai, China. *Cancer Epidemiol Biomarkers Prev* 2004:13:1772-80.

[127] Jacobs EJ, Connell CJ, McCullough ML, Chao A, Jonas CR, Rodriguez C, Calle EE, Thun MJ. Vitamin C, vitamin E, and multivitamin supplement use and stomach cancer mortality in the Cancer Prevention Study II cohort. *Cancer Epidemiol Biomarkers Prev* 2002; 11:35-41.

[128] Blot WJ, Li JY, Taylor PR, Guo W, Dawsey S, Wang GQ, Yang CS, Zheng SF, Gail M, Li GY. Nutrition intervention trials in Linxian, China: supplementation with specific vitamin/mineral combinations, cancer incidence, and disease-specific mortality in the general population. *J Natl Cancer Inst* 1993;85:1483-92.

[129] Epstein A. Thirty years of Epstein-Barr Virus. Epstein-Barr Virus Report 1994;l:3-4.

[130] Sasazuki S, Sasaki S, Tsubono Y, Okubo S, Hayashi M, Kakizoe T, Tsugane S. The effect of 5-year vitamin C supplementation on serum pepsinogen level and Helicobacter pylori infection. *Cancer Sci* 2003;94:378-82.

[131] Knight TM, Forman D, Al-Dabbagh SA, Doll R. Estimation of dietary intake of nitrate and nitrate in Great Britain. *Food Chem Toxicol* 1987; 25: 277-285.

[132] Pobel D, Riboli E, Cornee J, Hémon B, Guyader M. Nitrosamine, nitrate and nitrite in relation to gastric cancer: a case control study in Marseille, France. *Eur J Epidemiol* 1995; 11(1): 67–73.

[133] van Loon AJ, Botterweck AA, Goldbohm RA, Brants HA, van Klaveren JD, van den Brandt PA. Intake of nitrate and nitrite and the risk of gastric cancer: a prospective cohort study. *Br J Cancer* 1998; 78(1): 129–135.

[134] Knekt P, Jarvinen R, Dich J & Hakulinen T. Risk of colorectal and other gastro-intestinal cancers after exposure to nitrate, nitrite and N-nitroso compounds: a follow-up study. *Int J Cancer* 1999; 80(6): 852–856.

[135] Gonzalez CA, Pera G, Agudo A, Palli D, Krogh V, Vineis P, Tumino R, Panico S, Berglund G, Simán H, Nyrén O, et al. Smoking and the risk of gastric cancer in the European Prospective Investigation Into Cancer and Nutrition (EPIC). *Int J Cancer* 2003; 107: 629—634.

[136] Tredaniel J, Boffetta P, Buiatti E, Saracci R, Hirsch A. Tobacco smoking and gastric cancer: review and meta-analysis. *Int J Cancer* 1997; 72:565-573.

[137] Bagnardi V, Blangiardo M, La Vecchia C, Corrao G. A meta-analysis of alcohol drinking and cancer risk. *Br J Cancer* 2001; 85: 1700-1705.

[138] Fukayama M., Chong J.-M., and Kaizaki Y. Epstein-Barr virus and gastric carcinoma. *Gastric Cancer* (1998) 1: 104-114.

[139] Unakami M, Hara M, Fukuchi S, Akiyama H. Cancer of the gastric cardia and the habit of smoking. *Acta Pathol Jpn* 1989; 39:420-424.

[140] Palli D, Bianchi S, Decarli A, Cipriani F, Avellini C, Cocco P, Falcini F, Puntoni R, Russo A, Vindigni C. A case-control study of cancers of the gastric cardia in Italy. *Br J Cancer* 1992; 65: 263-266.

[141] Wu AH, Wan P & Bernstein L. A multiethnic population-based study of smoking, alcohol and body size and risk of adenocarcinomas of the stomach and esophagus (United States). *Cancer Causes Control* 2001; 12:721-732.

[142] Gammon MD, Schoenberg JB, Ahsan H, Risch HA, Vaughan TL, Chow WH, Rotterdam H, West AB, Dubrow R, Stanford JL, Mayne ST, Farrow DC, Niwa S, Blot WJ, Fraumeni JF Jr. Tobacco, alcohol, and socioeconomic status and adenocarcinomas of the esophagus and gastric cardia. *J Natl Cancer Inst* 1997; 89: 1277— 1284.

[143] Bagnardi V, Blangiardo M, La Vecchia C & Corrao G. Alcohol consumption and the risk of cancer: a metaanalysis. *Alcohol Res Health* 2001; 25(4): 263–270.

[144] Wang ZY, Cheng SJ, Zhou ZC, Athar M, Khan WA, Bickers DR, Mukhtar H. Antimutagenic activity of green tea polyphenols. *Mutat Res* 1989;223:273-85.

[145] Xu Y, Ho CT, Amin SG, Han C, Chung FL. Inhibition of tobacco- specific nitrosamine-induced lung tumorigenesis in A/J mice by green tea and its major polyphenols as antioxidants. *Cancer Res* 1992;52:3875-9.

[146] Wang ZY, Hong JY, Huang MT, Reuhl KR, Conney AH, Yang CS. Inhibition of N'-nitrosodiethylamine and 4-(methylnitrosamino)-l-(3-pyridyl)-l-butanone-induced tumorigenesis in A/J mice by green tea and black tea. *Cancer Res* 1992;52:1943-7.

[147] Yang CS, Maliakal P, Meng X. Inhibition of carcinogenesis by tea. *Annu Rev Pharmacol Toxicol* 2002;42:25-54.

[148] Moyers SB, Kumar NB. Green tea polyphenols and cancer chemoprevention: multiple mechanisms and endpoints for phase II trials. *Nutr Rev* 2004;62:204-11.

[149] Mukhtar H, Ahmad N. Tea polyphenols: prevention of cancer and optimizing health. *Am J Clin Nutr* 2000;71(suppl):698S-702S.

[150] Ji BT, Chow WH, Yang G, McLaughlin JK, Gao RN, Zheng W, Shu XO, Jin F, Fraumeni JF Jr, Gao YT. The influence of cigarette smoking, alcohol, and green tea consumption on the risk of carcinoma of the cardia and distal stomach in Shanghai, China. *Cancer* 1996;77:2449-57.

[151] Inoue M, Tajima K, Hirose K, Hamajima N, Takezaki T, Kuroishi T, Tominaga S. Tea and coffee consumption and the risk of digestive tract cancers: data from a comparative case-referent study in Japan. *Cancer Causes Control* 1998;9:209-16.

[152] Setiawan VW, Zhang ZF, Yu GP, Lu QY, Li YL, Lu ML, Wang MR, Guo CH, Yu SZ, Kurtz RC, Hsieh CC. Protective effect of green tea on the risks of chronic gastritis and stomach cancer. *Int J Cancer* 2001;92:600-4.

[153] Takezaki T, Gao CM, Wu JZ, Ding JH, Liu YT, Zhang Y, Li SP, Su P, Liu TK, Tajima K. Dietary protective and risk factors for esophageal and stomach cancers in a low-epidemic area for stomach cancer in Jiangsu Provance, China: comparison with those in a high-epidemic area. *Jpn J Cancer Res* 2001;92:1157-65.

[154] Tsubono Y, Nishino Y, Komatsu S, Hsieh CC, Kanemura S, Tsuji I, Nakatsuka H, Fukao A, Satoh H, Hisamichi S. Green tea and the risk of gastric cancer in Japan. *N Engl J Med* 2001;344:632-6.

[155] Hoshiyama Y, Kawaguchi T, Miura Y, Mizoue T, Tokui N. Yatsuya H, Sakata K, Kondo T, Kikuchi S, Toyoshima H, Hayakawa N, Tamakoshi A, Ohno Y, Yoshimura T; Japan Collaborative Cohort Study Group. A prospective study of stomach cancer death in relation to green tea consumption in Japan. *Br J Cancer* 2002;87: 309-13.

[156] Nagano J, Kono S, Preston DL, Mabuchi K. A prospective study of green tea consumption and cancer incidence, Hiroshima and Nagasaki, Japan. *Cancer Causes Control* 2001;15:501-8.

[157] Sasazuki S, Inoue M, Hanaoka T, Yamamoto S, Sobue T. Tsugane S. Green tea consumption and subsequent risk of gastric cancer by subsite: the JPHC study. *Cancer Causes Control* 2004; 15:483-91.

[158] Yang CS, Lee MJ, Chen L, Yang GY. Polyphenols as inhibitors of carcinogenesis. *Environ Health Perspect* 1997;105(suppl 4): 971-6.

[159] Khan MM, Goto R, Kobayashi K, Suzumura S, Nagata Y, Sonoda T, Sakauchi F, Washio M, Mori M. Dietary habits and cancer mortality among mid- die aged and older Japanese living in Hokkaido, Japan by cancer site and sex. *Asian Pac J Cancer Prev* 2004;5:58-65.

[160] Botelho F, Lunet N, Barros H. Coffee and gastric cancer: systematic review and meta-analysis. *Cad Saude Publica* 2006;22: 889-900.

[161] Tokunaga M, Land CE, Uemura Y, Tokudome T, Tanaka S, Sato E. Epstein-Barr virus in gastric carcinoma. *Am J Pathol* 1993;143:1250-4.

[162] Imai S, Koizumi S, Sugiura M, Tokunaga M, Uemura Y, Yamamoto N, Tanaka S, Sato E, Osato T. Gastric carcinoma: Monoclonal epithelial malignant cells expressing Epstein-Barr virus latent infection protein. *Proc Natl Acad Sci USA* 1994;91:9131-5.

[163] Nakamura S, Ueki T, Yao T, Ueyama T, Tsuneyoshi M. Epstein-Barr virus in gastric carcinoma with lymphoid stroma. Special reference to its detection by the polymerase chain reaction and in situ hybridization in 99 tumors, including a morphologic analysis. *Cancer (Phila)* 1994;73:2239-49.

[164] Yanai H, Takada K, Shimizu N, Mizugaki Y, Tada M, Okita K. Epstein-Barr virus infection in non-carcinomatous gastric epithelium. *J Pathol* 1997;183:293-8.

[165] Jing X, Nakamura Y, Nakamura M, Yokoi T, Shan L, Taniguchi E, Kakudo K. Detection of Epstein-Barr virus DNA in gastric carcinoma with lymphoid stroma. *Viral Immunol* 1997;10:49-58.

[166] Pagani A, Cerrato M, Bussolati G. Nonspecific in situ hybridization reaction in neuroendocrine cells and tumors of the gastrointestinal tract using oligonucleotide probes. *Diagn Mol Pathol* 1993;2:125-30.

[167] Matsunou H, Konishi F, Hori H, Ikeda T, Sasaki K, Hirose Y, Yamamichi N. Characteristics of Epstein-Barr virus-associated gastric carcinoma with lymphoid stroma in Japan. *Cancer (Phila)* 1996;77:1998-2004.

[168] Burke AP, Yen TSB, Shekitka KM, Sobin LH: Lymphoepithelial carcinoma of the stomach with Epstein-Barr virus demonstrated by polymerase chain reaction. *Mod Pathol* 1990;3:377-80.

[169] Watanabe H, Enjoji M, Imai T. Gastric carcinoma with lymphoid stroma: Its morphological characteristics and prognostic correlation. *Cancer* 1976;38:232-43.

[170] Chang KL, Chen YY, Shibata D, Weiss LM. Description of an in situ hybridization methodology for detection of Epstein-Barr virus RNA in paraffin-embedded tissues, with a survey of normal and neoplastic tissues. *Diagn Mol Pathol* 1992;l:246-55.

[171] Oda K, Tamaru J, Takenouchi T, Mikata A, Nonomura M, Saitoh N, Sarashina H, Nakajima N. Association of Epstein-Barr virus with gastric carcinoma with lymphoid stroma. *Am J Pathol* 1993;143:1063-71.

[172] Takano Y, Kato Y, Sugano H. Epstein-Barr virus-associated medullary carcinomas with lymphoid infiltration of the stomach. *Cancer Res Clin Oncol* 1994;120:303-8.

[173] Chong JM, Fukayama M, Hayashi Y, Takizawa T, Koike M, Konishi M, Kikuchi-Yanoshita R, Miyaki M. Microsatellite instability in the progression of gastric carcinoma. *Cancer Res* 1994;54:4595-7.

[174] Gulley ML, Pulitzer DR, Eagan PA, Schneider BG. Epstein-Barr virus infection is an early event in gastric carcinogenesis and is independent of bcl-2 expression and p53 accumulation. *Hum Pathol* 1996;27:20-7.

[175] Chong JM, Fukayama M, Hayashi Y, Funata N, Takizawa T, Koike M, Muraoka M, Kikuchi-Yanoshita R, Miyaki M, Mizuno S. Expression of CD44 variants in gastric carcinoma with or without Epstein-Barr virus. *Int J Cancer* 1997;74:450-4.

[176] Tashiro Y, Arikawa J, Itoh T, Tokunaga M. Clinico-pathologial findings of Epstein-Barr virus-related gastric cancer. In: Osato T, Takada K, Tokunaga M, editors. Epstein-Barr virus and human cancer. Tokyo: Japan Scientific Societies Press; 1998:87-97.

[177] Lertprasertuke N, Tsutsumi Y. Gastric carcinoma with lymphoid stroma. *Virchows Arch Pathol Anat* 1989;414:231-4.

[178] Ohfuji S, Osaki M, Tsujitani S, Ikeguchi M, Sairenji T, Ito H. Low frequency of apoptosis in Epstein-Barr virus-associated gastric carcinoma with lymphoid stroma. *Int J Cancer* 1996;68:710-5.

[179] Ojima H., Fukuda T, Nakajima T. and Nagamachi Y. Infrequent overexpression of p53 protein in Epstein-Barr virus-associated gastric carcinomas. *Jpn J. Cancer Res.* 1997; 88:262-266.

[180] Peek RM Jr, Blaser MJ: Helicobacter pylori and gastrointestinal tract adenocarcinomas. *Nat Rev Cancer* 2002; 2: 28–37.

[181] Marshall BJ, Windsor HM: The relation of Helicobacter pylori to gastric adenocarcinoma and lymphoma: pathophysiology, epidemiology, screening, clinical presentation, treatment, and prevention. *Med Clin North Am* 2005; 89: 313–344, viii. Review.

[182] Everhart JE: Recent developments in the epidemiology of Helicobacter pylori. *Gastroenterol Clin North Am* 2000; 29: 559–578.

[183] An international association between Helicobacter pylori infection and gastric cancer. The EUROGAST Study Group. *Lancet* 1993; 341: 1359–1362.

[184] Kikuchi S: Epidemiology of Helicobacter pylori and gastric cancer. *Gastric Cancer* 2002; 5: 6–15.

[185] Forman D, Newell DG, Fullerton F, Yarnell JW, Stacey AR, Wald N, Sitas F: Association between infection with Helicobacter pylori and risk of gastric cancer: evidence from a prospective investigation. *BMJ* 1991; 302:1302–1305.

[186] Nomura A, Stemmermann GN, Chyou PH, Kato I, Perez-Perez GI, Blaser MJ: Helicobacter pylori infection and gastric carcinoma among Japanese Americans in Hawaii. *N Engl J Med* 1991; 325: 1132–1136.

[187] Agha A, Graham DY: Evidence-based examination of the African enigma in relation to Helicobacter pylori infection. *Scand J Gastroenterol* 2005; 40: 523–529.

[188] Ito M., Tanaka S., Takata S., Oka S, Imagawa S, Ueda H, Egi Y, Kitadai Y, Yasui W, Yoshihara M, Haruma K, Chayama K. Morphological changes in human gastric tumours after eradication therapy of Helicobacter pylori in a short-term follow-up. *Aliment Pharmacol Ther* 2005; 21: 559–566.

[189] Saito K, Arai K, Mori M, Kobayashi R, Ohki I. Effect of Helicobacter pylori eradication on malignant transformation of gastric adenoma. *Gastrointestinal Endoscopy* 2000. 52(1):27-32.

[190] Uemura N, Mukai T, Okamoto S, Yamaguchi S, Mashiba H, Taniyama K, Sasaki N, Haruma K, Sumii K, Kajiyama G: Effect of Helicobacter pylori eradication on subsequent development of cancer after endoscopic resection of early gastric cancer. *Cancer Epidemiol Biomarkers Prev* 1997; 6: 639–642.

[191] Correa P: New strategies for the prevention of gastric cancer: Helicobacter pylori and genetic susceptibility. J Surg Oncol 2005; 90: 134–138.

[192] Fujioka T, Honda S, Tokieda M: Helicobacter pylori infection and gastric carcinoma in animal models. *J Gastroenterol Hepatol* 2000; 15(suppl):D55–D59.

[193] Honda S, Fujioka T, Tokieda M, Satoh R, Nishizono A, Nasu M: Development of Helicobacter pylori -induced gastric carcinoma in Mongolian gerbils. *Cancer Res* 1998; 58:4255.

[194] Sugiyama A, Maruta F, Ikeno T, Ishida K, Kawasaki S, Katsuyama T, Shimizu N, Tatematsu M: Helicobacter pylori infection enhances N-methyl-N-nitrosourea-induced stomach carcinogenesis in the Mongolian gerbil. *Cancer Res* 1998; 58: 2067–2069.

[195] Watanabe T, Tada M, Nagai H, Sasaki S, Nakao M: Helicobacter pylori infection induces gastric cancer in Mongolian gerbils. *Gastroenterology* 1998; 115: 642–648.

[196] Fox JG, Wang TC, Rogers AB, Poutahidis T, Ge Z, Taylor N, Dangler CA, Israel DA, Krishna U, Gaus K, Peek RM Jr: Host and microbial constituents influence Helicobacter pylori -induced cancer in a murine model of hypergastrinemia. *Gastroenterology* 2003; 124: 1879–1890.

[197] Nomura S, Baxter T, Yamaguchi H, Leys C, Vartapetian AB, Fox JG, Lee JR, Wang TC, Goldenring JR: Spasmolytic polypeptide expressing metaplasia to preneoplasia in H. felis -infected mice. *Gastroenterology* 2004;127: 582–594.

[198] Nagata J, Kijima H, Takagi A, Ito M, Goto K, Yamazaki H, Nakamura M, Mine T, Ueyama Y: Helicobacter pylori induces chronic active gastritis in p53-knockout mice. *Int J Mol Med* 2004; 13: 773–777.

[199] Cai X, Carlson J, Stoicov C, Li H, Wang TC, Houghton J: Helicobacter felis eradication restores normal architecture and inhibits gastric cancer progression in C57BL/6 mice. *Gastroenterology* 2005; 128: 1937–1952.

[200] Hatakeyama M: Oncogenic mechanisms of the Helicobacter pylori CagA protein. *Nat Rev Cancer* 2004;4:688-694.

[201] Azuma T, Yamazaki S, Yamakawa A, Ohtani M, Muramatsu A, Suto H, Ito Y, Dojo M, Yamazaki Y, Kuriyama M, Keida Y, Higashi H, Hatakeyama M: Association between diversity in the Src homology 2 domain-containing tyrosine phosphatase binding site of Helicobacter pylori CagA protein and gastric atrophy and cancer. *J Infect Dis* 2004; 189: 820-827.

[202] Glocker E, Lange C, Covacci A, Bereswill S, Kist M, Pahl HL: Proteins encoded by the cag pathogenicity island of Helicobacter pylori are required for NF-kappaB activation. *Infect Immun* 1998;66:2346-2348.

[203] Blaser MJ: Helicobacter pylori and gastrointestinal tract adenocarcinomas. *Nat Rev Cancer.* 2002;2:28-37.

[204] Karin M, Cao Y, Greten PR, Li ZW: NF-kappaB in cancer: From innocent bystander to major culprit. *Nat Rev Cancer.* 2002;2:301-310.

[205] Peek RM Jr: Events at the host-microbial interface of the gastrointestinal tract. IV. The pathogenesis of Helicobacter pylori persistence. *Am J Physiol Gastrointest Liver Physiol* 2005;289:G8-G12.

[206] Cover TL, Blanke SR: Helicobacter pylori VacA, a paradigm for toxin multifunctionality. *Nat Rev Microbiol* 2005;3:320-332.

[207] Yu J, Leung WK, Go MY, Chan MC, To KF, Ng EK, Chan FK, Ling TK, Chung SC, Sung JJ: Relationship between Helicobacter pylori babA2 status with gastric epithelial cell turnover and premalignant gastric lesions. *Gut* 2002;51:480-484.

[208] Ilver D, Arnqvist A, Ogren J, Prick IM, Ker-sulyte D, Incecik ET, Berg DE, Covacci A, Engstrand L, Boren T: Helicobacter pylori adhesin binding fucosylated histo-blood group antigens revealed by retagging. *Science* 1998;279:373-377.

[209] Segal ED, Shon J, Tompkins LS: Characterization of Helicobacter pylori urease mutants. *Infect Immun* 1992;60:1883-1889.

[210] Gobert AP, Mersey BD, Cheng Y, Blumberg DR, Newton JC, Wilson KT. Cutting edge: Urease release by Helicobacter pylori stimulates macrophage inducible nitric oxide synthase. *J Immunol* 2002;168:6002-6006.

[211] Zambon CF, Navaglia F, Basso D, Rugge M, Plebani M: Helicobacter pylori babA2, cagA, and si vacA genes work synergistically in causing intestinal metaplasia. *J Clin Pathol* 2003;56:287-291.

[212] Mahdavi J, Sonden B, Hurtig M, Olfat FO, Forsberg L, Roche N, Angstrom J, Larsson T, Teneberg S, Karlsson KA, Altraja S, Wadström T, Kersulyte D, Berg DE, Dubois A, Petersson C, Magnusson KE, Norberg T, Lindh F, Lundskog BB, Arnqvist A, Hammarström L, Borén T. Helicobacter pylori SabA adhesin in persistent infection and chronic inflammation. *Science* 2002;297:573-578.

[213] O' Brien DP, Israel DA, Krishna U, Romero-Gallo J, Nedrud J, Medof ME, Lin F, Redline R, Lublin DM, Nowicki BJ, Franco AT, Ogden S, Williams AD, Polk DB, Peek RM Jr. The role of decay-accelerating factor as a receptor for Helicobacter pylori and a mediator of gastric inflammation. *J Biol Chem* 2006;281: 13317-13323.

[214] Mandell L, Moran AP, Cocchiarella A, Houghton J, Taylor N, Fox JG, Wang TC, Kurt-Jones EA: Intact gram-negative Helicobacter pylori, Helicobacter felis, and Helicobacter hepaticus bacteria activate innate immunity via toll-like receptor 2 but not toll-like receptor 4. *Infect Immun* 2004;72: 6446-6454.

[215] Smythies LE, Waites KB, Lindsey JR, Harris PR, Ghiara P, Smith PD: Helicobacter pylori- induced mucosal inflammation is Th1 mediated and exacerbated in IL-4, but not IFN-gamma, gene-deficient mice. *J Immunol* 2000:165:1022-1029.

[216] Mitchell HM, Ally R, Wadee A, Wiseman M, Segal I: Major differences in the IgG subclass response to Helicobacter pylori in the first and third worlds. *Scand J Gastroenterol* 2002:37:517-522.

[217] El-Omar EM, Rabkin CS, Gammon MD, Vaughan TL, Risch HA, Schoenberg JB, Stanford JL, Mayne ST, Goedert J, Blot WJ, Fraumeni JF Jr, Chow WH: Increased risk of noncardia gastric cancer associated with proinflammatory cytokine gene polymorphisms. *Gastroenterology* 2003;124:1193-1120.

[218] El-Omar EM, Carrington M, Chow WH, McColl KE, Bream JH, Young HA, Herrera J, Lissowska J, Yuan CC, Rothman N, Lanyon G, Martin M, Fraumeni JF Jr, Rabkin CS: Interleukin-1 polymorphisms associated with increased risk of gastric cancer. *Nature* 2000; 404:398-402.

[219] El-Omar EM: The importance of interleukin 1beta in Helicobacter pylori associated disease. *Gut* 2001:48:743-747.

[220] Rad R, Prinz C, Neu B, Neuhofer M, Zeitner M, Voland P, Becker I, Schepp W, Gerhard M. Synergistic effect of Helicobacter pylori virulence factors and interleukin-1 polymorphisms for the development of severe histological changes in the gastric mucosa. *J Infect Dis* 2003;188: 272-281.

[221] Terres AM, Pajares JM, O' Toole D, Ahern S, Kelleher D: H. pylori infection is associated with downregulation of E-cadherin, a molecule involved in epithelial cell adhesion and proliferation control. *J Clin Pathol* 1998;51: 410-412.

[222] Chan AO, Lam SK, Wong BC, Kwong YL, Rashid A: Gene methylation in non-neoplas-tic mucosa of gastric cancer: Age or Helicobacter pylori related? *Am J Pathol* 2003;163: 370-371.

[223] Stoicov C, Saffari R, Cai X, Hasyagar C, Houghton J: Molecular biology of gastric cancer: Helicobacter infection and gastric adenocarcinoma: bacterial and host factors responsible for altered growth signaling. *Gene* 2004:341:1-17.

[224] Houghton J, Macera-Bloch LS, Harrison L, Kim KH, Korah RM: Tumor necrosis factor alpha and interleukin Ibeta up-regulate gastric mucosal Fas antigen expression in Helicobacter pylori infection. *Infect Immun* 2000:68:1189-1195.

[225] Lee KM, Lee DS, Yang JM, Ahn BM, Lee EH, Yoo JY, Kim YJ, Chung IS, Sun HS, Park DH: Effect of Helicobacter pylori on gastric epithelial cell kinetics and expression of apoptosis-related proteins in gastric carcinogenesis. *Korean J Gastroenterol* 2003;42:12-19.

[226] Fan X, Gunasena H, Cheng Z, Espejo R, Crowe SE, Ernst PB, Reyes VE: Helicobacter pylori urease binds to class II MHC on gastric epithelial cells and induces their apopto-sis. *J Immunol* 2000:165:1918-1924.

[227] Azuma T, Ito S, Sato F, Yamazaki Y, Miyaji H, Ito Y, Suto H, Kuriyama M, Kato T, Kohli Y: The role of the HLA-DQA1 gene in resistance to atrophic gastritis and gastric adenocarcinoma induced by Helicobacter pylori infection. *Cancer* 1998;82:1013-1018.

[228] Nagasako T, Sugiyama T, Mizushima T, Mi-ura Y, Kato M, Asaka M: Up-regulated SmadS mediates apoptosis of gastric epithelial cells induced by Helicobacter pylori in-fection. *J Biol Chem* 2003;278:4821-4825.

[229] Meyer-ter-Vehn T, Covacci A, Kist M, Pahl HL: Helicobacter pylori activates mitogen-activated protein kinase cascades and induces expression of the proto-oncogenes c-fos and c-jun. *J Biol Chem* 2000:275:16064-16072.

[230] Churin Y, Al- Ghoul L, Kepp O, Meyer TF, Birchmeier W, Naumann M: Helicobacter pylori CagA protein targets the c-Met receptor and enhances the motogenic response. *J Cell Biol* 2003;161:249-255.

[231] Keates S, Sougioultzis S, Keates AC, Zhao D, Peek RM Jr, Shaw LM, Kelly CP: cag+ Helicobacter pylori induce transactivation of the epidermal growth factor receptor in AGS gastric epithelial cells. *J Biol Chem* 2001;276: 48127-48134.

[232] Tuccillo C, Manzo BA, Nardone G, D' Argenio G, Rocco A, Di Popolo A, Delia VN, Staibano S, De Rosa G, Ricci V, Del Vecchio BC, Zar-rilli R, Romano M: Up-

regulation of heparin binding epidermal growth factor-like growth factor and amphiregulin expression in Helicobacter pylori-infected human gastric mucosa. *Dig Liver Dis* 2002;34:498-505.

[233] Wong BC, Wang WP, So WH, Shin VY, Wong WM, Fung FM, Liu ES, Hiu WM, Lam SK, Cho CH: Epidermal growth factor and its receptor in chronic active gastritis and gastroduodenal ulcer before and after Helicobacter pylori eradication. *Aliment Pharmacol Ther* 2001:15:1459-1465.

[234] Wang TC, Dangler CA, Chen D, Goldenring JR, Koh T, Raychowdhury R, Coffey RJ, Ito S, Varro A, Dockray GJ, Fox JG: Synergistic interaction between hypergastrinemia and Helicobacter infection in a mouse model of gastric cancer. *Gastroenterology* 2000;118: 36-47.

[235] Kinoshita Y, Ishihara S, Kadowaki Y, Fukui H, Chiba T: Reg protein is a unique growth factor of gastric mucosal cells. *J Gastroenterol* 2004;39:507-513.

[236] Romano M, Ricci V, Memoli A, Tuccillo C, Di Popolo A, Sommi P, Acquaviva AM, Del Vecchio Blanco C, Bruni CB, Zarrilli R: Helicobacter pylori up-regulates cyclooxygen-ase-2 mRNA expression and prostaglandin E2 synthesis in MKN 28 gastric mucosal cells in vitro. *J Biol Chem* 1998;273:28560-28563.

[237] Sawaoka H, Kawano S, Tsuji S, Tsuji M, Sun W, Gunawan ES, Hori M: Helicobacter pylori infection induces cyclooxygenase-2 expression in human gastric mucosa. *Prostaglandins Leukot Essent Fatty Acids* 1998;59:313-316.

[238] Fukumoto S, Ichihara T, Takada M, Kuroda Y: Expression of cyclooxygenases in Helicobacter pylori gastritis and residual gastritis after distal gastrectomy. *World J Surg* 2003; 27:145-148.

[239] Sung JJ, Leung WK, Go MY, To KF, Cheng AS, Ng EK, Chan FK: Cyclooxygenase-2 expression in Helicobacter pylori-associated premalignant and malignant gastric lesions. *Am J Pathol* 2000;157:729-735.

[240] Sun WH, Yu Q, Shen H, Ou XL, Cao DZ, Yu T, Qian C, Zhu F, Sun YL, Fu XL, Su H: Roles of Helicobacter pylori infection and cyclooxygenase-2 expression in gastric carcinogenesis. *World J Gastroenterol* 2004;10:2809-2133.

[241] Nardone G, Rocco A, Vaira D, Staibano S, Budillon A, Tatangelo F, Sciulli MG, Perna F, Salvatore G, Di Benedetto M, De Rosa G, Patrignani P: Expression of COX-2, mPGE-synthasel, MDR-1 (P-gp), and Bcl-xL: a molecular pathway of H pylori-related gastric carcinogenesis. *J Pathol* 2004;202:305-312.

[242] Pomorski T, Meyer TF, Naumann M: Helicobacter pylori-induced prostaglandin E(2) synthesis involves activation of cytosolic phospholipase A(2) in epithelial cells. *J Biol Chem* 2001:276:804-810.

[243] Jaiswal M, LaRusso NF, Gores GJ: Nitric oxide in gastrointestinal epithelial cell carcinogenesis: linking inflammation to oncogenesis. *Am J Physiol* 2001; 281:G626–G634.

[244] Rokkas T, Liatsos C, Petridou E, Papatheodorou G, Karameris A, Ladas SD, Raptis SA: Relationship of Helicobacter pylori CagA(+) status to gastric juice vitamin C levels. *Eur J Clin Invest* 1999:29:56-62.

[245] Sobala GM, Schorah CJ, Pignatelli B, Crabtree JE, Martin IG, Scott N, Quirke P: High gastric juice ascorbic acid concentrations in members of a gastric cancer family. *Carcinogenesis* 1993:14:291-292.

[246] Obst B, Wagner S, Sewing KF, Beil W: Helicobacter pylori causes DNA damage in gastric epithelial cells. Carcinogenesis 2000; 21: 1111–1115.

[247] Pignatelli B, Bancel B, Plummer M, Toyokuni S, Patricot LM, Ohshima H: Helicobacter pylori eradication attenuates oxidative stress in human gastric mucosa. *Am J Gastroenterol* 2001; 96: 1758–1766.

[248] Palli D, Saieva C, Gemma S, Masala G, Gomez-Miguel MJ, Luzzi I, D'Errico M, Matullo G, Ozzola G, Manetti R, Nesi G, Sera F, Zanna I, Dogliotti E, Testai E: GSTT1 and GSTM1 gene polymorphisms and gastric cancer in a high-risk Italian population. *Int J Cancer* 2005; 115: 284–289.

[249] Houghton J, Stoicov C, Nomura S, Rogers AB, Carlson J, Li H, Cai X, Fox JG, Goldenring JR, Wang TC: Gastric cancer originating from bone marrow-derived cells. *Science* 2004; 306: 1568–1571.

[250] Houghton J, Wang TC: Helicobacter pylori and gastric cancer: a new paradigm for inflammation-associated epithelial cancers. *Gastroenterology* 2005; 128: 1567–1578.

[251] Peek RM Jr, Crabtree JE: Helicobacter infection and gastric neoplasia. *J Pathol* 2006;208: 233-248.

[252] Wong BC, Lam SK, Wong WM, Chen JS, Zheng TT, Feng RE, Lai KC, Hu WH, Yuen ST, Leung SY, Fong DY, Ho J, Ching CK, Chen JS; China Gastric Cancer Study Group: Helicobacter pylori eradication to prevent gastric cancer in a high-risk region of China: a randomized controlled trial. *JAMA* 2004;291:187-194.

[253] Pritchard DM, Crabtree JE: Helicobacter pylori and gastric cancer. *Curr Opin Gastroenterol* 2006:22:62.

[254] Romano M, Ricci V, Zarrilli R: Mechanisms of disease: Helicobacter pylori-related gastric carcinogenesis: implications for chemoprevention. *Nat Clin Pract Gastroenterol Hepatol* 2006:3:622-632.

[255] Correa P. Helicobacter pylori and gastric carcinogenesis. *Am J Surg Pathol* 1995; 19: 837-3.

[256] Ming SC. Cellular and molecular pathology of gastric carcinoma and precursor lesions: a critical review. *Gastric Cancer* 1998; 1: 31-50.

[257] Asaka M, Sugiyama T, Nobuta A Kato M, Takeda H, Graham DY. Atrophic gastritis and intestinal metaplasia in Japan: results of a large multicenter study. *Helicobacter* 2001; 6: 294-9.

[258] Cheli R, Giacosa A, Pirasso A. Chronic gastritis: a dynamic process toward cancer. In: Ming, SC, ed. Precursor of Gastric Cancer. New York: Praeger Scientific, 1984: 117-29.

[259] Borchard F. Precancerous conditions and lesions of stomach. In: Rugge, M, Arslan-Pagnini, C, Di Mario, F, eds. Carcinoma gastrico e lesioni precancerose dello stomaco. Milano: EdizioniUnicopi, 1986: 175-210.

[260] Inoue M, Tajima K, Matsuura A, Suzuki T, Nakamura T, Ohashi K, Nakamura S, Tominaga S. Severity of chronic atrophic gastritis and subsequent gastric cancer occurrence: a 10-year prospective cohort study in Japan. *Cancer Lett* 2000; 161: 105-12.

[261] McColl KE, El-Omar E, Gillen D, Banerjee S. The role of Helicobacter pylori in the pathophysiology of duodenal ulcer disease and gastric cancer. *Semin Gastrointest Dis* 1997; 8:142-55.

[262] Leach SA, Thompson M, Hill M. Bacterially catalysed N-nitrosation reactions and their relative importance in the human stomach. *Carcinogenesis* 1987; 8: 1907-12.

[263] Lipkin M, Correa P, Mikol YB, Higgins PJ, Cuello C, Zarama G, Fontham E, Zavala D. Proliferative and antigenic modifications in human epithelial cells in chronic atrophic gastritis. *J Natl Cancer Inst* 1985; 75: 613-9.

[264] Konturek PC, Rembiasz K, Konturek SJ, Stachura J, Bielanski W, Galuschka K, Karcz D, Hahn EG. Gene expression of ornithine decarboxylase, cyclooxygenase-2, and gastrin in atrophic gastric mucosa infected with Helicobacter pylori before and after eradication therapy. *Dig Dis Sci* 2003; 48: 36-46.

[265] Heby O. Role of polyamines in the control of cell proliferation and differentiation. *Differentiation*. 1981;19(1):1-20.

[266] Patchett SE, Alstead EM, Butruk L, Przytulski K, Farthing MJ. Ornithine decarboxylase as a marker for premalignancy in the stomach. *Gut* 1995; 37: 13-6.

[267] Russo F, Linsalata M, Giorgio I, Caruso ML, Armentano R, Di Leo A. Polyamine levels and ODC activity in intestinal-type and diffuse-type gastric carcinoma. *Dig Dis Sci* 1997; 42: 576-9.

[268] Testino G, Valentini M, Cornaggia M, Testino R. Chronic atrophic gastritis and gastric cancer. *Dig Liver Dis* 2000; 32: 544.

[269] Leung WK, Sung JJ. Review article: intestinal metaplasia and gastric carcinogenesis. *Aliment Pharmacol Ther* 2002; 16: 1209-16.

[270] Shimoyama T, Fukuda S, Tanaka M, Nakaji S, Munakata A. Evaluation of the applicability of the gastric carcinoma risk index for intestinal type cancer in Japanese patients infected with Helicobacter pylori. *Virchows Arch* 2000; 436: 585-7.

[271] Jass JR, Filipe MI. Sulphomucins and precancerous lesions of the human stomach. *Histopathology* 1980; 4: 271-9.

[272] Ho SB, Shekels LL, Toribara NW, Kim YS, Lyftogt C, Cherwitz DL, Niehans GA. Mucin gene expression in normal, preneoplastic, and neoplastic human gastric epithelium. *Cancer Res* 1995; 55: 2681-90.

[273] Reis CA, David L, Correa P, Carneiro F, de Bolós C, Garcia E, Mandel U, Clausen H, Sobrinho-Simões M. Intestinal metaplasia of human stomach displays distinct patterns of mucin (MUC1, MUC2, MUC5AC, and MUC6) expression. *Cancer Res* 1999;59: 1003-7.

[274] Filipe MI, Munoz N, Matko I, Kato I, Pompe-Kirn V, Jutersek A, Teuchmann S, Benz M, Prijon T. Intestinal metaplasia types and the risk of gastric cancer: a cohort study in Slovenia. *Int J Cancer* 1994; 57: 324-9.

[275] Matsukura N, Suzuki K, Kawachi T, Aoyagi M, Sugimura T, Kitaoka H, Numajiri H, Shirota A, Itabashi M, Hirota T. Distribution of marker enzymes and mucin in intestinal metaplasia in human stomach and relation to complete and incomplete types of intestinal metaplasia to minute gastric carcinomas. *J Natl Cancer Inst* 1980; 65: 231-40.

[276] You WC, Li JY, Blot WJ, Chang YS, Jin ML, Gail MH, Zhang L, Liu WD, Ma JL, Hu YR, Mark SD, Correa P, Fraumeni JF Jr, Xu GW. Evolution of precancerous lesions in a rural Chinese population at high risk of gastric cancer. *Int J Cancer* 1999; 83: 615-9.

[277] Ohata H, Kitauchi S, Yoshimura N, Mugitani K, Iwane M, Nakamura H, Yoshikawa A, Yanaoka K, Arii K, Tamai H, Shimizu Y, Takeshita T, Mohara O, Ichinose M.

Progression of chronic atrophic gastritis associated with Helicobacter pylori infection increases risk of gastric cancer. *Int J Cancer* 2004; 109: 138-43.

[278] Cassaro M, Rugge M, Gutierrez O, Leandro G, Graham DY, Genta RM. Topographic patterns of intestinal metaplasia and gastric cancer. *Am J Gastroenterol* 2000; 95: 1431-8.

[279] Gong C, Mera R, Bravo JC, Ruiz B, Diaz-Escamilla R, Fontham ET, Correa P, Hunt JD. KRAS mutations predict progression of preneoplastic gastric lesions. *Cancer Epidemiol Biomarkers Prev* 1999; 8: 167-71.

[280] Leung WK, Kim JJ, Kim JG, Graham DY, Sepulveda AR. Microsatellite instability in gastric intestinal metaplasia in patients with and without gastric cancer. *Am J Pathol* 2000; 156: 537-43.

[281] Kang GH, Shim YH, Jung HY, Kim WH, Ro JY, Rhyu MG. CpG island methylation in premalignant stages of gastric carcinoma. *Cancer Res* 2001; 61: 2847-51.

[282] Shiao YH, Rugge M, Correa P, Lehmann HP, Scheer WD. p53 alteration in gastric precancerous lesions. *Am J Pathol* 1994; 144: 511-7.

[283] Yu J, Leung WK, Ng EK, To KF, Ebert MP, Go MY, Chan WY, Chan FK, Chung SC, Malfertheiner P, Sung JJ. Effect of Helicobacter pylori eradication on expression of cyclin D2 and p27 in gastric intestinal metaplasia. *Aliment Pharmacol Ther* 2001; 15: 1505-11.

[284] Chung IK, Hwang KY, Kim IH, Kim HS, Park SH, Lee MH, Kim CJ, Kim SJ. Helicobacter pylori and telomerase activity in intestinal metaplasia of the stomach. *Korean J Intern Med* 2002; 17: 227-33.

[285] Silberg DG, Furth EE, Taylor JK, Schuck T, Chiou T, Traber PG. CDX1 protein expression in normal, metaplastic, and neoplastic human alimentary tract epithelium. *Gastroenterology* 1997; 113:478-86.

[286] Satoh K, Mutoh H, Eda A, Yanaka I, Osawa H, Honda S, Kawata H, Kihira K, Sugano K. Aberrant expression of CDX2 in the gastric mucosa with and without intestinal metaplasia: effect of eradication of Helicobacter pylori. *Helicobacter* 2002; 7: 192-8.

[287] Hamamoto T, Yokozaki H, Semba S, Yasui W, Yunotani S, Miyazaki K, Tahara E. Altered microsatellites in incomplete-type intestinal metaplasia adjacent to primary gastric cancers. *J Clin Pathol* 1997; 50: 841-6.

[288] Ottini L, Palli D, Falchetti M, D'Amico C, Amorosi A, Saieva C, Calzolari A, Cimoli F, Tatarelli C, De Marchis L, Masala G, Mariani-Costantini R, Cama A. Microsatellite instability in gastric cancer is associated with tumor location and family history in a high-risk population from Tuscany. *Cancer Res* 1997; 57: 4523-9.

[289] Nardone G, Staibano S, Rocco A, Mezza E, D'armiento FP, Insabato L, Coppola A, Salvatore G, Lucariello A, Figura N, De Rosa G, Budillon G. Effect of Helicobacter pylori infection and its eradication on cell proliferation, DNA status, and oncogene expression in patients with chronic gastritis. *Gut* 1999; 44: 789-99.

[290] Brito MJ, Williams GT, Thompson H, Filipe MI. Expression of p53 in early (T1) gastric carcinoma and precancerous adjacent mucosa. *Gut* 1994; 35: 1697-700.

[291] Ochiai A, Yamauchi Y, Hirohashi S. p53 mutations in the non-neoplastic mucosa of the human stomach showing intestinal metaplasia. *Int J Cancer* 1996; 69: 28-33.

[292] Wu MS, Shun CT, Lee WC, Chen CJ, Wang HP, Lee WJ, Lin JT. Gastric cancer risk in relation to Helicobacter pylori infection and subtypes of intestinal metaplasia. *Br J Cancer* 1998; 78: 125-8.

[293] Fenoglio-Preiser C, Carneiro F, Correa P, et al. Gastric carcinoma. In: Hamilton, SR, Aaltonen, LA, eds. Pathology and Genetics, Tumors of the Digestive System. Lyon: IARC press, 2000: 39-52.

[294] Genta RM, Rugge M. Gastric precancerous lesions: heading for an international consensus. *Gut* 1999; 45: 15-8.

[295] Asaka M, Takeda H, Sugiyama T, Kato M. What role does Helicobacter pylori play in gastric cancer? *Gastroenterology* 1997; 113:856-60.

[296] Macartney JC, Camplejohn RS. DNA flow cytometry of histological material from dysplastic lesions of human gastric mucosa. *J Pathol* 1986; 150(2):113-8.

[297] Abdel-Wahab M, Attallah AM, Elshal MF, Eldousoky I, Zalata KR, el-Ghawalby NA, Gad el-Hak N, el-Ebidy G, Ezzat F. Correlation between endoscopy, histopathology, and DNA flow cytometry in patients with gastric dyspepsia. *Hepatogastroenterology* 1996; 43: 1313-20.

[298] Li J, Zhao A, Lu Y, Wang Y. Expression of p185erbB2 and p21ras in carcinoma, dysplasia, and intestinal metaplasia of the stomach: an immunohistochemical and in situ hybridization study. *Semin Surg Oncol* 1994; 10: 95-9.

[299] Sanz-Ortega J, Sanz-Esponera J, Caldes T, Gomez de la Concha E, Sobel ME, Merino MJ. LOH at the APC/MCC gene (5Q21) in gastric cancer and preneoplastic lesions. Prognostic implications. *Pathol Res Pract* 1996; 192: 1206-10.

[300] Glober GA, Cantrell EG, Doll R, Peto R. Interaction between ABO and rhesus blood groups, the site of origin of gastric cancers, and the age and sex of the patient. *Gut* 1971; 12: 570-3.

[301] Go MF. Review article: Natural history and epidemiology of Helicobacter pylori infection. *Aliment Pharmacol Ther* 2002; 16: 3-15.

[302] Asaka M, Kudo M, Kato M, Sugiyama T, Takeda H. Review article: Long-term Helicobacter pylori infection - from gastritis to gastric cancer. *Aliment Pharmacol Ther* 1998; 12: 9-15.

[303] Tahara E. Molecular biology of gastric cancer. *World J Surg* 1995; 19: 484-8.

[304] Perucho M. Cancer of the microsatellite mutator phenotype. *Biol Chem* 1996; 377: 675-84.

[305] Heyden JD, Martin IG, Cawkwell L. The role of microsatellite instability in gastric carcinoma. *Gut* 1998; 42: 300-3.

[306] Eshleman JR, Markowitz SD. Microsatellite instability in inherited and sporadic neoplasms. *Curr Opin Oncol* 1995; 7: 83-9.

[307] Huang JQ, Sridhar S, Chen Y, Hunt RH. Meta-analysis of the relationship between Helicobacter pylori seropositivity and gastric cancer. *Gastroenterology* 1998; 114: 1169-79.

[308] Tahara E. Molecular mechanism of stomach carcinogenesis. *J Cancer Res Clin Oncol* 1993;119:265-72.

[309] Yasui W, Oue N, Kuniyasu H, Ito R, Tahara E, Yokozaki H. Molecular diagnosis of gastric cancer: present and future. *Gastric Cancer* 2001;4:113-21.

[310] Ohgaki H, Yasui W, Yokota J. Genetic pathway to human cancer. In: Vainio H, Hietanen E, editors. Handbook of experimental pharmacology. Mechanisms in carcinogenesis and cancer reearch. Berlin Heidelberg New York Singapore Tokyo: Springer- Verlag; 2003. p. 25-39.

[311] Yokozaki H, Yasui W, Tahara E. Genetic and epigenetic changes in stomach cancer. *Int Rev Cytol* 2001;204:49-95.

[312] Yasui W, Oue N, Ono S, Mitani Y, Ito R, Nakayama H. Histone acetylation and gastrointestinal carcinogenesis. *Ann NY Acad Sci* 2003;983:220-31.

[313] Ebert MP, Fei G, Kahmann S, Muller O, Yu J, Sung JJ, Malfertheiner P. Increased beta-catenin mRNA levels and mutational alterations of the APC and beta-catenin gene are present in intestinal-type gastric cancer. *Carcinogenesis* 2002;23:87-91.

[314] Tamura G, Yin J, Wang S, Fleisher AS, Zou T, Abraham JM, Kong D, Smolinski KN, Wilson KT, James SP, Silverberg SG, Nishizuka S, Terashima M, Motoyama T, Meltzer SJ. E-Cadherin gene promoter hypermethylation in primary human gastric carcinomas. *J Natl Cancer Inst* 2000;92:569-73.

[315] Fiocca R, Luinetti O, Villani L, Mastracci L, Quilici P, Grillo F, Ranzani GN. Molecular mechanisms involved in the pathogenesis of gastric carcinoma: interactions between genetic alterations, cellular phenotype and cancer histotype. *Hepatogastroenterology* 2001;48:1523-30.

[316] El-Rifai W, Powell SM. Molecular biology of gastric cancer. *Semin Radiat Oncol* 2002;12:128-40.

[317] Ebert MP, Schandl L, Malfertheiner P. Helicobacter pylori infection and molecular changes in gastric carcinogenesis. *J Gastroenterol* 2002;37(Suppl 13):45-9.

[318] Kapadia CR. Gastric atrophy, metaplasia, and dysplasia: a clinical perspective. *J Clin Gastroenterol* 2003;36(5 Suppl):S29-36.

[319] Misdraji J, Lauwers GY. Gastric epithelial dysplasia. *Semin Diagn Pathol* 2002;19:20-30.

[320] Clouston AD. Timely topic: premalignant lesions associated with adenocarcinoma of the upper gastrointestinal tract. Pathology 2001;33:271-7.

[321] Zheng L., Wang L, Ajani J, Xie K. Molecular basis of gastric cancer. *Gastric Cancer* 2004;7: 61-77.

[322] Werner M, Becker KF, Keller G, Hofler H. Gastric adenocarcinoma: pathomorphology and molecular pathology. *J Cancer Res Clin Oncol* 2001;127:207-16.

[323] Miyoshi E, Haruma K, Hiyama T, Tanaka S, Yoshihara M. Shimamoto F, Chayama K. Microsatellite instability is a genetic marker for the development of multiple gastric cancers. *Int J Cancer* 2001;95:350-3.

[324] Hayden JD, Martin IG, Cawkwell L, Quirke P. The role of microsatellite instability in gastric carcinoma. *Gut* 1998;42:300- 3.

[325] Leung SY, Yuen ST, Chung LP, Chu KM, Chan AS, Ho JC. hMLH1 promoter methylation and lack of hMLH1 expression in sporadic gastric carcinomas with high-frequency microsatellite instability. *Cancer Res* 1999;59:159-64.

[326] Iacopetta BJ, Soong R, House AK, Hamelin R. Gastric carcinomas with microsatellite instability: clinical features and mutations to the TGF-beta type II receptor, IGFII receptor, and BAX genes. *J Pathol* 1999;187:428-32.

[327] Hailing KC, Harper J, Moskaluk CA, Thibodeau SN, Petroni OR, Yustein AS, Tosi P, Minacci C, Roviello F, Piva P, Hamilton SR, Jackson CE, Powell SM. Origin of microsatellite instability in gastric cancer. *Am J Pathol* 1999;155:205-11.

[328] Chan AO, Luk JM, Hui WM, Lam SK. Molecular biology of gastric carcinoma: from laboratory to bedside. *J Gastroenterol Hepatol* 1999;14:1150-60.

[329] Ranzani GN, Luinetti O, Padovan LS, Calistri D, Renault B. Burrel M, Amadori D, Fiocca R, Solcia E. p53 gene mutations and protein nuclear accumulation are early events in intestinal type gastric cancer but late events in diffuse type. *Cancer Epidemiol Biomarkers Prev* 1995;4:223-31.

[330] Wang JY, Lin SR, Hsieh JS, Hsu CH, Huang YS, Huang TJ. Mutations of p53 gene in gastric carcinoma in Taiwan. *Anticancer Res* 2001;21:513-20.

[331] Hollstein M, Shomer B, Greenblatt M, Soussi T, Hovig E, Montesano R, Harris CC. Somatic point mutations in the p53 gene of human tumors and cell lines: updated compilation. *Nucleic Acids Res* 1996;24:141-6.

[332] Fenoglio-Preiser CM, Wang J, Stemmermann GN, Noffsinger A. TP53 and gastric carcinoma: a review. *Hum Mutat* 2003;21:258-70.

[333] Imazeki F, Omata M, Nose H, Ohio M, Isono K. p53 gene mutations in gastric and esophageal cancers. *Gastroenterology* 1992;103:892-6.

[334] Kim JH, Takahashi T, Chiba I, Park JG, Birrer MJ, Roh JK, De Lee H, Kim JP, Minna JD, Gazdar AF. Occurrence of p53 gene abnormalities in gastric carcinoma tumors and cell lines. *Natl Cancer Inst* 1991;83:938-43.

[335] Yamada Y, Yoshida T, Hayashi K, Sekiya T, Yokota J. Hirohashi S, Nakatani K, Nakano H, Sugimura T, Terada M. p53 gene mutations in gastric cancer metastases and in gastric cancer cell lines derived from metastases. *Cancer Res* 1991;51:5800-5.

[336] Becker KF, Keller G, Hoefler H. The use of molecular biology in diagnosis and prognosis of gastric cancer. *Surg Oncol* 2000;9:5-11.

[337] Tahara E. Genetic alterations in human gastrointestinal cancers.*Cancer* 1995;75:1410-7.

[338] Horii A, Nakatsuru S, Miyoshi Y, Ichii S, Nagase H, Kato Y, Yanagisawa A, Nakamura Y. The APC gene, responsible for familial adenomatous polyposis, is mutated in human gastric cancer. *Cancer Res* 1992;52: 3231-3.

[339] Hanna NN, Mentzer RM Jr. Molecular genetics and management strategies in hereditary cancer syndromes. *J Ky Med Assoc* 2003;101:100-7.

[340] Hofler H, Becker KF. Molecular mechanisms of carcinogenesis in gastric cancer. *Recent Results Cancer Res* 2003;162:65-72.

[341] Hara T, Ooi A, Kobayashi M, Mai M, Yanagihara K, Nakanishi I. Amplification of c-myc, K-sam, and c-met in gastric cancers: detection by fluorescence in situ hybridization. *Lab Invest* 1998; 78:1143-53.

[342] Nakatsuru S, Yanagisawa A, Ichii S, Tahara E, Kato Y, Nakamura Y, Horii A. Somatic mutation of the APC gene in gastric cancer: frequent mutations in very well differentiated adenocarcinoma and signet-ring cell carcinoma. *Hum Mol Genet* 1992;l:559-63.

[343] Lee JH, Abraham SC, Kim HS, Nam JH, Choi C, Lee MC, Park CS, Juhng SW, Rashid A, Hamilton SR, Wu TT. Inverse relationship between APC gene mutation in gastric adenomas and development of adenocarcinoma. *Am J Pathol* 2002;161:611-8.

[344] Hsieh LL, Huang YC. Loss of heterozygosity of APC/MCC gene in differentiated and undifferentiated gastric carcinoma in Taiwan. *Cancer Lett* 1995;96:169-74.

[345] Munemitsu S, Albert I, Souza B, Rubinfeld B, Polakis P. Regulation of intracellular beta-catenin levels by the adenomatous polyposis coli (APC) tumor-suppressor protein. *Proc Natl Acad Sci USA* 1995;92:3046-3050.

[346] Peifer M. Signal transduction. Neither straight nor narrow. *Nature* 1999;400:213-5.

[347] Park WS, Oh RR, Park JY, Lee SH, Shin MS, Kim YS, Kim SY, Lee HK, Kim PJ, Oh ST, Yoo NJ, Lee JY. Frequent somatic mutations of the beta-catenin gene in intestinal-type gastric cancer. *Cancer Res* 1999;59:4257-60.

[348] Candidus S, Bischoff P, Becker KF, Hofler H. No evidence for mutations in alpha and beta-catenin genes in human gastric and breast carcinomas. *Cancer Res* 1996;56:49-52.

[349] Eads CA, Lord RV, Kurumboor SK, Wickramasinghe K.Skinner ML, Long TI, Peters JH, DeMeester TR, Danenberg KD, Danenberg PV, Laird PW, Skinner KA. Fields of aberrant CpG island hypermethylation in Barrett's esophagus and associated adeno-carcinoma. *Cancer Res* 2000;60:5021-6.

[350] Igaki H, Sasaki H, Tachimori Y, Kato H, Watanabe H, Kimura T, Harada Y, Sugimura T, Terada M. Mutation frequency of the p16/CDKN2 gene in primary cancers in the upper digestive tract. *Cancer Res* 1995;55:3421-3.

[351] Shim YH, Kang GH, Ro JY. Correlation of p16 hypermethylation with p16 protein loss in sporadic gastric carcinomas. *Lab Invest* 2000;80:689-95.

[352] Suzuki H, Itoh F, Toyota M, Kikuchi T, Kakiuchi H, Hinoda Y, Imai K. Distinct methylation pattern and microsatellite instability in sporadic gastric cancer. *Int J Cancer* 1999;83:309-13.

[353] Nakajima T, Akiyama Y, Shiraishi J, Arai T, Yanagisawa Y, Ara M, Fukuda Y, Sawabe M, Saitoh K, Kamiyama R, Hirokawa K, Yuasa Y. Age-related hypermethylation of the hMLH1 promoter in gastric cancers. *Int J Cancer* 2001;94:208-11.

[354] Leung WK, Yu J, Ng EK, To KF, Ma PK, Lee TL, Go MY, Chung SC, Sung JJ. Concurrent hypermethylation of multiple tumor-related genes in gastric carcinoma and adjacent normal tissues. *Cancer* 2001;91:2294-301.

[355] Oue N, Sentani K, Yokozaki H, Kitadai Y, Ito R, Yasui W. Promoter methylation status of the DNA repair genes hMLHl and MGMT in gastric carcinoma and metaplastic mucosa. *Pathobiology* 2001 ;69:143-9.

[356] Toyota M, Ahuja N, Ohe-Toyota M, Herman JG, Baylin SB, Issa JP. CpG island methylator phenotype in colorectal cancer. *Proc Natl Acad Sci USA* 1999;96:8681-6.

[357] Ohta M, Inoue H, Cotticelli MG, Kastury K, Baffa R, Palazzo J, Siprashvili Z, Mori M, McCue P, Druck T, Croce CM, Huebner K. The FHIT gene, spanning the chromosome 3p14.2 fragile site and renal carcinoma-associated t(3;8) breakpoint, is abnormal in digestive tract cancers. *Cell* 1996;84:587-97.

[358] Baffa R, Veronese ML, Santoro R, Mandes B, Palazzo JP, Rugge M, Santoro E, Croce CM, Huebner K. Loss of FHIT expression in gastric carcinoma. *Cancer Res* 1998;58:4708-14.

[359] Lee SH, Kim WH, Kim HK, Woo KM, Nam HS, Kim HS, Kim JG, Cho MH. Altered expression of the fragile histidine triad gene in primary gastric adenocarcinomas. *Biochem Biophys Res Commun* 2001; 284:850-5.

[360] Huiping C, Kristjansdottir S, Bergthorsson JT, Jonasson JG. Magnusson J, Egilsson V, Ingvarsson S. High frequency of LOH, MSI and abnormal expression of FHIT in gastric cancer. *Eur J Cancer* 2002;38:728-35.

[361] Uchino S, Tsuda H, Noguchi M, Yokota J, Terada M, Saito T, Kobayashi M, Sugimura T, Hirohashi S. Frequent loss of heterozygosity at the DCC locus in gastric cancer. *Cancer Res* 1992;52:3099-102.

[362] Yoshida Y, Itoh F, Endo T, Hinoda Y, Imai K. Decreased DCC mRNA expression in human gastric cancers is clinico-pathologically significant. *Int J Cancer* 1998;79:634-9.

[363] Tamura G. Molecular pathogenesis of adenoma and differentiated adenocarcinoma of the stomach. *Pathol Int* 1996;46:834-41.

[364] Graziano F, Cascinu S, Staccioli MP, Catalano V, Rossi MC. Baldelli AM, Giordani P, Muretto P, Catalano G. Potential role and chronology of abnormal expression of the Deleted in Colon Cancer (DCC) and the p53 proteins in the development of gastric cancer. *BMC Cancer* 2001;1:9-10.

[365] Park WS, Oh RR, Park JY, Lee JH, Shin MS, Kim HS, Lee HK, Kim YS, Kim SY, Lee SH, Yoo NJ, Lee JY. Somatic mutations of the trefoil factor family 1 gene in gastric cancer. *Gastroenterology* 2000;119:691-8.

[366] Bossenmeyer-Pourie C, Kantian R, Ribieras S, Wendling C, Stoll I, Thim L, Tomasetto C, Rio MC. The trefoil factor 1 participates in gastrointestinal cell differentiation by delaying Gl-S phase transition and reducing apoptosis. *J Cell Biol* 2002;157:761-70.

[367] Nogueira AM, Machado JC, Carneiro F, Reis CA, Gott P. Sobrinho-Simoes M. Patterns of expression of trefoil peptides and mucins in gastric polyps with and without malignant transformation. *J Pathol* 1999;187:541-8.

[368] Wu MS, Shun CT, Wang HP, Lee WJ, Wang TH, Lin JT. Loss of pS2 protein expression is an early event of intestinal-type gastric cancer. *Jpn J Cancer Res* 1998;89:278-82.

[369] Carneiro F, Sobrinho-Simoes M. The prognostic significance of amplification and overexpression of c-met and c-erb B-2 in human gastric carcinomas. *Cancer* 2000;88:238-40.

[370] Amemiya H, Kono K, Mori Y, Takahashi A, Ichihara F, Iizuka H, Sekikawa T, Matsumoto Y. High frequency of c-Met expression in gastric cancers producing alpha-fetoprotein. *Oncology* 2000;59:145-51.

[371] Zimovskii VF. Work experience of an allergology office. *Voen Med Zh* 1975;66-9.

[372] Park WS, Oh RR, Kim YS, Park JY, Shin MS, Lee HK, Lee SH, Yoo NJ, Lee JY. Absence of mutations in the kinase domain of the Met gene and frequent expression of Met and HGF/SF protein in primary gastric carcinomas. *APMIS* 2000;108:195-200.

[373] Ponzetto C, Giordano S, Peverali F, Delia Valle G, Abate ML. Vaula G, et al. c-met is amplified but not mutated in a cell line with an activated met tyrosine kinase. *Oncogene* 1991;6:553-9.

[374] Yu J, Miehlke S, Ebert MP, Hoffmann J, Breidert M, Alpen B, Starzynska T, Stolte Prof M, Malfertheiner P, Bayerdörffer E. Frequency of TPR-MET rearrangement in patients with gastric carcinoma and in first-degree relatives. *Cancer* 2000;88:1801-5.

[375] Ross JS, McKenna BJ. The HER-2/neu oncogene in tumors of the gastrointestinal tract. *Cancer Invest* 2001;19:554-68.

[376] Mizutani T, Onda M, Tokunaga A, Yamanaka N, Sugisaki Y.Relationship of C-erbB-2 protein expression and gene amplification to invasion and metastasis in human gastric cancer. *Cancer* 1993;72:2083-8.

[377] Allgayer H, Babic R, Gruetzner KU, Tarabichi A, Schildberg FW, Heiss MM. C-erbB-2 is of independent prognostic relevance in gastric cancer and is associated with the expression of tumor-associated protease systems. *J Clin Oncol* 2000;18:2201-9.

[378] Wang YL, Sheu BS, Yang HB, Lin PW, Chang YC. Overexpression of c-erb-B2 proteins in tumor and non-tumor parts of gastric adenocarcinoma - emphasis on its relation to H. pyloriinfection and clinicohistological characteristics. *Hepatogastroenterology* 2002;49:1172-6.

[379] Tateishi M, Toda T, Minamisono Y, Nagasaki S. Clinicopathological significance of c-erbB-2 protein expression in human gastric carcinoma. *J Surg Oncol* 1992;49:209-12.

[380] Rajevic U, Juvan R, Gazvoda B, Repse S, Komel R. Assessment of differential expression of oncogenes in gastric adenocarcinoma by fluorescent multiplex RT-PCR assay. *Pflugers Arch* 2001;442(6 Suppl l):R190-2.

[381] Yu J, Miehlke S, Ebert MP, Szokodi D, Wehvnignh B,Malfertheiner P, Ehninger G, Bayerdoerffer E. Expression of cyclin genes in human gastric cancer and in first degree relatives. *Chin Med J (Engl)* 2002;115:710-5.

[382] Kozma L, Kiss I, Hajdu J, Szentkereszty Z, Szakall S, Ember I.C-myc amplification and cluster analysis in human gastric carcinoma. *Anticancer Res* 2001;21:707-10.

[383] Katoh M. WNT2 and human gastrointestinal cancer (review). *Int J Mol Med* 2003;12:811-6.

[384] Czerniak B, Herz F, Gorczyca W, Koss LG. Expression of rasoncogene p21 protein in early gastric carcinoma and adjacentgastric epithelia. *Cancer* 1989;64:1467-73.

[385] Ohuchi N, Hand PH, Merlo G, Fujita J, Mariani-Costantini R. Thor A, Nose M, Callahan R, Schlom J. Enhanced expression of c-Ha-ras p21 in humanstomach adenocarcinomas denned by immunoassays using monoclonal antibodies and in situ hybridization. *Cancer Res* 1987;47:1413-20.

[386] Yamamoto T, Hattori T, Tahara E. Interaction between transforming growth factor alpha and c-Ha-ras p21 in progressionof human gastric carcinoma. *Pathol Res Pract* 1988;183:663-9.

[387] Spandidos DA, Karayiannis M, Yiagnisis M, Papadinitrion K. Field JK. Immunohistochemical analysis of the expression of thec-myc oncoprotein in human stomach cancers. *Digestion* 1991;50:127-34.

[388] Ninomiya I, Yonemura Y, Matsumoto H, Sugiyama K, KamataT, Miwa K, Miyazaki I, Shiku H. Expression of c-myc gene product in gastriccarcinoma. *Oncology* 1991;48:149-53.

[389] Kim NW, Piatyszek MA, Prowse KR, Harley CB, West MD, Ho PL, et al. Specific association of human telomerase activity with immortal cells and cancer. *Science* 1994;266:2011-5.

[390] Feakins RM, Nickols CD, Bidd H, Walton SJ. Abnormal expression of pRb, p16, and cyclin Dl in gastric adenocarcinoma and its lymph node metastases: relationship with pathological features and survival. *Hum Pathol* 2003;34:1276-82.

[391] Yasui W, Tahara E, Tahara H, Fujimoto J, Naka K, Nakayama J, Ishikawa F, Ide T, Tahara E. Immunohistochemical detection of human telomerase reverse transcriptase in normal and precancerous lesions of the stomach. *Jpn J Cancer Res* 1999;90:589-95.

[392] Kondo T, Oue N, Yoshida K, Mitani Y, Naka K, Nakayama H, Yasui W. Expression of POT1 is associated with tumor stage andtelomere length in gastric carcinoma. *Cancer Res* 2004;64:523-9.

[393] Takahashi Y, Cleary KR, Mai M, Kitadai Y, Bucana CD, Ellis LM. Significance of vessel count and vascular endothelial growthfactor and its receptor (KDR) in intestinal-type gastric cancer. *Clin Cancer Res* 1996;2:1679-84.

[394] Kitadai Y, Haruma K, Sumii K, Yamamoto S, Ue T, Yokozaki H, Yasui W, Ohmoto Y, Kajiyama G, Fidler IJ, Tahara E. Expression of IL-8 correlates with vascularity in human gastric carcinomas. *Am J Pathol* 1998;152:93-100.

[395] Takahashi Y, Bucana CD, Akagi Y, Liu W, Cleary KR, Mai M, Ellis LM. Significance of platelet-derived endothelial cell growth factor in the angiogenesis of human gastric cancer. *Clin CancerRes* 1998;4:429-34.

[396] Kido S, Kitadai Y, Hattori N, Haruma K, Kido T, Ohta M, Tanaka S, Yoshihara M, Sumii K, Ohmoto Y, Chayama **K**. Interleukin 8 and vascular endothelial growth factor — prognosticfactors in human gastric carcinoma? *Eur J Cancer* 2001 ;37:1482-7.

[397] Yasui W, Yokozaki H, Shimamoto F, Tahara H, Tahara E. Molecular-pathological diagnosis of gastrointestinal tissues and its contribution to cancer histopathology. *Pathol Int* 1999;49:763-74.

[398] Xiangming C, Natsugoe S, Takao S, Hokita S, Tanabe G, Baba M, Kuroshima K, Aikou T. The cooperative role of p27 and cyclin E in the prognosis of advanced gastric carcinoma. *Cancer* 2000;89:1214—9.

[399] Tsujie M, Yamamoto H, Tomita N, Sugita Y, Ohue M, Sakita I, Tamaki Y, Sekimoto M, Doki Y, Inoue M, Matsuura N, Monden T, Shiozaki H, Monden M.et al. Expression of tumor supressor gene p16 (INK4) products in primary gastric cancer. *Oncology* 2000;58:126-36.

[400] Fondevila C, Metges JP, Fuster J, Grau JJ, Palacin A, Castells A, Volant A, Pera M. p53 and VEGF expression are independent predictors oftumor recurrence and survival following curative resection of gastric cancer. *Br J Cancer* 2004;90:206-15.

[401] Pinto-de-Sousa J, Silva F, David L, Leitao D, Seixas M, Pimenta A, Cardoso-de-Oliveira M. Clinicopathological significance and survival influence of p53 protein expression in gastric carcinoma. *Histopathology* 2004;44:323-31.

[402] Joo YE, Rew JS, Choi SK, Bom HS, Park CS, Kim SJ. Expression of e-cadherin and catenins in early gastric cancer. J ClinGastroenterol 2002;35:35-42.

[403] Takeichi M. Cadherin cell adhesion receptors as a morphogenetic regulator. *Science* 1991;251:1451-7.

[404] Mingchao, Devereux TR, Stockton P, Sun K, Sills RC, Clayton N, Portier M, Flake G. Loss of E-cadherin expression in gastric intestinal metaplasia and later stage p53 altered expression in gastric carcinogenesis. *Exp Toxicol Pathol* 2001;53:237-46.

[405] Shimada Y, Yamasaki S, Hashimoto Y, Ito T, Kawamura J, Soma T, Ino Y, Nakanishi Y, Sakamoto M, Hirohashi S, Imamura M. Clinical significance of dysadherin expression in gastric cancer patients. *Clin Cancer Res* 2004;10:2818-23.

[406] Chan AO, Lam SK, Chu KM, Lam CM, Kwok E, Leung SY, Yuen ST, Law SY, Hui WM, Lai KC, Wong CY, Hu HC, Lai CL, Wong J. Soluble E-cadherin is a valid prognostic marker in gastric carcinoma. *Gut* 2001;48:808-11.

[407] Yamauchi K, Uehara Y, Kitamura N, Nakane Y, Hioki K. Increased expression of CD44v6 mRNA significantly correlates with distant metastasis and prognosis in gastric cancer. *Int J Cancer* 1998;79:256-62.

[408] Saito H, Tsujitani S, Katano K, Ikeguchi M, Maeta M, Kaibara N. Serum concentration of CD44 variant 6 and its relation to prognosis in patients with gastric carcinoma. *Cancer* 1998;83:1094-101.

[409] Mayer B, Jauch KW, Gunthert U, Figdor CG, Schildberg FW, Funke I, Johnson JP. De-novo expression of CD44 and survival in gastric cancer. *Lancet* 1993;342:1019-22.

[410] Yamashita K, Azumano I, Mai M, Okada Y. Expression and tissue localization of matrix metalloproteinase 7 (matrilysin) inhuman gastric carcinomas. Implications for vessel invasion andmetastasis. *Int J Cancer* 1998;79:187-94.

[411] Inoue T, Yashiro M, Nishimura S, Maeda K, Sawada T, Ogawa Y, Sowa M, Chung KH. Matrix metalloproteinase-1 expression is a prognostic factor for patients with advanced gastric cancer. *Int J Mol Med* 1999;4:73-7.

[412] Mori M, Mimori K, Shiraishi T, Fujie T, Baba K, Kusumoto H, Haraguchi M, Ueo H, Akiyoshi T. Analysis of MT1-MMP and MMP2 expression in human gastric cancers. *Int J Cancer* 1997;74:316-21.

[413] Mimori K, Mori M, Shiraishi T, Fujie T, Baba K, Haraguchi M, Abe R, Ueo H, Akiyoshi T. Clinical significance of tissue inhibitor of metalloproteinase expression in gastric carcinoma. *Br J Cancer* 1997;76:531-6.

[414] Nathan C. Nitric oxide as a secretory product of mammaliancells. *FASEB J* 1992;6:3051-64.

[415] Moncada S, Higgs A. The L-arginine-nitric oxide pathway. *N Engl J Med* 1993;329:2002-12.

[416] Ambs S, Hussain SP, Harris CC. Interactive effects of nitricoxide and the p53 tumor suppressor gene in carcinogenesis and tumor progression. *FASEB J* 1997;ll:443-8.

[417] Fukumura D, Jain RK. Role of nitric oxide in angiogenesis andmicrocirculation in tumors. *Cancer Metastasis Rev* 1998;17:77-89.

[418] Tamir S, Tannenbaum SR. The role of nitric oxide (NO) in thecarcinogenic process. *Biochim Biophys Acta* 1996;1288:F31-6.

[419] Wink DA, Vodovotz Y, Laval J, Laval F, Dewhirst MW. Mitchell JB. The multifaceted roles of nitric oxide in cancer. *Carcinogenesis* 1998;19:711-21.

[420] Wang B, Wei D, Crum VE, Richardson EL, Xiong HH, Luo Y, Huang S, Abbruzzese JL, Xie K. A novel model system for studying the double-edged roles ofnitric oxide production in pancreatic cancer growth and metastasis. *Oncogene* 2003 ;22:1771-82.

[421] Xie K, Huang S. Contribution of nitric oxide-mediated apoptosisto cancer metastasis inefficiency. *Free Radic Biol Med* 2003; 34:969-86.

[422] Shi Q, Huang S, Jiang W, Kutach LS, Ananthaswamy HN, XieK. Direct correlation between nitric oxide synthase II inducibility and metastatic ability of UV-2237 murine fibrosarcoma cells carrying mutant p53. *Cancer Res* 1999;59:2072-5.

[423] Hibbs JB Jr, Taintor RR, Vavrin Z. Macrophage cytotoxicity: role for L-arginine deiminase and imino nitrogen oxidation to nitrite. *Science* 1987;235:473-6.

[424] Thomsen LL, Miles DW, Happerfield L, Bobrow LG, KnowlesRG, Moncada S. Nitric oxide synthase activity in human breastcancer. *Br J Cancer* 1995;72:41-4.

[425] Cobbs CS, Brenman JE, Aldape KD, Bredt DS, Israel MA. Expression of nitric oxide synthase in human central nervoussystem tumors. *Cancer Res* 1995;55:727-30.

[426] Leibovich SJ, Polverini PJ, Fong TW, Harlow LA, Koch AE. Production of angiogenic activity by human monocytes requires an L-arginine/nitric oxide-synthase-dependent effector mechanism. *Proc Natl Acad Sci USA* 1994;91:4190-4.

[427] Schmidt HH, Walter U. NO at work. *Cell* 1994;78:919-25.

[428] Jenkins DC, Charles IG, Thomsen LL, Moss DW, Holmes LS, Baylis SA, Rhodes P, Westmore K, Emson PC, Moncada S. Roles of nitric oxide in tumor growth. *Proc Natl Acad Sci USA* 1995;92:4392-6.

[429] Leung DW, Cachianes G, Kuang WJ, Goeddel DV, Ferrara N. Vascular endothelial growth factor is a secreted angiogenic mito-gen. *Science* 1989;246:1306-9.

[430] Senger DR, Perruzzi CA, Feder J, Dvorak HF. A highly conserved vascular permeability factor secreted by a variety ofhuman and rodent tumor cell lines. *Cancer Res* 1986;46:5629-32.

[431] Rajnakova A, Moochhala S, Goh PM, Ngoi S. Expression of nitric oxide synthase, cyclooxygenase, and p53 in different stages of human gastric cancer. *Cancer Lett* 2001;172:177-85.

[432] Rajnakova A, Goh PM, Chan ST, Ngoi SS, Alponat A.Moochhala S. Expression of differential nitric oxide synthase isoforms in human normal gastric mucosa and gastric cancer tissue. *Carcinogenesis* 1997;18:1841-5.

[433] Koh E, Noh SH, Lee YD, Lee HY, Han JW, Lee HW, Hong S. Differential expression of nitric oxide synthase in human stomach cancer. *Cancer Lett* 1999;146:173-80.

[434] Goto T, Haruma K, Kitadai Y, Ito M, Yoshihara M, Sumii K, Hayakawa N, Kajiyama G. Enhanced expression of inducible nitric oxide synthase and nitrotyrosine in gastric mucosa of gastric cancer patients. *Clin Cancer Res* 1999;5:1411-5.

[435] Holian O, Wahid S, Atten MJ, Attar BM. Inhibition of gastriccancer cell proliferation by resveratrol: role of nitric oxide. *AmJ Physiol Gastrointest Liver Physiol* 2002;282:G809-16.

[436] Feng CW, Wang LD, Jiao LH, Liu B, Zheng S, Xie XJ. Expression of p53, inducible nitric oxide synthase and vascular endothelial growth factor in gastric precancerous and cancerous lesions: correlation with clinical features. *BMC Cancer* 2002;2:8.

[437] Khare PD, Liao S, Hirose Y, Kuroki M, Fujimura S, YamauchiY, Miyajima-Uchida H, Kuroki M. Tumor growth suppression by a retroviral vector displaying scFv antibody to CEA and carrying the iNOS gene. *Anticancer Res* 2002;22:2443-6.

[438] Van Rees BP, Saukkonen K, Ristimaki A, Polkowski W, Tytgat ON, Drillenburg P, Offerhaus GJ. Cyclooxygenase-2 expression duringcarcinogenesis in the human stomach. *J Pathol* 2002;196:171-9.

[439] Van Rees BP, Ristimaki A. Cyclooxygenase-2 in carcinogenesisof the gastrointestinal tract. *Scand J Gastroenterol* 2001;36:897-903.

[440] Lim HY, Joo HJ, Choi JH, Yi JW, Yang MS, Cho DY, Kim HS, Nam DK, Lee KB, Kim HC. Increased expression of cyclooxygenase-2 protein in human gastric carcinoma. *Clin Cancer Res* 2000;6:519-25.

[441] Saukkonen K, Nieminen O, van Rees B, Vilkki S, Harkonen M, Juhola M, Mecklin JP, Sipponen P, Ristimäki A. Expression of cyclooxygenase-2 in dysplasia of the stomach and in intestinal-type gastric adenocarcinoma. *Clin Cancer Res* 2001;7:1923-31.

[442] Lee TL, Leung WK, Lau JY, Tong JH, Ng EK, Chan FK, Chung SC, Sung JJ, To KF. Inverse association between cyclooxygenase-2 overexpression and microsatellite instability in gastric cancer. *Cancer Lett* 2001;168:133-40.

[443] Murata H, Kawano S, Tsuji S, Tsuji M, Sawaoka H, Kimura Y, Shiozaki H, Hori M. Cyclooxygenase-2 overexpression enhances lymphatic invasion and metastasis in human gastric carcinoma. *Am J Gastroenterol* 1999; 94:451-5.

[444] Song SH, Jong HS, Choi HH, Inoue H, Tanabe T, Kim NK, Bang YJ. Transcriptional silencing of cyclooxygenase-2 by hyper-methylation of the 5' CpG island in human gastric carcinoma cells. *Cancer Res* 2001;61:4628-35.

[445] Kim H, Lim JW, Kim KH. Helicobacter pylori-induced expression of interleukin-8 and cyclooxygenase-2 in AGS gastricepithelial cells: mediation by nuclear factor-kappaB. *Scand J Gastroenterol* 2001;36:706-16.

[446] Akhtar M, Cheng Y, Magno RM, Ashktorab H, Smoot DT. Meltzer SJ, et al. Promoter methylation regulates Helicobacter pylori-stimulated cyclooxygenase-2 expression in gastric epithelial cells. *Cancer Res* 2001;61:2399-403.

[447] McCarthy CJ, Crofford LJ, Greenson J, Scheiman JM. Cyclooxygenase-2 expression in gastric antral mucosa beforeand after eradication of Helicobacter pylori infection. *Am J Gastroenterol* 1999;94:1218-23.

[448] Fukuda Y, Kurihara N, Imoto I, Yasui K, Yoshida M, Yanagihara K, Park JG, Nakamura Y, Inazawa J. CD44 is a potential target of amplificationwithin the 11p13 amplicon detected in gastric cancer cell lines. *Genes Chromosomes Cancer* 2000;29:315-24.

[449] Iizuka N, Tangoku A, Hazama S, Yoshino S, Mori N, Oka M. Nm23-Hl gene as a molecular switch between the free-floating and adherent states of gastric cancer cells. *Cancer Lett* 2001;174:65-71.

[450] Kawasaki K, Hayashi Y, Wang Y, Suzuki S, Morita Y, Nakamura T, Narita K, Doe W, Itoh H, Kuroda Y. Expression of urokinase-type plasminogen activator receptor and plasminogen activator inhibitor-1 in gastric cancer. *J Gastroenterol Hepatol* 1998;13:936-44.

[451] Karlsson KA. The human gastric colonizer Helicobacter pylori: a challenge for host-parasite glycobiology. *Glycobiology* 2000;10:761-71.

[452] Almeida R, Silva E, Santos-Silva F, Silberg DG, Wang J, De Bolos C, David L. Expression of intestine-specific transcription factors, CDX1 and CDX2, in intestinal metaplasia and gastric carcinomas. *J Pathol* 2003;199:36-40.

[453] Yu Y, Zhang YC, Zhang WZ, Shen LS, Hertzog P, Wilson TJ, Xu DK. Ets1 as a marker of malignant potential in gastric carcinoma. *World J Gastroenterol* 2003;9:2154-9.

[454] Tsutsumi S, Kuwano H, Asao T, Nagashima K, Shimura T, Mochiki E. Expression of Ets-1 angiogenesis-related protein in gastric cancer. *Cancer Lett* 2000;160:45-50.

[455] Sasaki N, Morisaki T, Hashizume K, Yao T, Tsuneyoshi M, Noshiro H, Nakamura K, Yamanaka T, Uchiyama A, Tanaka M, Katano M. Nuclear factor-kappaB p65 (ReIA) transcription factor is constitutively activated in human gastric carcinoma tissue. *Clin Cancer Res* 2001;7:4136-42.

[456] Wang L, Wei D, Huang S, Peng Z, Le X, Wu TT, Yao J, Ajani J, Xie K. Transcription factor Sp1 expression is a significant predictor of survival in human gastric cancer. *Clin Cancer Res* 2003; 9:6371-80.

[457] Mitani Y, Oue N, Hamai Y, Aung PP, Matsumura S, Nakayama H, Kamata N, Yasui W. Histone H3 acetylation is associated with reduced p21WAF1/CIP1 expression in gastric carcinoma. *J Pathol* 2005;205:65-73.

[458] Suzuki T, Kuniyasu H, Hayashi K, Naka K, Yokozaki H, Ono S, Ishikawa T, Tahara E, Yasui W. Effect of trichostatin A on cell growth and expression of cell cycle- and apoptosis-related molecules in human gastric and oral carcinoma cell lines. *Int J Cancer* 2000;88:992-7.

[459] Oue N, Motoshita J, Yokozaki H, Hayashi K, Tahara E, Taniyama K, Matsusaki K, Yasui W. Distinct promoter hypermethylation of p16ink4a, CDH1, and RAR-beta in

intestinal, diffuse-adherent, and diffuse-scattered type gastric carcinoma. *J Pathol* 2002;198:55-9.

[460] Oshimo Y, Oue N, Mitani Y, Nakayama H, Kitadai Y, Yoshida K, Ito Y, Chayama K, Yasui W. Frequent loss of RUNX3 expression by promoter hypermethylation in gastric carcinoma. *Pathobiology* 2004;71:137-43.

[461] Oue N, Shigeishi H, Kuniyasu H, Yokozaki H, Kuraoka K, Ito R, Yasui W. Promoter methylation of MGMT is associated with protein loss in gastric carcinomas. *Int J Cancer* 2001;93:805-9.

[462] Oue N, Matsumura S, Nakayama H, Kitadai Y, Taniyama K.Matsusaki K, Yasui W. Expression of the TSP-1 gene and its association with promoter hypermethylation in gastric carcinomas. *Oncology* 2003;64:423-9.

[463] Hamai Y, Oue N, Mitani Y, Nakayama H, Ito R, Matsusaki K, Yoshida K, Toge T, Yasui W. DNA methylation and histone acetylation status of HLTF gene are associated with reduced expression in gastric carcinoma. *Cancer* Sci 2003;94:692-8.

[464] Oshimo Y, Oue N, Mitani Y, Nakayama H, Kitadai Y, Yoshida K, Chayama K, Yasui W. Frequent epigenetic inactivation of RIZ1 by promoter hypermethylation in human gastric carcinoma. *Int J Cancer* 2004;110:212-8.

[465] Oshimo Y, Kuraoka K, Nakayama H, Kitadai Y, Yoshida K. Chayama K, et al. Epigenetic inactivation of SOCS-1 by CpG island hypermethylation in human gastric carcinoma. *Int J Cancer* 2004;112:212-8.

[466] Toyota M, Ahuja N, Suzuki H, Itoh F, Ohe-Toyota M, Imai K, Baylin SB, Issa JP. Aberrant methylation in gastric cancer associated with the CpG island methylator phenotype. *Cancer Res* 1999;59:5438-42.

[467] Yasui W, Oue N, Aung PP, Matsumura S, Shutoh M, Nakayama H. Molecular-pathological prognostic factors of gastric cancer: a review. *Gastric Cancer* 2005;8(2):86-94.

[468] Gonzalez CA, Sala N, Capella G. Genetic susceptibility and gastric cancer risk. *Int J Cancer* 2002;100:249-60.

[469] Kuraoka K, Oue N, Matsumura S, Hamai Y, Ito R, Nakayama H, Yasui W. A single nucleotide polymorphism in the transmembrane domain coding region of HER-2 is associated with development and malignant phenotype of gastric cancer. *Int J Cancer* 2003;107:593-6.

[470] Kuraoka K, Oue N, Yokozaki H, Kitadai Y, Ito R, Nakayama H, Yasui W. Correlation of a single nucleotide polymorphism in the E-cadherin gene promoter with tumorigenesis and progression ofgastric carcinoma in Japan. *Int J Oncol* 2003;23:421-7.

[471] Matsumura S, Oue N, Kitadai Y, Chayama K, Yoshida K.Yamaguchi Y, Toge T, Imai K, Nakachi K, Yasui W. A single nucleotide polymorphism in the MMP-1 promoter is correlated with histological differentiation ofgastric cancer. *J Cancer Res Clin Oncol* 2004;130:259-65.

[472] Matsumura S, Oue N, Nakayama H, Kitadai Y, Yoshida K.Yamaguchi Y, Imai K, Nakachi K, Matsusaki K, Chayama K, Yasui W. A single nucleotide polymorphism of theMMP9 promoter affects tumor progression and invasive phenotype of gastric cancer. *J Cancer Res Clin Oncol* 2005;131:19-25.

[473] Wu MS, Huang SP, Chang YT, Lin MT, Shun CT, Chang MC, Wang HP, Chen CJ, Lin JT. Association of the -160 C —> A promoter polymorphism ofthe E-cadherin gene with gastric carcinoma risk. *Cancer* 2002; 94:1443-8.

[474] Pharoah PD, Oliveira C, Machado JC, Keller G, Vogelsang H. Laux H, Becker KF, Hahn H, Paproski SM, Brown LA, Caldas C, Huntsman D. CDH1 c-160a promoter polymorphism is not associated with risk of stomach cancer. *Int J Cancer* 2002;101:196-7.

[475] Shiotani A, Iishi H, Uedo N, Ishiguro S, Tatsuta M, Nakae Y, Kumamoto M, Merchant JL. Evidence that loss of sonic hedgehog is an indicator of Helicobacter pylori-induced atrophic gastritis progressing to gastric cancer. *Am J Gastroenterol* 100: 581–587, 2005.

[476] Van den Brink GR. Hedgehog signaling in development and homeostasis of the gastrointestinal tract. *Physiol Rev* 2007;87: 1343–1375.

[477] Shiotani A, Kamada T, Yamanaka Y, Manabe N, Kusunoki H, Hata J, Haruma K. Sonic hedgehog and CDX2 expression in the stomach. *Journal of Gastroenterology and Hepatology.* 2008. – Vol. 23, Suppl. 2; S161–S166.

[478] Shiotani A, Iishi H, Uedo N, Ishiguro S, Tatsuta M, Nakae Y, Kumamoto M, Merchant JL. Evidence that loss of sonic hedgehog is an indicator of Helicobacter pylori-induced atrophic gastritis progressing to gastric cancer. *Am. J. Gastroenterol.* 2005;100: 581–7.

[479] El-Zaatari M, Tobias A, Grabowska AM, Kumari R, Scotting PJ, Kaye P, Atherton J, Clarke PA, Powe DG, Watson SA. De-regulation of the sonic hedgehog pathway in the InsGas mouse model of gastric carcinogenesis. *Br J Cancer* 2007; 96 :1855–1861.

[480] Zavros Y. The Adventures of Sonic Hedgehog in Development and Repair. IV. Sonic hedgehog processing, secretion, and function in the stomach *Am J Physiol Gastrointest Liver Physiol* 2008;294: G1105–G1108.

[481] Weissman IL. Stem cells: units of development, units of regeneration, and units in evolution. *Cell.* 2000 Jan 7;100(1):157-68.

[482] Murphy MJ, Wilson A, Trumpp A. More than just proliferation: Myc function in stem cells. *Trends Cell Biol* 2005 Mar;15(3):128-37.

[483] Blanpain C, Horsley V, Fuchs E. Epithelial stem cells: turning over new leaves. *Cell* 2007;128: 445–458.

[484] Trumpp A., and Wiestler O. D. Mechanisms of Disease: cancer stem cells—targeting the evil twin. *Nat Clin Pract Oncol.* June 2008 Vol 5 No 6: 337-347.

[485] Gao L, Nieters A, Brenner H. Meta-analysis: tumour invasion-related genetic polymorphisms and gastric cancer susceptibility. *Aliment Pharmacol Ther* 2008; 28: 565–573.

[486] Roberts-Thomson IC, Butler WJ. Polymorphism and gastric cancer. *J Gastroenterol Hepatol* 2005; 20: 793–4.

[487] Hamajima N, Naito M, Kondo T, Goto Y. Genetic factors involved in the development of Helicobacter pylori-related gastric cancer. *Cancer Sci* 2006; 97: 1129–38.

[488] Collins FS, Morgan M, Patrinos A. The human genome project: lessons from large-scale biology. *Science* 2003; 300: 286-90.

[489] Collins FS, Green ED, Guttmacher AE, Guyer MS. A vision for the future of genomic research. *Nature* 2003; 422: 835-47.

[490] Lee D. H., Hahm K.-B. Inflammatory cytokine gene polymorphisms and gastric cancer *J. Gastroenterol. Hepatol.* 2008;23:1470-1472.

[491] Hurme M, Lahdenpohja N, Santtila S. Gene polymorphisms of interleukin-1 and 10 in infectious and autoimmune diseases. *Ann. Med.* 1998; 30: 469-73.

[492] Tarlow JK, Blakemore AI, Lennard A, Solari R, Hughes HN, Steinkasserer A, Duff GW. Polymorphism in human IL-1 receptor antagonist gene intron 2 is caused by variable numbers of an 86-bp tandem repeat. *Hum. Genet.* 1993; 91: 403-4.

[493] Wallace JL, Cucala M, Mugridge K, Parente L. Secretagogue-specific effects of interleukin-1 on gastric acid secretion. *Am. J. Physiol.* 1991; 261: G559-64.

[494] Furuta T, El-Omar EM, Xiao F, Shirai N, Takashima M, Sugimura H. Interleukin 1beta polymorphisms increase risk of hypochlorhydria and atrophic gastritis and reduce risk of duodenal ulcer recurrence in Japan. *Gastroenterology* 2002; 123: 92-105.

[495] Garza-Gonzalez E, Bosques-Padilla FJ, EL-Omar E, Hold G, Tijerina-Menchaca R, Maldonado-Garza HJ, Pérez-Pérez GI. Role of the polymorphic IL-1B, IL-IRN and TNF-A genes in distal gastric cancer in Mexico. *Int. J. Cancer* 2005; 114: 237-41.

[496] Camargo MC, Mera R, Correa P, Peek RM Jr, Fontham ET, Goodman KJ, Piazuelo MB, Sicinschi L, Zabaleta J, Schneider BG. Interleukin-1beta and interleukin-1 receptor antagonist gene polymorphisms and gastric cancer: a meta-analysis. *Cancer Epidemiol Biomarkers Prev.* 2006; 15: 1674-87.

[497] Wang P, Xia HH, Zhang JY, Dai LP, Xu XQ, Wang KJ. Association of interleukin-1 gene polymorphisms with gastric cancer: a meta-analysis. *Int. J. Cancer* 2007; 120: 552-62.

[498] Lu W, Pan K, Zhang L, Lin D, Miao X, You W. Genetic polymorphisms of interleukin (IL)-IB, IL-IRN, IL-8, IL-10 and tumor necrosis factor (alpha) and risk of gastric cancer in Chinese population. *Carcinogenesis* 2005; 26: 631-6.

[499] Garcia-Gonzalez MA, Lanas A, Quintero E, Nicolás D, Parra-Blanco A, Strunk M, Benito R, Angel Simón M, et al. Gastric cancer susceptibility is not linked to pro- and anti-inflammatory cytokine gene polymorphisms in whites: a Nationwide Multicenter Study in Spain. *Am. J. Gastroenterol.* 2007; 102: 1893-5.

[500] Shin WG, Jang JS, Kim HS, Kim SJ, Kim KH, Jang MK, Lee JH, Kim HJ, Kim HY. Polymorphisms of interleukin-1 and interleukin-2 genes in patients with gastric cancer in Korea. *J Gastroenterol Hepatol* 2008; 23: 1567-73.

[501] Houghton J.M., Wang T. C. Role of Bone Marrow–Derived Cells in Gastric Adenocarcinoma. In: The Biology of Gastric Cancers (Editors Timothy C. Wang, James G. Fox, Andrew S. Giraud). Springer, 2009: 561-586.

[502] Bjornson C., Reitze R., Reynolds B., Magli M., and Vescovi A. Turning brain into blood: a hematopoietic fate adopted by neural stem cells in vivo. *Science* 1999; 283:534–537.

[503] Clarke D., Johansson C., Wilbertz J., Veress B., Nilsson E., Karlstrom H., Lendahl U., and Frisen J.. Generalized potential of adult neural stem cells. *Science* 2000;288:1660–1663.

[504] Harris J.R., Brown G.A.J., Jorgensen M., Kaushal S., Ellis E.A., Grant M.B., and Scott E.W. Bone marrow-derived cells home to and regenerate retinal pigment epithelium after injury. *Invest Ophthalmol Vis Sci* 2006;47(5):2108–2113.

[505] Vassilopoulos G., Wang P.R., and Russell D.W. Transplanted bone marrow regenerates liver by cell fusion. *Nature* 2003;422(6934):901–904.

[506] Kaplan R.N., Riba R.D., Zacharoulis S., Bramley A.H., Vincent L., Costa C., MacDonald D.D., Jin D.K., Shido K., Kerns S.A., Zhu Z., Hicklin D., Wu Y., Port J.L.,

Altorki N., Port E.R., Ruggero D., Shmelkov S.V., Jensen K.K., Rafii S., and Lyden D. VEGFR1-positive haematopoietic bone marrow progenitors initiate the pre-metastatic niche. *Nature* 2005;438(7069):820–827.

[507] Boivin G.P., Washington K., Yang K., Ward J.M., Pretlow T.P., Russell R., Besselsen D.G., Godfrey V.L., Doetschman T., Dove W.F., Pitot H.C., Halberg R.B., Itzkowitz S.H., Groden J., and Coffey R.J. Pathology of mouse models of intestinal cancer: consensus report and recommendations. *Gastroenterology* 2003; 124:762–777.

[508] Wang T.C., Goldenring J.R., Dangler C., Ito S., Mueller A., Jeon W.K., Koh T.J., and Fox J.G. Mice lacking secretory phospholipase A2 show altered apoptosis and differentiation with Helicobacter felis infection. *Gastroenterology* 1999; 114:675–689.

[509] Li H.C., Stoicov C., Rogers A.B., and Houghton J.M. Stem cells and cancer: evidence for bone marrow stem cells in epithelial cancers. *World J Gastroenterol* 2006;12(3):363–371.

[510] McDonald SA, Greaves LC, Gutierrez-Gonzalez L, Rodriguez-Justo M, Deheragoda M, Leedham SJ, Taylor RW, Lee CY, Preston SL, Lovell M, Hunt T, Elia G, Oukrif D, Harrison R, Novelli MR, Mitchell I, Stoker DL, Turnbull DM, Jankowski JA, Wright NA. Mechanisms of Field Cancerization in the Human Stomach: The Expansion and Spread of Mutated Gastric Stem Cells. *Gastroenterology* 2008;134:500–510.

[511] Tatematsu M, Tsukamoto T, Inada K. Stem cells and gastric cancer: role of gastric and intestinal mixed intestinal metaplasia. *Cancer Sci* 2003;94:135–141.

[512] Hattori T, Fjuita S. Fractographic study on the growth and multiplication of the gastric gland of the hamster. The gland division cycle. *Cell Tissue Res* 1974;153:145–149.

[513] Inada K, Nakanishi H, Fujimitsu Y, Shimizu N, Ichinose M, Miki K, Nakamura S, Tatematsu M. Gastric and intestinal mixed and solely intestinal types of intestinal metaplasia in the human stomach. *Pathol Int* 1997;47:831-41.

[514] Gutierrez-Gonzalez L., Wright N.A. Biology of intestinal metaplasia in 2008: More than a simple phenotypic alteration. *Dig Liver Dis*. 2008; 40: 510-522.

[515] Tsukamoto T, Mizoshita T, Tatematsu M. Gastric-and-intestinal mixed-type intestinal metaplasia: aberrant expression of transcription factors and stem cell intestinalization. *Gastric Cancer* 2006;9:156-66.

[516] Nam KT, Varro A, Coffey RJ, Goldenring JR. Potentiation of oxyntic atrophy-induced gastric metaplasia in amphiregulin-deficient mice. *Gastroenterology* 2007;132:1804-19.

[517] Schmidt PH, Lee JR, Joshi V, Playford RJ, Poulsom R, Wright NA, Goldenring JR. Identification of a metaplastic cell lineage associated with human gastric adenocarcinoma. Lab Invest 1999;79:639-46.

[518] Wright NA, Poulsom R, Stamp GW, Hall PA, Jeffery RE, Longcroft JM, Rio MC, Tomasetto C, Chambon P. Epidermal growth factor (EGF/URO) induces expression of regulatory peptides in damaged human gastrointestinal tissues. *J Pathol* 1990;162:279-84.

[519] Wright NA, Pike C, Elia G. Induction of a novel epidermal growth factor-secreting cell lineage by mucosal ulceration in human gastrointestinal stem cells. *Nature* 1990;343:82-5.

[520] Giraud AS. Metaplasia as a premalignant pathology in the stomach. *Gastroenterology* 2007; 132:2053-6.

[521] Goldenring JR, Nomura S. Differentiation of the gastric mucosa III. Animal models of oxyntic atrophy and metaplasia. *Am J Physiol Gastrointest Liver Physiol* 2006;291:G999-1004.

[522] Ogawa M, Nomura S, Varro A, Wang TC, Goldenring JR. Altered metaplastic response of waved-2 EGF receptor mutant mice to acute oxyntic atrophy. *Am J Physiol Gastrointest Liver Physiol* 2006;290:G793-804.

[523] Chaves P, Crespo M, Ribeiro C, Laranjeira C, Pereira AD, Suspiro A, Cardoso P, Leitão CN, Soares J. Chromosomal analysis of Barrett's cells: demonstration of instability and detection of the metaplastic lineage involved. *Mod Pathol* 2007;20:788-96.

[524] Nardone G, Rocco A, Budillon G. Molecular alteration of gastric carcinoma. *Minerva Gastroenterol Dietol* 2002;48:189-93.

[525] Rocco A, Caruso R, Toracchio S, Rigoli L, Verginelli F, Catalano T, Neri M, Curia MC, Ottini L, Agnese V, Bazan V, Russo A, Pantuso G, Colucci G, Mariani-Costantini R, Nardone G. Gastric adenomas: relationship between clinicopathological findings, Helicobacter pylori infection, APC mutations and COX-2 expression. *Ann Oncol* 2006;17, Suppl 7:vii103-8.

[526] Silberg DG, Sullivan J, Kang E, Swain GP, Moffett J, Sund NJ, Sackett SD, Kaestner KH. Cdx2 ectopic expression induces gastric intestinal metaplasia in transgenic mice. *Gastroenterology* 2002;122:689-96.

[527] Mutoh H, Hakamata Y, Sato K, Eda A, Yanaka I, Honda S, Osawa H, Kaneko Y, Sugano K. Conversion of gastric mucosa to intestinal metaplasia in Cdx2-expressing transgenic mice. *Biochem Biophys Res Commun* 2002;294:470-9.

[528] Nozaki K, Ogawa M, Williams JA, Lafleur BJ, Ng V, Drapkin RI, Mills JC, Konieczny SF, Nomura S, Goldenring JR. A Molecular Signature of Gastric Metaplasia Arising in Response to Acute Parietal Cell Loss. *Gastroenterology* 2008;134:511–522.

[529] Karam SM, Leblond CP. Dynamics of epithelial cells in the corpus of the mouse stomach. III. Inward migration of neck cells followed by progressive transformation into zymogenic cells. *Anat Rec* 1993;236:297–313.

[530] Ramsey VG, Doherty JM, Chen CC, Stappenbeck TS, Konieczny SF, Mills JC. The maturation of mucus-secreting gastric epithelial progenitors into digestive-enzyme secreting zymogenic cells requires Mist1. *Development* 2007;134:211–222.

[531] Nomura S, Yamaguchi H, Ogawa M, Wang TC, Lee JR, Goldenring JR. Alterations in gastric mucosal lineages induced by acute oxyntic atrophy in wild type and gastrin deficient mice. *Am J Physiol* 2004;288:G362–G375.

[532] Means AL, Meszoely IM, Suzuki K, Miyamoto Y, Rustgi AK, Coffey RJ Jr, Wright CV, Stoffers DA, Leach SD. Pancreatic epithelial plasticity mediated by acinar cell transdifferentiation and generation of nestin-positive intermediates. *Development* 2005; 132:3767–3776.

[533] Zhu L, Shi G, Schmidt CM, Hruban RH, Konieczny SF. Acinar cells contribute to the molecular heterogeneity of pancreatic intraepithelial neoplasia. *Am J Pathol* 2007;171:263–273.

[534] Shajan P., Beglinger C. Helicobacter pylori and Gastric Cancer: The Causal Relationship. *Digestion* 2007;75:25-35.

In: Gastric Cancer: Diagnosis, Early Prevention, and Treatment   ISBN 978-1-61668-313-9
Editor: V. D. Pasechnikov, pp.119-149   © 2010 Nova Science Publishers, Inc.

Chapter III

PATHOLOGY OF GASTRIC CANCER, PRECANCEROUS CONDITIONS AND PRECANCEROUS MUCOSAL LESIONS

Massimo Rugge[1-2], Sergey Chukov[3], Victor Pasechnikov[4], Donato Nitti[5] and David Y Graham[2]

[1]Department of Diagnostic Sciences & Special Therapies - Pathology Unit, University of Padova, Italy
[2]Department of Medicine, Veterans Affairs Medical Center and Baylor College of Medicine Houston, Texas USA
[3]Department of Pathology, State Medical Academy of Stavropol, Russian Federation
[4]Department of Therapy, State Medical Academy of Stavropol, Russian Federation
[5]Department of Oncology & Surgical Sciences; Surgery Unit, University of Padova, Italy

ABSTRACT

This chapter considers the pathology of gastric cancer (GC) and its precursor lesions. The aim of the Authors is to provide basic information on the natural history of both precancerous and cancerous lesions, and their clinical context, and on the diagnostic issues and prognostic implications providing the biological rationale for their follow-up and treatment.

Over the last 25 years, a growing body of evidence has shown that full-blown cancer is the final step along a lengthy pathway, which includes a progressive accumulation of genotypic and phenotypic changes – and sporadic gastric cancer is no exception [1, 2].

Less than 10% of stomach cancers are inherited. The genetic factors involved in familial gastric malignancies remain largely unknown, though specific, well characterized mutations are involved in a subset of patients. Families harboring germ-line *E-cadherin* truncating mutations (with an autosomal dominant pattern of inheritance) have a high prevalence of diffuse-type GC. Other hereditary conditions predisposing to

GC include familial adenomatous polyposis (FAP), hereditary non-polyposis colorectal cancer, and Li-Fraumeni's and Peutz-Jeghers' syndromes [3-5].

The majority of GCs are sporadic. Most of them are triggered by long-standing inflammatory conditions (due primarily to infectious, but also to chemical agents) resulting in a largely-unknown interplay of phenotypic and molecular derangements. Such a natural history was initially highlighted by Pelayo Correa and is currently known as the multistage cascade of gastric oncogenesis (Figure 1). This chapter will describe each of the single phenotypic steps along this biological pathway [1, 2].

PRECANCEROUS CONDITIONS AND PRECANCEROUS LESIONS WITHIN THE GASTRIC MUCOSA

As in other areas of the gastrointestinal tract, so too within the gastric mucosa, a basic distinction is drawn between precancerous *conditions* and precancerous *lesions*. According to Basil Morson, a precancerous condition "... is best regarded as a clinical state associated with a significantly increased risk of cancer, whereas a precancerous lesion is a histopathological abnormality in which cancer is more likely to occur ... In many clinical conditions with an increased risk of cancer, there is also an identifiable precancerous lesion, but this is not invariably so." [6].

PRECANCEROUS (NON-HEREDITARY) CONDITIONS

Clinical situations carrying an increased risk of GC include: a) environmental atrophic gastritis; b) autoimmune atrophic gastritis; c) peptic (gastric) ulcer; d) gastric mucosal hyperplasia (diffuse or focal-polypoid). All these situations are primarily non-hereditary (though a genetic predisposition has been claimed for some of them); hereditary syndromes should be considered as a separate category (see above).

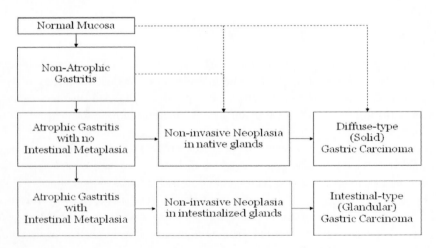

Figure 1. Gastric cancerogenesis according to Pelayo Correa.

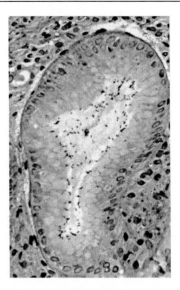

Figure 2. *Helicobacter pylori* within the lumen of a gastric gland (Warthin-Starry stain).

Atrophic (Environmental) Gastritis

Any long-standing gastric mucosal inflammation (with or without atrophic changes) is associated with a greater risk of cancer [7, 8]. The risk of developing intestinal-type (or *epidemic*) GC, however, is significantly higher in cases of atrophic gastritis. The etiology of atrophy is due mainly to environmental agents, and *Helicobacter pylori* (*H.pylori*) is the most prevalent etiological agent worldwide (Figure 2) [9]. Both in the population and in single patient, interactions between bacterial and host-related factors modulate the risk of atrophy [10]. Other environmental agents carry a significantly lower risk of atrophic transformation. The etiology of atrophy with the second highest incidence is primarily host-related and represented by autoimmune gastritis. *H.pylori*-related and autoimmune gastritis may co-exist and that is when the risk of cancer becomes most likely.

Atrophy assessment and grading is based on histology, but non-invasive tests (pepsinogens I [PgI] and II [PgII], and gastrin 17 serology) have also proved reliable indicators of mucosal atrophy. Several studies have consistently shown that PgI and/or the PgI/PgII ratio are valid markers of atrophic (corpus) gastritis. Low plasma levels of gastrin-17 are associated with both antral atrophy and severe pan-atrophy, and both these conditions also feature a low PgI and PgI/PgII ratio. Raised plasma levels of gastrin-17 are characteristically detected in atrophic (autoimmune) corpus gastritis [15]. The serological profile of gastric mucosal atrophy may thus offer useful information for screening patients before considering invasive (and more expensive) diagnostic procedures (endoscopy with biopsy sampling) [16-18].

The endoscopic detection of atrophic changes (and even advanced precancerous alterations) is inconsistent (except in Japan), so atrophy assessment relies on histology and its reliable assessment demands the use of a validated endoscopic biopsy sampling protocol. Assuming that different extents and topographical distributions of atrophy express different clinico-biological situations (associated with different cancer risks), the Houston-updated

Sydney System established that multiple biopsy samples are needed to explore the different mucosal compartments [19]. Different biopsy sampling protocols have been proposed, but they all recommend exploring both the oxyntic and the antral mucosa. The *incisura angularis* is also considered for the purpose of establishing the earliest onset of any atrophic-metaplastic transformation (Figure 3) [20, 21]. In this setting, and even more in the histological assessment of more advanced precancerous lesions (*i.e.* non-invasive neoplasia), additional specimens should be obtained (any endoscopically visible focal lesions has to be additionally sampled) (Figure 3).

In the gastric mucosa, atrophy is defined as the "loss of appropriate glands" [22, 23]. Different phenotypes of atrophic transformation may be seen:

- Disappearance or evident shrinkage of glandular units, replaced by fibrosis. At both corpus and antrum levels, such a situation results in a reduced glandular mass, but no changes are seen in the native cell phenotype (Figure 4A);
- Metaplastic replacement of the native glands by glands featuring a new cellular commitment (i.e. intestinal and/or pseudo-pyloric metaplasia) (Figure 4B);. The number of glands is not necessarily lower, but the metaplastic replacement of the original glandular units results in a reduced population of native glands ("appropriate" for the compartment considered). Such a condition is also basically consistent with the definition of "loss of appropriate glands".

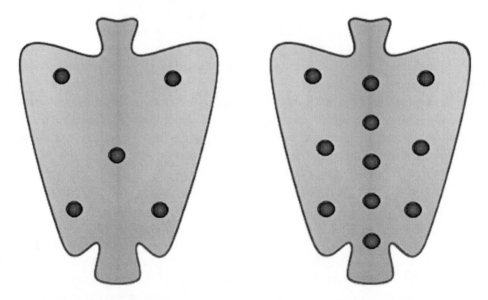

Figure 3. Gastric mucosa biopsy sampling protocols (stomach is open along the greater curve). On the left, the biopsy sampling basically applied in all procedures for assessing the stomach; on the right, an example of the (more extensive) sampling adopted in the follow-up of non-invasive neoplasia (any focal lesion has to be additionally sampled).

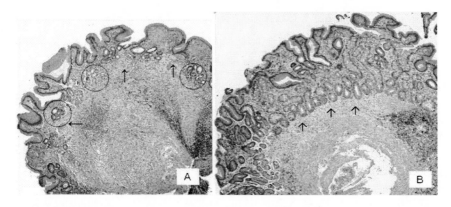

Figure 4. A. Atrophy in antral mucosa: evident loss of appropriate glands replaced by fibrosis of the lamina propria. "Surviving" native mucosecreting glandular structures (circles) are embedded in a fibrous stroma (↑).

B. Atrophy in antral mucosa: The native antral (mucosecreting) glands are replaced by metaplastic glandular structures ("loss of appropriate glands"). Metaplastic goblet and Paneth cells (↑) are shown.

Pseudo-pyloric metaplasia will be extensively discussed in the paragraph dedicated to autoimmune atrophic gastritis (which is its most typical clinico-pathological setting).

As for intestinal metaplasia (IM), different subtypes of intestinalization have been distinguished, based on whether the metaplastic epithelium phenotype resembles that of the large bowel mucosa (colonic type IM) or of the small bowel mucosa (small-intestinal type IM) (Figure 5); [24-26]. These two main types of intestinalization may be further classified according to their histochemical type (sialomucins and sulfomucins as assessed by high iron diamine [HID] histochemistry) and the cellular location (in goblet and/or columnar cells) of the mucin products. The risk of cancer is believed to increase from Type I to Type III IM (Table 1) [27, 28].

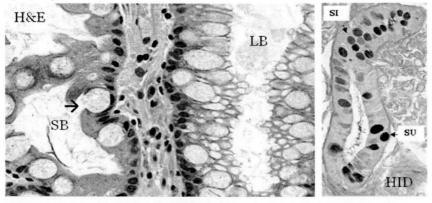

Figure 5. Intestinal metaplasia (IM) in tow adjacent glands of stomach mucosa. On the left side, the H&E stain shows goblet cells (↑) similar to those of the small bowel ("small bowel type" [SB]). On the right side, the metaplastic transformation realizes the phenotype of the large bowel glands (no brush-border is detectable= "colonic type" [LB]).

The High Iron Diamine (HID) histochemical reaction shows blue goblet cells containing sialomucins (SI) and brown goblet cells containing sulfomucins (SU).

Table 1. intestinal Metaplasia Phenotypes

Intestinal metaplasia	Hematoxylin-eosin	PAS & HID
Type I (complete, mature, small bowel type)	Columnar cells (non-secreting, mature, absorptive)	Neutral mucins (PAS+ve)
	Goblet cells	Sialomucins
Type II (incomplete, immature, large bowel type)	Columnar cells (secreting, immature, non-absorptive)	Neutral mucins (PAS+ve), sulfomucins
	Goblet cells	Sialomucins + sulfomucins
Type III (incomplete, immature, large bowel type)	Columnar cells (secreting, immature, non-absorptive)	Sulfomucins
	Goblet cells	Sialomucins + Sulfomucins

The more extensive the mucosal intestinalization, the more Type III IM is represented, and the greater the extent of Type III metaplasia, the higher the risk of intestinal-type gastric cancer.

Sometimes (and particularly in *H.pylori*-associated gastritis), severe inflammation makes it impossible to determine whether glands that "appear to be lost" are merely obscured by the inflammatory infiltrate or have genuinely disappeared. In such cases, the final atrophy assessment should be deferred until a post-therapy re-evaluation can be performed (*e.g.* after eradicating *H. pylori* infection) and a temporary classification of "high grade inflammation precluding atrophy assessment" (or "indefinite for atrophy") is used (though this category is not meant to represent a biological entity).

In tune with the above-mentioned criteria, an international group of gastrointestinal pathologists (the Atrophy Club) arranged the histological spectrum of atrophic changes into a formal classification (Table 2). After testing it in real cases, the inter-observer consistency in recognizing/scoring the atrophic lesions was judged to be more than adequate [22].

Table 2. Atrophy in gastric mucosa

0. Absent				
1. Indefinite				
2. Present	Histological type	Location		Histological grading
		Antrum	Corpus	
	2.1 Metaplastic	Key lesion: Intestinal metaplasia	Key lesion: Intestinal metaplasia, Pseudopyloric metaplasia	2.1.1 Mild (G1)
				2.1.2 Moderate (G2)
				2.1.3 Severe (G3)
	2.2 Non-Metaplastic	Key lesion: Disappearance of glands; Fibrosis of lamina propria		2.1.1 Mild (G1)
				2.1.2 Moderate (G2)
				2.1.3 Severe (G3)

Autoimmune Gastritis

Autoimmune gastritis is due to an immunomediated selective destruction of the parietal cells, so the inflammation is restricted to the specialized (oxyntic) mucosa. The serological detection of anti-parietal-cell auto antibodies represents the serological marker of this disease, but its pathogenesis is still not clear (the potential responsibility of anti-intrinsic factor antibodies has been also suggested). The immunomediated destruction of the parietal cells (the source of intrinsic factor) results in pernicious anemia.

Both atrophic phenotypes, with and without metaplastic epithelial transformation, may be featured in autoimmune gastritis. The non-metaplastic variant has already been described. In the metaplastic variant, there may be two histotypes of metaplastic glands.

Pseudo-pyloric metaplasia of the native corpus epithelia is characterized by antral-like (metaplastic) mucosa obtained from what was anatomically corpus mucosa. In such cases, it is particularly important to inform the pathologist about the location from where biopsy specimens were obtained (to avoid the fact that the antral-like mucosa is in fact metaplastic epithelia escaping the pathologist's attention). The original oxyntic commitment of a pseudo-pyloric metaplastic epithelium is revealed by its immunostaining positive for pepsinogen I, which is only found in the corpus mucosa. Intestinal metaplasia (see above) is believed to arise in previously-antralized (pseudo-pyloric metaplasia) oxyntic glands.

Histological Reporting on Atrophic Gastritis

The Sydney System and its Houston-updated version attempt to provide a scoring system to help pathologists grade the severity of different histological variables belonging to the spectrum of gastritis, and mucosal atrophy among them [19]. The Sydney matrix was unable to produce a clear biopsy reporting format that was easy for clinicians and patients to understand, and that unequivocally ranked the cancer risk of a given case of gastritis. A sizeable body of literature has confirmed that the extent/location of gastric atrophy (and the metaplastic subtype in particular) correlates consistently with the cancer risk [2, 9, 29-31]. Based on these findings, an International Group of Gastroenterologists and Pathologists (Operative Link on Gastritis Assessment [OLGA]) recently proposed a histological gastritis staging system designed to enable a plain ranking of the severity of disease of the stomach as a whole [32, 33]. The OLGA system uses the biopsy sampling protocol suggested by the Sydney System and considers gastric atrophy as the key lesion for assessing disease progression (and its related cancer risk).

In each of the 2 mucosal compartments (mucosecreting and oxyntic), an overall atrophy score expresses the percentage of compartmental atrophic changes. Using this strategy, an overall atrophy score is obtained that separately summarizes the scores for the antrum/incisura and the corpus mucosa: the OLGA stage results from the combination of the overall "antrum score" with the overall "corpus score". Visual Analog scales (VAS) have been provided to enable a consistent assessment of the OLGA staging system [34]. The OLGA histology report also includes the etiological information obtainable from the tissue samples available (*i.e. H.pylori* infection; autoimmune disease, *etc.*) (Figure 6).

Atrophy Score		Corpus			
		No Atrophy (score 0)	Mild Atrophy (score 1)	Moderate Atrophy (score 2)	Severe Atrophy (score 3)
A n t r u m	No Atrophy (score 0) (including *incisura angularis*)	STAGE 0	STAGE I	STAGE II	STAGE II
	Mild Atrophy (score 1) (including *incisura angularis*)	STAGE I	STAGE I	STAGE II	STAGE III
	Moderate Atrophy (score 2) (including *incisura angularis*)	STAGE II	STAGE II	STAGE III	STAGE IV
	Severe Atrophy (score 3) (including *incisura angularis*)	STAGE III	STAGE III	STAGE IV	STAGE IV

Figure 6. The OLGA Staging for gastritis.

Chronic Gastric Ulcer

Chronic gastric ulcer is the focal marker of a disease affecting the whole stomach, and this means that chronic gastric ulcer occurs mostly in (cancer-prone) atrophic mucosa [30, 35, 36].

Epithelial dysplasia at the margins of chronic gastric ulcers should be considered the most reliable indicator of an ulcer-specific increased risk of cancer. Such a situation is infrequent, however, and the epithelial lesions surrounding the ulcer crater frequently show hyperplastic (reparative) changes, sometime consistent with the histological category of "indefinite for non-invasive neoplasia".

The definition of "ulcer-cancer" (*i.e.* adenocarcinoma developing in an existing peptic ulcer) requires both reliable evidence of a chronic ulcer existing prior to the malignancy and proof of neoplastic changes (invasive or non-invasive) at the edge of the ulcer [37].

When any chronic gastric ulcer is first detected endoscopically, it should prudentially be suspected of being neoplastic, until histology proves otherwise. Such a clinical suspicion provides the rationale for the biopsy sampling protocol. The edge of the ulcer should be extensively "drilled" to obtain multiple biopsy samples. Because chronic ulcer is just one part of a stomach disease, the biopsy protocol should always include obtaining specimens from oxyntic, *angularis* and antral mucosa (as recommended for assessing gastritis).

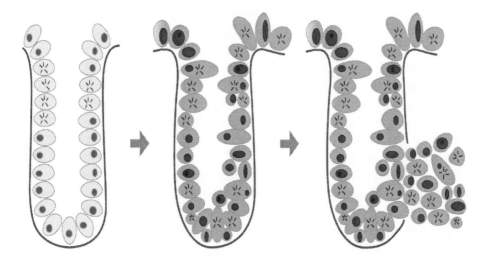

Figure 7. Multistep gastric oncogenesis: from a native gastric gland (first glandular unit on the left) to a neoplastic intra-glandular (synonym: intra-epithelial) transformation (i.e.: Non-invasive Neoplasia). In the third gland, neoplastic epithelia spread into the lamina propria (the broken continuity of basal membrane is represented).

Diseases Associated with Mucosal Hyperplasia (Be it Diffuse or Focal-polypoid)

Gastric mucosal hyperplasia may be focal (e.g. hyperplastic polyps) or diffuse (Ménétrier's disease). Non-invasive neoplastic foci may occur in both conditions and are believed to be the main determinant in establishing their cancer risk, so the magnitude of the risk depends on the prevalence of non-invasive neoplasia.

The available information on the incidence of diffuse gastric mucosal hyperplasia is inconsistent. The figures generally include Ménétrier's disease and hypertrophic gastropathy (with or without protein loss); accounts of gastric cancers associated with such diseases are largely anecdotal.

Focal/polypoid hyperplasia rarely (if ever) arises in a normal stomach [38, 39]. A comprehensive list of the polypoid lesions arising within the gastric mucosa is given in table 3. In a recent retrospective study, Dirschmid et al. [40] showed that hyperplastic polyps of the stomach can be considered as a precancerous condition depending on the different diseases coexisting with the polypoid lesions (*i.e.* autoimmune gastritis and *Helicobacter pylori* gastritis).

Focal hyperplastic lesions include three major situations, i.e. hyperplastic polyps, hamartomatous polyps, and the so-called gastritis cystica profunda.

Hyperplastic polyps account for 70-80% of all gastric polyps [41]. Their overall malignant potential is very low (less than 2%). The occurrence of dysplasia reportedly ranges from 1% to 20% and it is more frequent in larger polyps [40, 42]. Genetic analysis suggests that simultaneous large gastric hyperplastic polyps have a clonal origin and may therefore be considered as neoplastic. Furthermore, hyperplastic polyps may have a replication error phenotype that has been linked to cancer [43].

Fundic gland polyps (also known as oxyntic polyps) are polypoid hyperplastic lesions that have recently come to light; they are clinically associated with long-term treatment with proton pump inhibitors. Fundic polyps are frequently multiple and sometimes occur throughout the oxyntic mucosa. The cancer risk associated with all these conditions ranges from low to nil (with the exception of cases with a syndromic predisposition to GC) [44-46].

Gastritis cystica profunda is a particular (mainly focal/polypoid) hyperplastic lesion seen close to the anastomoses in patients who have undergone partial gastrectomy (Billroth II) for benign diseases. The foveolar epithelium becomes hyperplastic and mucosecreting (dilated) glands are displaced in the submucosa. The concomitant hyperplasia of the muscularis mucosa may contribute to the derangement of the normal mucosal architecture. Non-invasive neoplastic changes can sometimes be detected in both native foveolar and/or intestinalized epithelia (usually more than 10 years after the partial gastrectomy). Non-invasive neoplasia may underlie the increased risk of carcinoma, the incidence of which is 3 times higher in gastric remnants than in intact stomachs [47].

Table 3. Gastric polyps and polypoid lesions

Neoplastic
-Adenoma (sporadic or syndromic)
-Carcinoma (primary or metastatic)
-Carcinoid (different histotypes and different clinical behaviors)
Hyperplastic/Inflammatory
-Gastritis-related (infectious or chemical [reflux or NSAIDs])
-Polypoid hyperplasia near stomas, ulcers (including gastritis cystica profunda)
-Inflammatory fibroid polyp
-Xanthelasma
-Fundic gland polyp
Hamartomatous/Syndromic
-Peutz-Jehgers
-Juvenile
-Cowden's disease
-Pancreatic heterotopia
-Brunner glands
Non-Epithelial
-GIST
-Smooth muscle tumors (different, benign and malignant histotypes)
-Vascular tumors (different, benign and malignant histotypes)
-Neural tumors (different, benign and malignant histotypes)
-Lymphoid (benign [lymphoid hyperplasia] and malignant [lymphoma])
-Adipose

PRECANCEROUS LESIONS

Gastric Non-Invasive Neoplasia (Dysplasia): Definition and Morphology

Gastric adenocarcinoma may coexist with cyto-architectural changes in the adjacent glands, showing a degree of (de-)differentiation somewhere between that of the native mucosa and that of the cancer. For such phenotypic alterations, the Western literature has adopted the definition of dysplasia [6, 48-56], while Japanese authors speak of borderline lesions, atypical epithelium, or group 3 lesions [57-59]. The topographical contiguity and morphological similarity of the dysplasia and carcinoma have prompted the hypothesis that the two lesions are "biologically related". As for the nature of this biological relationship, dysplastic lesions have been considered as either: a) alterations coexisting with or in reaction to an adjacent neoplasm (*i.e.* para-cancerous lesions); or b) dedifferentiated lesions with a potential for acquiring the biological features (e.g. local invasiveness, metastases) typical of full-blown adenocarcinoma (*i.e.* pre-cancerous lesions).

Gastric dysplasia was originally defined exclusively on the basis of its morphological appearance [6] (Table 4), but in the last fifteen years molecular studies have detected a number of genotypic alterations common to gastric dysplasia and GC; both the cytohistological abnormalities and the "mutated" molecular profile qualify the dysplastic epithelia as neoplastic. Considering the phenotypic and genotypic similarities between dysplastic and neoplastic epithelia, the distinction between dysplasia and invasive GC lies essentially in the fact that carcinoma is associated with histological proof of invasiveness (infiltration of the *lamina propria* that is lacking, by definition, in dysplasia) (Figures 7, 8). In much the same way as for advanced precancerous lesions developing in non-glandular mucosa, gastric dysplasia has also been defined as an intraepithelial/intraglandular neoplasia (*i.e.* confined by the dysplastic glands' basal membrane). The continuity/integrity of the dysplastic glands' basal membrane separates the epithelia from the stroma (i.e. the *lamina propria*), and the continuity of such a wall prevents the stromal invasion required for any metastatic implant.

Dysplasia is characterized by three basic morphological features: i) epithelial atypia; ii) abnormal epithelial differentiation; and iii) a disrupted mucosal architecture [6]. Different combinations of these phenotypic changes have contributed to dysplasia being arranged on a three-tiered scale: mild, moderate and severe.

In 1998, an international group of European, Japanese, and North American pathologists proposed an original classification of advanced precancerous gastric lesions; the proposal was later adopted by the authoritative World Health Organization Agency [31, 60]. Table 5 shows this *Padova International Classification*, which replaces the term dysplasia with *non-invasive neoplasia* (NiN), thereby emphasizing the biological juxtaposition of non-invasive and invasive neoplastic lesions. Both the Padova classification and the WHO Agency grade non-invasive neoplasia on a two-tiered scale (low- and high-grade) (Figure 8). In histology reports on biopsy samples, 2 additional categories can be recorded, i.e. "indefinite for NiN", and "NiN coexisting with suspected invasive adenocarcinoma". Both these diagnostic labels are not biological entities and should respectively be applied: (a) when hyperplastic lesions are indistinguishable from neoplastic intraepithelial changes; and (b) when microglandular structures, possibly infiltrating the lamina propria, coexist with non-invasive neoplasia.

Table 4. Phenotypic changes and histological grading of advanced gastric precancerous lesions

B Morson *et al.* (1980)	WHO-2000 & Padova international (2000)
Mild dysplasia **Disorganized mucosal architecture**: mild irregularity of mucosal architecture (back to back glands). Budding and branching of crypts. Possible papillary growth. **Abnormal differentiation**: reduced number of goblet and Paneth cells **Cellular atypia**: Mild. Nuclear stratification with increased nuclear-cytoplasmic ratio.	**Low-grade NON-invasive (synonim: Intraepithelial) Neoplasia** Slight mucosal architecture abnormality with "expanding" adenomatous growth. Budding, branching, and ectasia of glandular structures. Possibly, papillary growth. Decreased differentiation of superficial epithelia. Mucous depletion of columnar cells coexists with few or no goblet and/or Paneth cells. Cigar-like, pseudo-stratified nuclei. Abnormal nuclear-cytoplasmic ratio. Increased mitotic activity (mitosis detectable all throughout the length of the glandular structure: proliferative compartment expansion).
Moderate dysplasia **Disorganized mucosal architecture**: intermediate between mild and severe dysplasia. **Abnormal differentiation**: intermediate between mild and severe dysplasia. **Cellular atypia**: intermediate between mild and severe.	
Severe dysplasia **Disorganized mucosal architecture**: severe irregularity of mucosal architecture (back to back glands). Diffuse budding and branching of crypts. Possible papillary growth. **Abnormal differentiation**: cells population virtually consistent only of columnar epithelia; both goblet and Paneth cells are virtually absent. **Cellular atypia**: severe.	**High-grade NON-invasive (synonim: Intraepithelial) Neoplasia** Severe mucosal architecture abnormality, coexisting with glandular adenomatous growth. Severe budding, branching and ectasia of glandular structures. Papillary growth. Absence of superficial differentiation. Columnar epithelia with severe mucous depletion. goblet and/or Paneth cells are absent. Cigar-like, pseudo-stratified nuclei, with abnormal nuclear-cytoplasmic ratio and prominent nucleoli. High-grade mitotic activity (all throughout the length of the glandular structures); atypical mitotic figures.

Table 5. The Padova International Classification of gastric non-invasive neoplasia

1 Negative for non-invasive neoplasia (NiN)	
2 Indefinite for non-invasive neoplasia	
	2.1 - Foveolar hyperproliferation
	2.2 - Hyperproliferative intestinal metaplasia
3 Non-invasive neoplasia (NiN)	
	3.1 - Low-grade non-invasive neoplasia
	3.2 - High-grade non-invasive neoplasia
4 non-invasive neoplasia coexisting with features suggesting invasive carcinoma	
5 Invasive adenocarcinoma of the stomach	

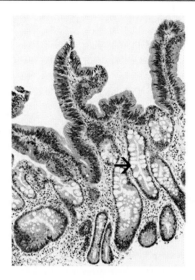

Figue 8. High-grade non-invasive Neoplasia (HG-NiN): Columnar epithelia (with atypical cigar like, pseudo-stratified nuclei) organized in papillary structures. The non-neoplastic epithelia are intestinalized (goblet cells ↑).

When tested by the international group of pathologists that proposed it, the Padova International classification demonstrated an adequate reproducibility [60].

Non-invasive Neoplasia (NiN): Progression to Invasive Cancer and (Possible) Reversion

According to Correa's hypothesis, non-invasive neoplasia is the most advanced phenotypic change before early invasive gastric cancer sets in. Japanese and some European studies suggest, however, that the starting point for any neoplastic transformation lies in the gland's proliferative zone (gland's neck), where metaplasia, dysplasia and adenocarcinoma my arise coincidentally. Such a theory basically denies the possibility of precancerous lesions being detected and phenotypically characterized in the stomach [61-63].

In Western countries, where the onset of gastric cancer is considered the final step in a long-standing oncogenic process, NiN is generally assumed to be a reliable marker of a greater risk of GC [52]. In industrialized countries, the declining incidence of GC coincides with a declining prevalence of precancerous gastric lesions [64, 65].

Both low- and high-grade NiN may progress to GC, and the different prognostic significance of high- and low-grade lesions has been validated in prospective studies [66, 67]. The high rate of cancer progression associated with high-grade NiN makes this lesion a candidate for surgical treatment. It is worth noting that, when NiN was followed up prospectively, 75% of GCs were diagnosed in their initial stage [WHO pTNM: stage I], suggesting that following up NiN is a valid strategy for the secondary prevention of GC [66-68].

Excluding (rare) cases of it developing in the stomach's native glands, NiN usually arises from intestinalized epithelia; this is consistent with the hypothesis that field cancerization is in fact atrophy (with or without intestinal metaplasia) [69, 70]. The morphogenesis of IM is still far from being fully elucidated. Recent evidence shows that genetic mutations and/or epigenetic modifications in gastric stem cells may result in a "mutated glandular unit", which may either convert back to its native phenotype or eventually turn into a neoplastic cell, through further mutational events [71].

Epigenetic and/or somatic changes in the intestine-specific Homebox genes (i.e. *CDX1* and *CDX2*) have been accused of being responsible (or co-responsible) for metaplastic changes [72, 73]. Given the potential reversibility of epigenetic changes, the regression of gastric IM (and low-grade NiN, at least) is biologically plausible, rather like the "decarcinogenesis" achieved in large bowel adenomas by administering anti-inflammatory drugs.

The regression of metaplastic (and even dysplastic) changes has been demonstrated by long-term follow-up studies applying different chemopreventive strategies [29, 74]. A recent long-term follow-up trial also showed that *H.pylori* eradication significantly modified the natural history of advanced precancerous lesions: when the pathological outcome of low-grade NiN was compared between *H.pylori*-infected (follow-up: mean 43 months, range 12-160 months) and *H.pylori*-eradicated patients (follow-up: mean 37 months, range 12-119 months), *H.pylori* eradication was associated with a significantly lower risk of evolution into high-grade NiN or GC [75].

Molecular Pathology of Non-Invasive Neoplasia of the Stomach

Molecular typing of gastric NiN has reinforced the conviction that these lesions belong to the same biological spectrum as their invasive counterpart. The most accepted current theory suggests that non-invasive neoplastic cells derive from previously-intestinalized (metaplastic) epithelia. More recently, the stem-cell nature of this cancer-oriented cell was pointed out: in fact, an experimental model of chronic *H.pylori*-related gastritis demonstrated that bone marrow–derived cells may home onto the injured gastric glands, where they can eventually acquire a neoplastic (phenotypic and molecular) profile [76]. The role of stem cells in gastric oncogenesis needs to be further explored [70].

There are still no molecular markers available, however, to enable the distinction between atypical hyperplastic lesions and low-grade NiN, or between high-grade NiN and early invasive neoplasia (*i.e.* invasive/infiltrating intramucosal GC).

Table 6. Molecular abnormalities associated with non-invasive neoplasia and EGC

Cell cycle regulator	Adenoma*	Superficial carcinoma*
Cyclin E (IHC expression)	8/182	11/47 (§)
p16 (reduced IHC expression)	not determined	3/38
p21 (reduced IHC expression)	32/144	25/45
p27 (reduced IHC expression)	1/11	3/20

* According to the Japanese classification of gastric carcinoma [13].

IHC= immunohistochemical assessment.

(§) significantly different prevalence between adenoma and carcinoma.

The molecular profile of preneoplastic stomach lesions is variable. It is not clear whether this heterogeneity is due to: a) the biological profiles of the lesions *per se;* b) the different molecular biology methods used in the published studies; or c) differences in the histological criteria adopted to classify the histological lesions. Caution is warranted in accepting descriptions of the molecular changes associated with NiN, also because information on the molecular profile of precancerous lesions often results from the analysis of only a few cases. The genetic and epigenetic changes reported in gastric neoplastic non-invasive (as well as invasive) precancerous lesions may affect the *DNA repair system* genes, tumor suppressor genes, oncogenes, cell cycle regulators, growth factors, and adhesion molecules [77-81].

a) Genetic Instability

Microsatellite instability (MSI) has been demonstrated in both IM and adenomas ("dysplastic" flat or polypoid lesions) [82]. In IM, the mutant phenotype has been associated with type III-IM [83], whereas in flat or polypoid dysplastic lesions (*adenomas* according to the Japanese classification system), MSI has been associated more frequently with dysplastic lesions coexisting with invasive cancer [84, 85]. In a recent study, MSI was documented in 11 (20%) of 55 consecutive Italian patients with gastric NiN and no coexisting GC (indefinite for NiN in 29 cases; low-grade NiN in 17; high-grade NiN in 9), showing that changes in the DNA repair system have to be considered among the early molecular events in gastric carcinogenesis [79].

b) Tumor Suppressor Gene Changes

p53 alterations have been found throughout the spectrum of histological lesions involved in the process of gastric oncogenesis. Loss of heterozygosis at the *p53 locus* was demonstrated in 14% of a series of metaplastic lesions and in 22% of gastric adenomas [86]. In a longitudinal study, Sakurai *et al.* showed that *missense* mutations are associated with dysplastic lesions that evolve into carcinoma [87]. Somatic mutations of the *APC* gene have been found in 6% of incomplete type IM and in proportions varying between 20% and 42% of adenomatous lesions [88]. *APC* mutations were documented in 76% of 78 cases of flat/raised dysplasia unassociated with adenocarcinoma, and in 3% of flat/raised dysplastic lesions coexisting with full-blown adenocarcinoma [86]. *Nonsense* or *frameshift APC* and *p53* mutations have been associated with high-grade adenomas, whereas *silent* mutations are more often associated with low-grade atypical lesions [88, 89]. Epigenetic changes (methylation) in *pS2* (considered a tumor suppressor involved specifically in gastric carcinogenesis) give rise to a more limited expression of the corresponding protein. *pS2* expression is reduced in IM and completely lacking in dysplastic lesions [90].

c) Oncogene Changes

c-met, K-sam and *c-erb2* alterations have been found in full-blown gastric carcinomas, but little information is available on any such alterations in precancerous lesions.

d) Cell Cycle Regulators

p15, p16, p21 and p27 are cyclin-dependent kinase inhibitor proteins and are consequently involved in cell cycle regulation, acting as suppressors of neoplastic growth. Cyclin E is involved in regulating the G1/S phase of the cell cycle. Changes in both cyclin-dependent kinase and cyclin E have been observed in precancerous lesions and full-blown carcinomas (Table 6) [91].

e) Adhesion Molecules

Cell adhesion molecules (e-cadherin, p-cadherin, alpha-catenin) can act as tumor growth suppressors. A reduced expression of E-cadherin has been documented in invasive neoplasms with various degrees of differentiation, but no unequivocal data are currently available on the gene's expression in pre-invasive lesions [92]. CD44 is considered important in regulating cell-to-cell interactions. Aberrant CD44 transcripts have been found in IM, but no information is available on the expression of this molecule in more advanced lesions [93].

Non-invasive Neoplasia in Clinical Practice: Follow-up Strategies

No evidence-based guidelines are available as yet to support a specific clinical strategy in response to a histological diagnosis of gastric NiN. The Japanese experience cannot be wholly exported to the Western world because the two areas do not share the same diagnostic criteria. Even in the recent *Vienna classification*, the presence or absence of stromal invasion is not believed to discriminate between preneoplastic lesions and GC, (as considered in Western tradition) [94-96].

On the basis of current knowledge, the following recommendations may be considered for the clinical management of non-invasive neoplasia:

1. The low prevalence of NiN and the different risk of invasive GC associated with different grades of NiN make it necessary for a histological diagnosis to be validated by a second opinion [66, 97];
2. In patients informed of the cancer risk associated with low-grade NiN, an annual follow-up seems sufficient to monitor the clinical-biological course of their lesions. Patient compliance with repeated endoscopic procedures is crucial [98];
3. Endoscopic follow-up must include extensive sampling of the gastric mucosa. Since most histological lesions have no macroscopic counterpart, biopsy sampling must be extensive and standardized (with additional, *not* alternative, biopsies being taken from any focal lesions) [68, 69]. The endoscopic procedure must be handled by a specialist with the necessary awareness and expertise;
4. The risk of low-grade lesions progressing to high-grade lesions or cancer is higher in a setting of extensive IM [97, 99];
5. When low-grade NiN coexists with *H.pylori* infection, eradication reduces the risk of progression [75];
6. The strong likelihood of high-grade NiN being associated with or progressing to GC, makes resection indicated. Until endoscopic mucosal resection (EMR) has become widespread in the Western world, gastric resection remains the only viable option.

GASTRIC CANCER

Gastric epithelial malignancies are usually adenocarcinomas. Two morphological variants of GC are distinguished according to the cancer's location (proximal *versus* distal) and histology (glandular *versus* solid). Albeit with significant exceptions, intestinal-type GC is located distally, while diffuse carcinoma tends to arise in the proximal stomach.

As mentioned in the chapter on epidemiology, the prevalence of the GC's location differs significantly in different epidemiological contexts: at macro-epidemiological level, it can be assumed that the prevalence of proximally-located diffuse GC rises with increasing socio-economic status (and vice versa).

The distinction between proximal GC and adenocarcinoma arising in the distal esophagus is debatable. The international gastric cancer association distinguishes true esophageal adenocarcinoma (Type I) from GCs arising in the cardia (Type II), or sub-cardial mucosa (Type III). The consistency of such a distinction is limited by the fact that all these cancers are generally detected in an advanced stage, by which time the anatomical landmarks have been destroyed by cancer growth [100]. Inconsistent results have likewise been achieved on applying immunohistochemical profiling to distinguish esophageal from gastric adenocarcinoma.

Depending on its local growth, gastric carcinoma is divided into two stages, i.e. early and advanced [101, 102].

Early Gastric Cancer

In 1962, the Japanese Society of Gastroenterological Endoscopy defined early gastric cancer (EGC) as epithelial malignancy limited to the mucosa or submucosa, irrespective of any presence of lymph node metastases [103].

While the definition of EGC is accepted worldwide, its histological assessment differs significantly in the hands of between Asian and all other pathologists: an Asian diagnosis of EGC does not necessarily demand histological proof of neoplastic invasion of the lamina propria, as required in Western countries. As a consequence, only a subgroup of Asian cases of ECG (those associated with stromal invasion) is identified consistently by Eastern and Western pathologists.

Given this discrepancy in its histological classification and the different strategies devoted to preventing secondary GC (extensively applied in Asian countries), the prevalence of EGC differs significantly in Western and Far Eastern populations. In particular, while almost 50% of GCs detected in Japan are staged as early, their prevalence amounts to less than 5% in Western countries. Accordingly, the 5-year survival rates are significantly lower (87% *versus* 92%) and the rates of lymph node metastases being detected at the initial diagnosis are significantly higher (20% *versus* 5%) in non-Asian than in Asian populations [104].

EGC is usually located along the lesser curvature, but almost 15% of early adenocarcinomas reveal multiple (synchronous) locations. According to the Japanese Research Society for gastric cancer, three major types of EGCs are endoscopically and/or grossly distinguishable (Type I, Type IIa-b-c; Type III) (Figure 9) [57].

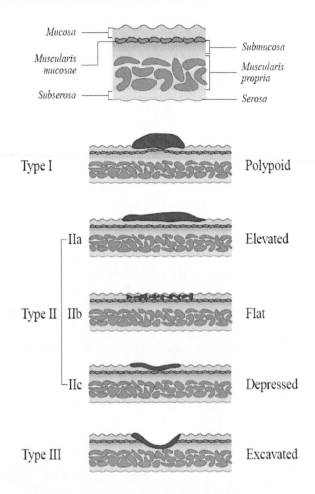

Figure 9. Macroscopic classification of Early Gastric Cancer (normal anatomical layers of gastric wall are also shown).

The finding of metastatic nodes is not in conflict with the definition of EGC. In the Japanese literature, the prevalence of EGC-associated nodal metastases ranges between 15% and 30%, and correlates significantly with the depth of parietal infiltration [105]. The immunohistochemical and molecular assessment of nodal status increases the prevalence of both micrometastases and isolated tumor cells [105, 106].

Advanced Gastric Cancer

There is evidence to show that "although EGC shows a relatively long natural history..., it progresses to the advanced stage with time and leads to death ... if left untreated." Longitudinal studies have demonstrated that almost 50% of EGCs progress to an invasive stage within 4 years [107, 108].

Gross Pathology

In according with Bormann and -with minor modifications- with the Japanese Research Society for Gastric Cancer), four major types of GC are grossly distinguishable: polypoid, fungating, ulcerated, and infiltrating (Figure 10) [57, 109]: polypoid GC produces a neoplastic mass protruding into the lumen, while the definition of fungating cancer is applied to polypoid GC that have undergone extensive central necrosis/ulceration; ulcerated cancers basically look like peptic ulcers with raised edges, and infiltrating tumors have a plaque-like appearance with desmoplastic intraparietal growth. The polypoid variant is the least prevalent (less than 10% of cases), while a fungating growth is considered the most frequent (up to 35%). The clinical impact of the Bormann's or any other macroscopic classifications of GC is minimal and they basically have no prognostic implications in the pathologist's assessment of resected stomachs [101, 102].

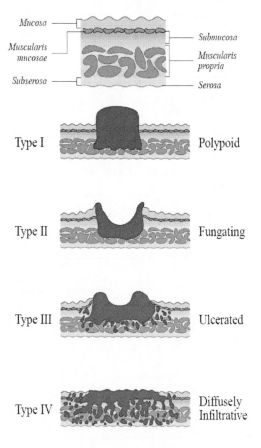

Figure 10. Macroscopic types of advanced gastric cancer (normal anatomical layers of gastric wall are also shown).
Type I: Polypoid, sharply demarcated tumor usually with a wide base; Type II: Ulcerated cancer infiltrating the surrounding wall; Type III: diffusely infiltrating cancer (ulcer is not a typical feature); Type IV: Diffusely infiltrating cancer. The Japanese Classification of Gastric carcinoma also consider a Type V variant that can not be classified into any of the above Types.

Table 7. Advanced gastric cancer: Histological classifications

Author(s) Histotypes	Basic morphology
P Lauren (1965)	
Intestinal	Glandular structures (variable differentiation). Most frequently coexisting with intestinal metaplasia. Most frequent in GC "endemic" areas
Diffuse	Solid or discohesive growth (also with mucous lakes). No extensive gastric mucosa intestinalization coexists
Mixed Diffuse & Intestinal	Coexisting Intestinal and Diffuse features
RM Mulligan (1972)	
Intestinal Cell cancer	Glandular structures (variable differentiation) lined by columnar epithelium (indistinct cellular margins; pseudostratified (cigar-like) nuclei. Most frequently coexisting with intestinal metaplasia
Pyloro-Cardiac cancer	Glandular structures (variable differentiation) lined by clear columnar/ epithelium with distinct cellular borders; rounded basal or central nuclei
Mucus cell carcinoma	Signet ring cells with mucous lakes
SC Ming (1977)	
Expanding	Neoplasia growths "*en mass*", rounded, well defined interface separates neoplasia from adjacent tissues. Most frequently arranged in well defined glandular structures. Intestinal metaplasia frequently coexists
Infiltrative	Neoplasia growths as single cells or small neoplastic clusters infiltrating the surrounding tissue with no well defined interface separating neoplasia from adjacent tissues. Most frequently solid or microglandular
J Jass (1980)	
Intestinal Type	Extensive IM coexisting with adenocarcinoma; Expanding Growth. Tubular differentiation. Acid mucins predominate
Gastric Type	Little or no IM coexisting with adenocarcinoma; Infiltrating growth, Neutral mucins predominate
N Goseki (1992)	
Group I	Tubular differentiation-well; Mucus in cytoplasm-poor
Group II	Tubular differentiation-well; Mucus in cytoplasm-rich
Group III	Tubular differentiation-poor; Mucus in cytoplasm-poor
Group IV	Tubular differentiation-poor; Mucus in cytoplasm-rich
WHO (2000)	
Tubular carcinoma	Tubules or acinar structures variable in size. Columnar eosinophilic epithelia with pseudostratified cigar-like nuclei and/or clear cells (nests, tubular or papillary arrangement. Mostly expanding growth, becoming infiltrative in less differentiated variants. Cytology atypia from low to high-grade (poorly differentiated variant is called solid carcinoma). When prominent lymphoid stroma is present the definition of medullary (or adenocarcinoma with lymphoid stroma)

		cancer is applied
	Papillary carcinoma	Exophytic cancers with fibrovascular finger-like structures lined by cylindrical/cuboidal cells. Variable cellular atypia. Demarcation from surrounding tissue is variable (infiltrating or expanding growth pattern).
	Mucinous carcinoma	More than 50% of the tumor consists of extracellular mucinous lakes. Two major patterns: glands lined by columnar mucous-secreting cells; cell clusters floating in mucinous lakes.
	Signet-ring cancer cell	More than 50% of the tumor consists of signet-ring cells (isolated or small nests). Mostly infiltrative growth. Desmoplasia may be prominent.
	Others	Adenosquamous carcinoma; Squamous cell carcinoma; Mixed adenocarcinoma-carcinoid; Parietal cell carcinoma; Paneth cell rich adenocarcinoma; Hepatoid adenocarcinoma; Carcinoma with osseous stromal metaplasia; Undifferentiated carcinoma; Small cell carcinoma; Choriocarcinoma; Endodermal sinus tumor; Embryonal carcinoma.

More important is the cancer's topographical location. Cancers arising in the proximal stomach are the least prevalent the world over, but they are being seen with increasing frequency in Europe and North America. Their distinction into cancer Types I, II and III has already been mentioned [100]. Cancers of the distal stomach are the most prevalent everywhere. The location of the gastric epithelial malignancy may reflect the cancer's etiology and have therapeutic implications.

Histology

Gastric cancers are histologically heterogeneous and their classification is generally based on the most prevalent histological component (tubules, papillae, mucous lakes, solid nests/islands, undifferentiated epithelia) (Figure 11). Cancer histology has been used as a prognostic parameter or biological variable in speculations concerning gastric oncogenesis [110-113]. Some of the several classifications proposed link cancer's morphology to both the biology of the oncogenic process and the prognosis. The most referenced histological classifications are listed in Table 7 [101, 102, 114-118].

In 2000, the authoritative WHO Agency proposed a descriptive classification of gastric epithelial malignancies [31]. Extensive illustrations of each histological phenotype are readily accessible in the original WHO publication. Consistently with this WHO classification, the different cancer histotypes are listed in Table 7 along with a summary of their main histological features.

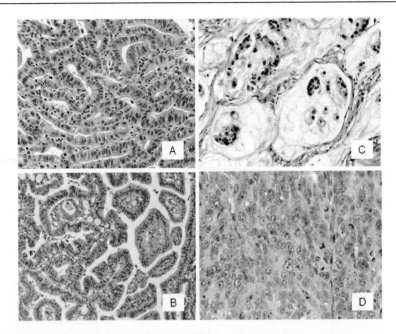

Figure 11. Histology of Gastric Cancer (H&E stain): a) well differentiated tubular adenocarcinoma (Intestinal type according to Lauren's classification); b) Papillary adenocarcinoma (Intestinal type according to Lauren's classification); c) Mucinous gastric adenocarcinoma (neoplastic epithelia floating into mucous lakes); d) Poorly differentiated (solid) adenocarcinoma

Local and Metastatic Spread

After its initial (early) growth, GC progressively expands within the gastric wall until it reaches the serous layer. Albeit with major exceptions, the tumor's phenotype varies according to its depth of infiltration in the wall and, generally speaking, the cancer phenotype is all the more dedifferentiated, the deeper the infiltration [119].

The rich lymphatic network of the gastric mucosa enables lymph node metastases to develop early on - in fact, they may be detected already in EGC (see EGC definition above). Whatever the cancer stage, the histological detection of lymphatic vessels invasion is the only independent predictor of lymph node metastases [120].

In cases of pN0 cancer, isolated tumor cells may be seen in regional lymph nodes; for the time being, we have no evidence of the prognostic value, if any, of such isolated tumor cells (ITC) [121]. Conflicting results have also emerged from studies on the prognostic impact of circulating GC cells [122].

The number of metastatic lymph nodes is considered prognostically relevant and no fewer than 15 nodes are required for reliable pathological staging (pTNM). As in other GI cancers, it has been suggested that the GC's prognosis depends on the number of lymph nodes considered, which in turn depends on the extent of the surgical *toilette* [D1 *versus* D2 *versus* D3 lymphadenectomy] and the accuracy of post-surgical lymph node harvesting [123-127].

Table 8. TNM classification of gastric tumours (WHO 2000)

T= Primary Tumour		M= distant metastasis				
TX	Primary tumor cannot be assessed	**MX**	distant metastasis can not be assessed			
T0	No evidence of tumor	**M0**	no distant metastasis			
Tis	Intraepithelial tumor (= Carcinoma *in situ* = Non-invasive Neoplasia)	**M1**	distant metastasis present			
T1	Tumour invades lamina propria or submucosa	**Stage Grouping**				
T2	Tumour invades muscularis propria or subserosa					
T3	Tumour penetrates serosa (visceral peritoneum) without invasion of adjacent structures					
T4	Tumour invades adjacent structures	**STAGE 0**	**Tis/N0**			**M0**
N= regional lymph node metastasis		**STAGE IA**	**T1/N0**			**M0**
Nx	Regional lymph nodes cannot be assessed					
N0	No regional lymph node metastasis	**STAGE IB**	**T1/N1**	**T2/N0**	**T1/N2**	**M0**
N1	Metastasis in 1 to 6 regional lymph nodes					
N2	Metastasis in 7 to 15 regional lymph nodes	**STAGE II**	**T1/N2**	**T2/N1**	**T3/N0**	**M0**
N3	Metastasis in more than 15 regional lymph nodes					
		STAGE IIIA	**T2/N2**	**T3/N1**	**T4/N0**	**M0**
		STAGE IIIB	**T3/N2**			**M0**
		STAGE IV	**T4/N1-N2-N3**			**M0**
			T1-2-3/N3			**M0**
			Any T/N			**M1**

Extranodal metastatic implants are strongly influenced by gender, age and histological phenotype. Intestinal-type GC, which typically arises in the distal stomach of older (male) patients, are more likely to develop liver metastases. Diffuse cancers of the proximal stomach (in both genders) reveal early peritoneal diffusion. Ovarian metastases are known as Krukenberg tumors [101, 102]. Transperitoneal spread can also be responsible for uterine metastases (both parietal and mucosal).

Gastric Cancer Staging

After curative resection, the 5-year overall survival rates in Western countries are 35% or less, and by 10 years after surgery, no more than 15% of GC patients are still alive. The 5-year survival rates differs significantly by cancer stage [128]; the most frequently-used staging system is the one produced by the AJCC [129] (Table 8). In 1998, Siewert et al. showed the prognostic impact of the ratio of metastatic to removed nodes [130]: this was subsequently confirmed by various authors and prompted the proposal to modify conventional pTNM-staging to create a "pTRM-system", where the original N (node) category is replaced by the more informative ratio of metastatic to removed lymph nodes [131-136].

REFERENCES

[1]   Correa, P. A human model of gastric carcinogenesis. *Cancer Res* 1988; 48: 3554-3560.

[2]   Correa, P. The biological model of gastric carcinogenesis. *IARC Sci Publ* 2004: 301-310.

[3]   Humar, B, Blair, V, Charlton, A, et al. E-Cadherin Deficiency Initiates Gastric Signet-Ring Cell Carcinoma in Mice and Man. *Cancer Res* 2009.

[4]   Barber, M, Murrell, A, Ito, Y, et al. Mechanisms and sequelae of E-cadherin silencing in hereditary diffuse gastric cancer. *J Pathol* 2008; 216: 295-306.

[5]   Huntsman, DG, Carneiro, F, Lewis, FR, et al. Early gastric cancer in young, asymptomatic carriers of germ-line E-cadherin mutations. *N Engl J Med* 2001; 344: 1904-1909.

[6]   Morson, BC, Sobin, LH, Grundmann, E, et al. Precancerous conditions and epithelial dysplasia in the stomach. *J Clin Pathol* 1980; 33: 711-721.

[7]   Correa, P. Chronic gastritis: a clinico-pathological classification. *Am J Gastroenterol* 1988; 83: 504-509.

[8]   Correa, P. The epidemiology and pathogenesis of chronic gastritis: three etiologic entites. *Front Gastrointest Res* 1980; 6: 98-108.

[9]   Uemura, N, Okamoto, S, Yamamoto, S, et al. Helicobacter pylori infection and the development of gastric cancer. *N Engl J Med* 2001; 345: 784-789.

[10]   Amieva, MR and El-Omar, EM. Host-bacterial interactions in Helicobacter pylori infection. *Gastroenterology* 2008; 134: 306-323.

[11]   Broutet, N, Plebani, M, Sakarovitch, C, et al. Pepsinogen A, pepsinogen C, and gastrin as markers of atrophic chronic gastritis in European dyspeptics. *Br J Cancer* 2003; 88: 1239-1247.

[12]   Miki, K, Morita, M, Sasajima, M, et al. Usefulness of gastric cancer screening using the serum pepsinogen test method. *Am J Gastroenterol* 2003; 98: 735-739.

[13]   Dinis-Ribeiro, M, da Costa-Pereira, A, Lopes, C, et al. Validity of serum pepsinogen I/II ratio for the diagnosis of gastric epithelial dysplasia and intestinal metaplasia during the follow-up of patients at risk for intestinal-type gastric adenocarcinoma. *Neoplasia* 2004; 6: 449-456.

[14] Dinis-Ribeiro, M, Yamaki, G, Miki, K, et al. Meta-analysis on the validity of pepsinogen test for gastric carcinoma, dysplasia or chronic atrophic gastritis screening. *J Med Screen* 2004; 11: 141-147.

[15] Sipponen, P and Graham, DY. Importance of atrophic gastritis in diagnostics and prevention of gastric cancer: application of plasma biomarkers. *Scand J Gastroenterol* 2007; 42: 2-10.

[16] Pasechnikov, VD, Chukov, SZ, Kotelevets, SM, et al. Invasive and non-invasive diagnosis of Helicobacter pylori-associated atrophic gastritis: a comparative study. *Scand J Gastroenterol* 2005; 40: 297-301.

[17] Ren, JS, Kamangar, F, Qiao, YL, et al. Serum pepsinogens and risk of gastric and esophageal cancers in the General Population Nutrition Intervention Trial cohort. *Gut* 2009.

[18] di Mario, F and Cavallaro, LG. Non-invasive tests in gastric diseases. *Dig Liver Dis* 2008; 40: 523-530.

[19] Dixon, MF, Genta, RM, Yardley, JH, et al. Classification and grading of gastritis. The updated Sydney System. International Workshop on the Histopathology of Gastritis, Houston 1994. *Am J Surg Pathol* 1996; 20: 1161-1181.

[20] Mastracci, L, Bruno, S, Spaggiari, P, et al. The impact of biopsy number and site on the accuracy of intestinal metaplasia detection in the stomach. A morphometric study based on virtual biopsies. *Dig Liver Dis* 2008; 40: 632-640.

[21] Graham, DY, Kato, M, and Asaka, M. Gastric endoscopy in the 21st century: appropriate use of an invasive procedure in the era of non-invasive testing. *Dig Liver Dis* 2008; 40: 497-503.

[22] Rugge, M, Correa, P, Dixon, MF, et al. Gastric mucosal atrophy: interobserver consistency using new criteria for classification and grading. *Aliment Pharmacol Ther* 2002; 16: 1249-1259.

[23] Ruiz, B, Garay, J, Johnson, W, et al. Morphometric assessment of gastric antral atrophy: comparison with visual evaluation. *Histopathology* 2001; 39: 235-242.

[24] Jass, JR and Filipe, MI. Sulphomucins and precancerous lesions of the human stomach. *Histopathology* 1980; 4: 271-279.

[25] Jass, JR and Filipe, MI. The mucin profiles of normal gastric mucosa, intestinal metaplasia and its variants and gastric carcinoma. *Histochem J* 1981; 13: 931-939.

[26] El-Zimaity, HM, Ramchatesingh, J, Saeed, MA, et al. Gastric intestinal metaplasia: subtypes and natural history. *J Clin Pathol* 2001; 54: 679-683.

[27] Pagnini, CA and Bozzola, L. Precancerous significance of colonic type intestinal metaplasia. *Tumori* 1981; 67: 113-116.

[28] Pagnini, CA, Farini, R, Cardin, F, et al. Gastric epithelial dysplasia and sulphomucin-type intestinal metaplasia. *Tumori* 1983; 69: 355-357.

[29] Correa, P, Fontham, ET, Bravo, JC, et al. Chemoprevention of gastric dysplasia: randomized trial of antioxidant supplements and anti-helicobacter pylori therapy. *J Natl Cancer Inst* 2000; 92: 1881-1888.

[30] Graham, DY. Helicobacter pylori infection in the pathogenesis of duodenal ulcer and gastric cancer: a model. *Gastroenterology* 1997; 113: 1983-1991.

[31] Fenoglio-Preiser, CM, Carneiro F, Correa P, Guildford P, Lambert R, Megraud F, Munoz N, Powell SM, Rugge M, Sasako M, Stolte M, Watanabe H Gastric carcinoma.

In: S. R. Hamilton, Aaltonen LA (ed.), Pathology & Genetics, *Tumors of the Digestive System.*, pp. 39-52. Lyon: IARC Press, 2000.

[32] Rugge, M and Genta, RM. Staging gastritis: an international proposal. *Gastroenterology* 2005; 129: 1807-1808.

[33] Sipponen, P and Stolte, M. Clinical impact of routine biopsies of the gastric antrum and body. *Endoscopy* 1997; 29: 671-678.

[34] Rugge, M, Correa, P, Di Mario, F, et al. OLGA staging for gastritis: a tutorial. *Dig Liver Dis* 2008; 40: 650-658.

[35] Pang, SH, Leung, WK, and Graham, DY. Ulcers and gastritis. *Endoscopy* 2008; 40: 136-139.

[36] Sung, JJ, Kuipers, EJ, and El-Serag, HB. Systematic review: update on the global incidence and prevalence of peptic ulcer disease. *Aliment Pharmacol Ther* 2009.

[37] Sugano, H, Nakamura, K, and Kato, Y. Pathological studies of human gastric cancer. *Acta Pathol Jpn* 1982; 32 Suppl 2: 329-347.

[38] Stolte, M. Hyperplastic polyps of the stomach: associations with histologic patterns of gastritis and gastric atrophy. *Am J Surg Pathol* 2001; 25: 1342-1344.

[39] Abraham, SC, Park, SJ, Lee, JH, et al. Genetic alterations in gastric adenomas of intestinal and foveolar phenotypes. *Mod Pathol* 2003; 16: 786-795.

[40] Dirschmid, K, Platz-Baudin, C, and Stolte, M. Why is the hyperplastic polyp a marker for the precancerous condition of the gastric mucosa? *Virchows Arch* 2006; 448: 80-84.

[41] Oberhuber, G and Stolte, M. Gastric polyps: an update of their pathology and biological significance. *Virchows Arch* 2000; 437: 581-590.

[42] Genta, RM Gastric Lumps and Bumps: No Polyp is an Island. Rodger C. *Haggitt Gastrointestinal Pathology Society. In:* USCAP Annual Meeting, 2004.

[43] Muehldorfer, SM, Stolte, M, Martus, P, et al. Diagnostic accuracy of forceps biopsy versus polypectomy for gastric polyps: a prospective multicentre study. *Gut* 2002; 50: 465-470.

[44] Graham, DY and Genta, RM. Long-term proton pump inhibitor use and gastrointestinal cancer. *Curr Gastroenterol Rep* 2008; 10: 543-547.

[45] Borch, K, Skarsgard, J, Franzen, L, et al. Benign gastric polyps: morphological and functional origin. *Dig Dis Sci* 2003; 48: 1292-1297.

[46] Garrean, S, Hering, J, Saied, A, et al. Gastric adenocarcinoma arising from fundic gland polyps in a patient with familial adenomatous polyposis syndrome. *Am Surg* 2008; 74: 79-83.

[47] MacDonald, WC and Owen, DA. Gastric carcinoma after surgical treatment of peptic ulcer: an analysis of morphologic features and a comparison with cancer in the nonoperated stomach. *Cancer* 2001; 91: 1732-1738.

[48] Grundmann, E. Histologic types and possible initial stages in early gastric carcinoma. *Beitr Pathol* 1975; 154: 256-280.

[49] Oehlert, W, Keller, P, Henke, M, et al. [Gastric mucosal dysplasias: what is their clinical significance (author's transl)]. *Dtsch Med Wochenschr* 1975; 100: 1950-1956.

[50] Jass, JR. A classification of gastric dysplasia. *Histopathology* 1983; 7: 181-193.

[51] Ming, SC, Bajtai, A, Correa, P, et al. Gastric dysplasia. Significance and pathologic criteria. *Cancer* 1984; 54: 1794-1801.

[52] Riddell, RH. Premalignant and early malignant lesions in the gastrointestinal tract: definitions, terminology, and problems. *Am J Gastroenterol* 1996; 91: 864-872.

[53]   Goldstein, NS and Lewin, KJ. Gastric epithelial dysplasia and adenoma: historical review and histological criteria for grading. *Hum Pathol* 1997; 28: 127-133.

[54]   Lewin, KJ. Nomenclature problems of gastrointestinal epithelial neoplasia. *Am J Surg Pathol* 1998; 22: 1043-1047.

[55]   Riddell, RH and Iwafuchi, M. Problems arising from eastern and western classification systems for gastrointestinal dysplasia and carcinoma: are they resolvable? *Histopathology* 1998; 33: 197-202.

[56]   Lauwers, GY and Riddell, RH. Gastric epithelial dysplasia. *Gut* 1999; 45: 784-790.

[57]   *Japanese classification of gastric carcinoma.* Tokyo: Kanehara & Company, Ltd, 1995.

[58]   Takagi, K, Kumakura, K, Sugano, H, et al. [Polypoid lesions of the stomach-with special reference to atypical epithelial lesions]. *Gan No Rinsho* 1967; 13: 809-817.

[59]   Nagayo, T. Histological diagnosis of biopsied gastric mucosae with special reference to that of borderline lesions. *Gann Monogr* 1971; 11: 245-256.

[60]   Rugge, M, Correa, P, Dixon, MF, et al. Gastric dysplasia: the Padova international classification. *Am J Surg Pathol* 2000; 24: 167-176.

[61]   Kirchner, T, Muller, S, Hattori, T, et al. Metaplasia, intraepithelial neoplasia and early cancer of the stomach are related to dedifferentiated epithelial cells defined by cytokeratin-7 expression in gastritis. *Virchows Arch* 2001; 439: 512-522.

[62]   Hattori, T. Development of adenocarcinomas in the stomach. *Cancer* 1986; 57: 1528-1534.

[63]   Srivastava, A and Lauwers, GY. Gastric epithelial dysplasia: the Western perspective. *Dig Liver Dis* 2008; 40: 641-649.

[64]   de Vries, AC, Meijer, GA, Looman, CW, et al. Epidemiological trends of pre-malignant gastric lesions: a long-term nationwide study in the Netherlands. *Gut* 2007; 56: 1665-1670.

[65]   Rugge, M. Secondary prevention of gastric cancer. *Gut* 2007; 56: 1646-1647.

[66]   Rugge, M, Farinati, F, Baffa, R, et al. Gastric epithelial dysplasia in the natural history of gastric cancer: a multicenter prospective follow-up study. Interdisciplinary Group on Gastric Epithelial Dysplasia. *Gastroenterology* 1994; 107: 1288-1296.

[67]   Rugge, M, Cassaro, M, Di Mario, F, et al. The long term outcome of gastric non-invasive neoplasia. *Gut* 2003; 52: 1111-1116.

[68]   Rugge, M, Cassaro, M, Pennelli, G, et al. Pathology and cost effectiveness of endoscopy surveillance for premalignant gastric lesions. *Gut* 2003; 52: 453-454.

[69]   Garcia, SB, Park, HS, Novelli, M, et al. Field cancerization, clonality, and epithelial stem cells: the spread of mutated clones in epithelial sheets. *J Pathol* 1999; 187: 61-81.

[70]   Karam, SM. Cellular origin of gastric cancer. *Ann N Y Acad Sci* 2008; 1138: 162-168.

[71]   McDonald, SA, Greaves, LC, Gutierrez-Gonzalez, L, et al. Mechanisms of field cancerization in the human stomach: the expansion and spread of mutated gastric stem cells. *Gastroenterology* 2008; 134: 500-510.

[72]   Bai, YQ, Yamamoto, H, Akiyama, Y, et al. Ectopic expression of homeodomain protein CDX2 in intestinal metaplasia and carcinomas of the stomach. *Cancer Lett* 2002; 176: 47-55.

[73]   Rugge, M, Ingravallo, G, Farinati, F, et al. Re: CDX2 homeotic gene expression in gastric noninvasive neoplasia. *Am J Surg Pathol* 2004; 28: 834-835; author reply 835.

[74]   Mera, R, Fontham, ET, Bravo, LE, et al. Long term follow up of patients treated for Helicobacter pylori infection. *Gut* 2005; 54: 1536-1540.

[75]   Rugge, M, Russo, VM, and Guido, M. Review article: what have we learnt from gastric biopsy? *Aliment Pharmacol Ther* 2003; 17 Suppl 2: 68-74.

[76]   Houghton, J, Stoicov, C, Nomura, S, et al. Gastric cancer originating from bone marrow-derived cells. *Science* 2004; 306: 1568-1571.

[77]   El-Rifai, W and Powell, SM. Molecular biology of gastric cancer. *Semin Radiat Oncol* 2002; 12: 128-140.

[78]   Carneiro, F, Oliveira, C, Leite, M, et al. Molecular targets and biological modifiers in gastric cancer. *Semin Diagn Pathol* 2008; 25: 274-287.

[79]   Rugge, M, Bersani, G, Bertorelle, R, et al. Microsatellite instability and gastric non-invasive neoplasia in a high risk population in Cesena, Italy. *J Clin Pathol* 2005; 58: 805-810.

[80]   Jin, Z, Tamura G, Honda T, Motoyama T. Molecular and cellular phenotypic profiles of gastric noninvasive neoplasia. *Lab Invest* 2002; 82: 1637-1645.

[81]   Homma, N, Tamura G, Honda T, Jin Z, Ohmura K, Kawata S, Motoyama T. Hypermethylation of Chfr and hMLH1 in gastric noninvasive and early invasive neoplasias. *Virchows Arch* 2005; 446: 120-126.

[82]   Chong, JM, Fukayama, M, Hayashi, Y, et al. Microsatellite instability in the progression of gastric carcinoma. *Cancer Res* 1994; 54: 4595-4597.

[83]   Seruca, R, Santos, NR, David, L, et al. Sporadic gastric carcinomas with microsatellite instability display a particular clinicopathologic profile. *Int J Cancer* 1995; 64: 32-36.

[84]   Isogaki, J, Shinmura, K, Yin, W, et al. Microsatellite instability and K-ras mutations in gastric adenomas, with reference to associated gastric cancers. *Cancer Detect Prev* 1999; 23: 204-214.

[85]   Lee, JH, Abraham, SC, Kim, HS, et al. Inverse relationship between APC gene mutation in gastric adenomas and development of adenocarcinoma. *Am J Pathol* 2002; 161: 611-618.

[86]   Semba, S, Yokozaki, H, Yamamoto, S, et al. Microsatellite instability in precancerous lesions and adenocarcinomas of the stomach. *Cancer* 1996; 77: 1620-1627.

[87]   Sakurai, S, Sano, T, and Nakajima, T. Clinicopathological and molecular biological studies of gastric adenomas with special reference to p53 abnormality. *Pathol Int* 1995; 45: 51-57.

[88]   Tamura, G, Maesawa, C, Suzuki, Y, et al. Mutations of the APC gene occur during early stages of gastric adenoma development. *Cancer Res* 1994; 54: 1149-1151.

[89]   Tohdo, H, Yokozaki, H, Haruma, K, et al. p53 gene mutations in gastric adenomas. *Virchows Arch B Cell Pathol Incl Mol Pathol* 1993; 63: 191-195.

[90]   Lefebvre, O, Chenard, MP, Masson, R, et al. Gastric mucosa abnormalities and tumorigenesis in mice lacking the pS2 trefoil protein. *Science* 1996; 274: 259-262.

[91]   Tahara, E, Yokozaki H, Yasui W. Stomach-genetic and epigenetic alterations of preneoplastic and neoplastic lesions. *In:* S. Srivastava, Henson DE, Gazdar A (ed.), *Molecular pathology of early cancer.* Ohmsha, Amsterdam, Berlin, Oxford, Tokyo, Washington DC: AIOS-press, 1999.

[92]   Becker, KF, Atkinson, MJ, Reich, U, et al. E-cadherin gene mutations provide clues to diffuse type gastric carcinomas. *Cancer Res* 1994; 54: 3845-3852.

[93]   Higashikawa, K, Yokozaki, H, Ue, T, et al. Evaluation of CD44 transcription variants in human digestive tract carcinomas and normal tissues. *Int J Cancer* 1996; 66: 11-17.

[94]   Schlemper, RJ, Riddell, RH, Kato, Y, et al. The Vienna classification of gastrointestinal epithelial neoplasia. *Gut* 2000; 47: 251-255.

[95]   Genta, RM and Rugge, M. Gastric precancerous lesions: heading for an international consensus. *Gut* 1999; 45 Suppl 1: I5-8.

[96]   Genta, RM and Rugge, M. Review article: pre-neoplastic states of the gastric mucosa - a practical approach for the perplexed clinician. *Aliment Pharmacol Ther* 2001; 15 Suppl 1: 43-50.

[97]   Rugge, M, Leandro, G, Farinati, F, et al. Gastric epithelial dysplasia. How clinicopathologic background relates to management. *Cancer* 1995; 76: 376-382.

[98]   Weinstein, WM and Goldstein, NS. Gastric dysplasia and its management. *Gastroenterology* 1994; 107: 1543-1545.

[99]   Rugge, M, Meggio, A, Pennelli, G, et al. Gastritis staging in clinical practice: the OLGA staging system. *Gut* 2007; 56: 631-636.

[100] Siewert, JR and Stein, HJ. Classification of adenocarcinoma of the oesophagogastric junction. *Br J Surg* 1998; 85: 1457-1459.

[101] Ozde, R, Goldblum J. *Surgical Pathology of the GI Tract, Liver, Biliary Tract, and Pancreas*. Philadelphia: Saunders, 2008.

[102] Fenoglio-Preiser, CM, Isaacson PG, Lantz PE, Noffsinger AE, Stemmermann GN. *Gastrointestinal Pathology: An Atlas and Text*. New York: Lippincott Williams & Wilkins, 2007.

[103] Murakami, T. Pathomorphological diagnosis - definition and gross classification of early gastric cancer. *GANN Monograph on Cancer Research* 1971; 11: 53-55.

[104] Ono, H. Early gastric cancer: diagnosis, pathology, treatment techniques and treatment outcomes. *Eur J Gastroenterol Hepatol* 2006; 18: 863-866.

[105] Son, HJ, Song, SY, Kim, S, et al. Characteristics of submucosal gastric carcinoma with lymph node metastatic disease. *Histopathology* 2005; 46: 158-165.

[106] Arigami, T, Natsugoe, S, Uenosono, Y, et al. Vascular endothelial growth factor-C and -D expression correlates with lymph node micrometastasis in pN0 early gastric cancer. *J Surg Oncol* 2009; 99: 148-153.

[107] Tsukuma, H, Oshima, A, Narahara, H, et al. Natural history of early gastric cancer: a non-concurrent, long term, follow up study. *Gut* 2000; 47: 618-621.

[108] Nitti, D, Mocellin, S, Marchet, A, et al. Recent advances in conventional and molecular prognostic factors for gastric carcinoma. *Surg Oncol Clin N Am* 2008; 17: 467-483, vii.

[109] Borrmann, R Geshwulste des Magens und Duodenums. *In:* L. O. e. Henke F (ed.), *Handbuch der Speziellen Pathologischen Anatomie und Histologie*. Berlin: Springer-Verlag, 1926.

[110] Arslan Pagnini, C and Rugge, M. Gastric cancer: problems in histogenesis. *Histopathology* 1983; 7: 699-706.

[111] Pagnini, CA and Rugge, M. Advanced gastric cancer and prognosis. *Virchows Arch A Pathol Anat Histopathol* 1985; 406: 213-221.

[112] Dixon, MF, Martin, IG, Sue-Ling, HM, et al. Goseki grading in gastric cancer: comparison with existing systems of grading and its reproducibility. *Histopathology 1994; 25: 309-316.*

[113] MacDonald, WC, Owen, DA, and Le, N. Chronic advanced gastric cancer: clinicopathologic analysis of survival data. *Hum Pathol* 2008; 39: 641-649.

[114] Goseki, N, Takizawa, T, and Koike, M. Differences in the mode of the extension of gastric cancer classified by histological type: new histological classification of gastric carcinoma. *Gut* 1992; 33: 606-612.

[115] Ming, SC. Gastric carcinoma. A pathobiological classification. *Cancer* 1977; 39: 2475-2485.

[116] Mulligan, RM. Histogenesis and biologic behavior of gastric carcinoma. *Pathol Annu* 1972; 7: 349-415.

[117] Jass, JR. Role of intestinal metaplasia in the histogenesis of gastric carcinoma. *J Clin Pathol* 1980; 33: 801-810.

[118] Lauren, P. The Two Histological Main Types of Gastric Carcinoma: Diffuse and So-Called Intestinal-Type Carcinoma: an Attempt at a Histo-Clinical Classification. *Acta Pathol Microbiol Scand* 1965; 64: 31-49.

[119] Nakamura, T, Yao, T, Kabashima, A, et al. Loss of phenotypic expression is related to tumour progression in early gastric differentiated adenocarcinoma. *Histopathology* 2005; 47: 357-367.

[120] Morita, H, Ishikawa, Y, Akishima-Fukasawa, Y, et al. Histopathological predictor for regional lymph node metastasis in gastric cancer. *Virchows Arch* 2009; 454: 143-151.

[121] Fukagawa, T, Sasako, M, Shimoda, T, et al. The prognostic impact of isolated tumor cells in lymph nodes of T2N0 gastric cancer: comparison of American and Japanese gastric cancer patients. *Ann Surg Oncol* 2009; 16: 609-613.

[122] Hanisch, E, Hottenrott, C, and Roukos, DH. Circulating cancer cells: could they be used in the clinic as recurrence markers for gastric and colorectal cancer? *Ann Surg Oncol* 2009; 16: 778-779; author reply 780-772.

[123] Gilbert, SM and Hollenbeck, BK. Limitations of lymph node counts as a measure of therapy. *J Natl Compr Canc Netw* 2009; 7: 58-61.

[124] Coburn, NG. Lymph nodes and gastric cancer. *J Surg Oncol* 2009; 99: 199-206.

[125] Verlato, G, Roviello, F, Marchet, A, et al. Indexes of surgical quality in gastric cancer surgery: experience of an Italian network. *Ann Surg Oncol* 2009; 16: 594-602.

[126] Sasako, M, Sano, T, Yamamoto, S, et al. D2 lymphadenectomy alone or with para-aortic nodal dissection for gastric cancer. *N Engl J Med* 2008; 359: 453-462.

[127] Aurello, P, D'Angelo, F, Rossi, S, et al. Classification of lymph node metastases from gastric cancer: comparison between N-site and N-number systems. Our experience and review of the literature. *Am Surg* 2007; 73: 359-366.

[128] Shiraishi, N, Sato, K, Yasuda, K, et al. Multivariate prognostic study on large gastric cancer. *J Surg Oncol* 2007; 96: 14-18.

[129] Sobin, LH, Wittekind C, ed. *TNM classification of malignant tumours,* 6th edition. New York: Wiley-Liss, 2002.

[130] Siewert, JR, Bottcher, K, Stein, HJ, et al. Relevant prognostic factors in gastric cancer: ten-year results of the German Gastric Cancer Study. *Ann Surg* 1998; 228: 449-461.

[131] Nitti, D, Marchet, A, Olivieri, M, et al. Ratio between metastatic and examined lymph nodes is an independent prognostic factor after D2 resection for gastric cancer: analysis of a large European monoinstitutional experience. *Ann Surg Oncol* 2003; 10: 1077-1085.

[132] Rodriguez Santiago, JM, Munoz, E, Marti, M, et al. Metastatic lymph node ratio as a prognostic factor in gastric cancer. *Eur J Surg Oncol* 2005; 31: 59-66.

[133] Cheong, JH, Hyung, WJ, Shen, JG, et al. The N ratio predicts recurrence and poor prognosis in patients with node-positive early gastric cancer. *Ann Surg Oncol* 2006; 13: 377-385.

[134] Liu, C, Lu, P, Lu, Y, et al. Clinical implications of metastatic lymph node ratio in gastric cancer. *BMC Cancer* 2007; 7: 200.

[135] Celen, O, Yildirim, E, and Berberoglu, U. Prognostic impact of positive lymph node ratio in gastric carcinoma. *J Surg Oncol* 2007; 96: 95-101.

[136] Kunisaki, C, Makino, H, Akiyama, H, et al. Clinical significance of the metastatic lymph-node ratio in early gastric cancer. *J Gastrointest Surg* 2008; 12: 542-549.

In: Gastric Cancer: Diagnosis, Early Prevention, and Treatment   ISBN 978-1-61668-313-9
Editor: V. D. Pasechnikov, pp. 151-172   © 2010 Nova Science Publishers, Inc.

Chapter IV

STRATEGIES FOR SCREENING AND EARLY DETECTION OF GASTRIC CANCER

Victor Pasechnikov[1], Sergey Chukov[2], Pentti Sipponen[3]
[1]Department of Therapy, State Medical Academy of Stavropol, Russian Federation
[2]Department of Pathology, State Medical Academy of Stavropol, Russian Federation
[3]Department of Pathology, University of Helsinki, Finland

ABSTRACT

Detection of the Early Gasric Cancer allows us to achieve the high levels of survival of the patients. Thus, we need the screening method(s) which would provide the information for the gastroenterologists about the very early stages of cancer, or, better, about the obvious precancerous changes of the gastric mucosa. The ideal screening method should be non-invasive and non-expensive, and, in the same time, it should have high sensitivity and specificity. This Chapter contains the description of the known methods of screening Gastric Cancer and Precancer, as well as the results of the authors' own experience in the testing the non-invasive screening method for detection of the gastric precancerous changes.

Gastric cancer remains the second biggest cause of cancer death worldwide [1]. Early detection of gastric cancer is vital. Whereas advanced gastric cancer has a poor prognosis, early gastric cancer (EGC) represents a potentially curable stage in the natural history of the disease. Gastrectomy with lymph node dissection in particular has provided an excellent therapeutic outcome for EGC, achieving 5- year survival rates higher than 90% [2]. In addition, early detection might increase the number of patients whose lesion can be treated endoscopically [3, 4, 5].

It has been estimated that EGC progresses to advanced gastric cancer after a median period of 37 months [6]. During this time span EGC proceeds from the asymptomatic and undetectable stage to the asymptomatic but detectable one, and finally to the symptomatic and detectable stage [7]. Patients with advanced cancer typically have severe anemia and malnutrition and sometimes stenotic symptoms at either the pylorus or the cardia. Although no symptoms are caused directly by the tumor itself in EGCs, patients with EGC may develop symptoms, mainly those related to peptic ulcers occurring inside the cancerous mucosa [8-20]. In most cases, gastric cancer is preceded for decades by persistent chronic active gastritis. This became clear in the 1960s and 1970s, when endoscopic biopsy sampling became possible and various excellent cohort studies on the dynamics of gastritis were performed, in particular in Scandinavia and the Baltic States. It appeared that the anatomy and function of the gastric mucosa normally remained unchanged throughout life, unless chronic active gastritis was present [21]. The most common cause of gastritis was unknown at that time, but later it appeared to be Helicobacter pylori colonization. Chronic H. pylori gastritis eventually leads in more than half of the affected subjects to gradual loss of glandular structures with its specialized cells and a collapse of the reticulin skeleton of the mucosa, a condition of atrophic gastritis [22]. As a result, the glandular layer of the mucosa becomes thinner, and glands are replaced by fibrosis and intestinal metaplasia. The major clinical importance of this condition is that it significantly increases the risk for the intestinal type of gastric cancer. This risk may be elevated up to 90 fold in subjects with severe atrophic gastritis throughout the complete stomach [23]. The annual incidence of gastric cancer among patients with atrophic gastritis varied in cohort studies between 0.3 and 1.0% [24].

Invasive cancer is the final step in a cascade of morphological changes which have been defined as multistep oncogenesis [25,26]. These changes are represented histopathologically by superficial gastritis leading to multifocal atrophy, intestinal metaplasia and, finally, dysplasia/cancer [25]. The pathological changes, atrophy and intestinal metaplasia (IM), which have been accepted as precancerous conditions [25], are the serious consequences of H pylori associated infection which are developing at the relatively early stages when the patient can be successfully treated. M. Rugge et al. [27] have summarized the four major biopsy-based contributions to the current knowledge of non-neoplastic gastric diseases: (i) the in vivo definition of gastritis; (ii) the recognition of the clinicopathological patterns of gastritis; (iii) the morphological links between gastritis and stomach cancer; and finally (iv) the recent information on the possible reversibility of early or advanced precancerous gastric lesions. Difficulties in search of proofs that H.pylori-associated chronic atrophic gastritis is undoubtedly precancerous condition are caused by difficulties in clinical diagnosis of gastritis and by uncertainty of concept of atrophy.

The definition and clinical diagnosis of gastritis have always been a known problem. The reason is the absence of characteristic symptoms different from those in patients with other upper gastrointestinal tract disorders. For this reason, gastritis is mainly diagnosed by pathologists, endoscopists, or radiologists rather than clinicians.

Considering a problem of gastric cancer, it is necessary to distinguish the prognostic value of different types of chronic gastritis. Some types rather tend to further development of peptic ulcer disease, whereas others are obviously precancerous state. This different prognosis is of so much importance that allowed to P. Sipponen [28] to recognize so-called "ulcer phenotype" and "cancer phenotype" of gastritis.

According to this division, cumulative risk of peptic ulcer is highest among subjects in whom the H. pylori gastritis occurs in association with nonatrophic corpus mucosa and in whom the gastritis is antrally predominant ("ulcer phenotype"). It was estimated that, among middle-aged men with H. pylori-related nonatrophic gastritis, 20% to 30% may achieve a symptomatic duodenal ulcer (DU) or gastric ulcer (GU) during their lifetime [29]. The another phenotype of gastritis, which is typical in patients with gastric cancer (in those with gastric cancer of intestinal-type, in particular), is often an extensive, multifocal, and advanced atrophic gastritis that is either of H. pylori or autoimmune origin [23,30,31]. Atrophy and metaplasia are seen in biopsies from both antrum and corpus but are particularly prominent in the biopsies from small curvature and incisura angularis [31]. In atrophic gastritis with autoimmune background, atrophy is limited to the corpus in most of the cases and the antrum is normal. In addition to the cases with multifocal atrophic gastritis, the cancer risk is also increased in patients in whom the atrophic gastritis and metaplasia are advanced but limited to the antrum or corpus [23,32]. The retrospective case control studies [23] suggest that atrophic gastritis of the antrum and corpus are independent risk factors for gastric cancer and that the risk of gastric cancer exponentially increases with increasing grade of atrophy. The cancer risk is highest among patients in whom the atrophic gastritis is severe and in whom the atrophy is extensive (i.e., atrophic gastritis occurs in both the antrum and corpus). Among such subjects with a severe "panatrophy" (severe atrophy in both the antrum and corpus), the cancer risk has been estimated to be 90-fold as compared with risk in patients with normal, healthy stomachs [23].

As it was reviewed by P. Sipponen [28], endoscopic biopsies provide information on the type, grade, and extent of inflammation, atrophy, and intestinal metaplasia in the stomach, which may be helpful and, sometimes, is even critical in a proper diagnosis of gastric disorders on an evidence-based basis [33-36]. Classification of gastritis and atrophic gastritis with endoscopic inspection only, without information obtained from the biopsy specimens, may result in errors, both in over- and under-diagnosis of gastritis, and in false conclusions of the status of the gastric mucosa. Even in experienced hands [37], only 83% of patients diagnosed to have "gastritis" by endoscopic inspection showed inflammation in histology. Correspondingly, 17% of patients diagnosed to have healthy mucosa, in fact, had gastritis in histology. The risk of misdiagnosis further increases in less experienced hands and in the presence of atrophic gastritis, in particular.

With the increasing grade and extent of atrophic gastritis, infection itself tends to burn out and the colonization of the mucosa with helicobacter organisms may be minimal. In these cases, the absence of bacteria in biopsy specimens or negative urease biopsy test, or even negative breath test or negative antigen stool test, does not exclude the presence of on-going H. pylori infection and positive H. pylori serology [38,39]. However, microscopy provides significant information on the mucosal status also in these cases. The rationale of gastric biopsy sampling is based upon the fact that inflammation, atrophy (loss of mucosal glands) and intestinal metaplasia are quite widely distributed lesions in the stomach when present and, particularly, when advanced. Therefore, the gastritis-related lesions can be diagnosed with a reasonable degree of reliability by the biopsy specimens [38,40]. Correct interpretation of the histologic appearances requires that five parameters be noted and semiquantitatively graded into three positive categories (mild, moderate, or severe) and separately recorded from biopsies from the antrum and corpus [41]. These five parameters are chronic inflammation (mononuclear inflammation), "activity" (acute, polymorphonuclear inflammation), atrophy (loss of normal glands), intestinal metaplasia, and colonization of biopsies with H. pylori organisms in nonmetaplastic areas of the epithelium [40-42].

How can we reveal the gastric mucosal atrophy in a concrete person, among those suffering from dyspepsia, without the performance of invasive procedure? How can we be sure that our dyspeptic patient is not a "precancerous" patient, i.e., the patient suffering from chronic atrophic gastritis with probable intestinal metaplasia and dysplasia of gastric mucosal epithelium? The answer is – we should have a screening method for diagnosis of atrophic gastritis.

The original definition of screening was done by the UK National Screening Committee [43,44]: Screening is the systematic application of a test or enquiry to identify individuals at sufficient risk of a specific disorder to warrant further investigation or direct preventive action, amongst persons who have not sought medical attention on account of symptoms of that disorder.

The requirements of cancer screening programs differ among countries due to differences in cancer incidence and mortality. In Japan, although the incidence and mortality of gastric cancer have decreased in the last decade, gastric cancer screening is a major issue because the incidence and mortality remain high [45]. Around 1960, gastric cancer screening using photofluorography was started in Miyagi prefecture, and this approach has been adopted nationwide. A national mass screening program for gastric cancer has been active for about 50 years in Japan employing mostly photofluorography [46-51]. This involves double-contrast barium meal studies of the stomach, with seven principal views. With the establishment of the Japanese Society of Gastric Mass Survey in 1962 (later renamed Gastroenterological Mass Survey), the program has spread throughout the country. Cohort and case-control studies generally show a decrease in the mortality risk from gastric cancer because of this program [48]. In 1983, under the Health Service Law for the Aged, gastric cancer screening was introduced for all residents aged 40 years and over. In 2004, 4.4 million inhabitants participated in gastric cancer screening; the screening rate has been around 13% [52]. In Japan, the research group for cancer screening recommended six cancer screening programs in 2001 [53]. Photofluorography was recommended for gastric cancer screening based on the results of several case–control and cohort studies. Although photofluorography screening has been mandated in population-based screening as public policy, other methods including endoscopy, serum pepsinogen testing and Helicobacter pylori antibody testing have been used mainly in the clinical setting for opportunistic screening.

From the 1980s it became evident that esophagogastroduodenoscopy (EGD) was promising in the earlier detection of gastric cancer because of its ability to detect subtle mucosal abnormalities better than radiography. Therefore, endoscopic screening was expected to be an alternative strategy to radiography. Its accuracy is higher, and it enables simultaneous biopsy for histological confirmation of malignancy [54,55]. Nowadays the so-called gastritis-like type of early gastric cancer is increasing in Japan [56,57]. This type of EGC cannot be identified by radiological investigation, so suspicions of its existence are generated during endoscopy and confirmed only by pathology. Furthermore, earlier detection of gastric malignancies increases the possibility of a successful endoscopic treatment instead of surgery [58]. Although the positive predictive value of radiographic screening for gastric cancer organized by the government is only 1%–2%, its sensitivity is 70%–90% [48]. Unfortunately, only 20% of the eligible population aged <40 years accept this governmental screening program [59]. On the other hand, it is believed that each year more than 6 million people are examined by either radiography or EGD outside of the mass screening program. According to the Survey of Medical Care Activities in Public Health Insurance 2004, more than 7.8 million people are examined annually by EGD in Japan. With a population of 85 million <20 years old, 9% of Japanese undergo EGD every year [60]. The explanation for this trend is that endoscopic examination is widely considered to be more accurate for detecting EGC [54,55]. According to the 4th and 5th National Cancer Surveys in Japan [59], gastric cancer (including the advanced cases) is most commonly detected in outpatient clinics, whereas only 6.0% is identified by the government-based mass screening program and 4.6% by private health assessment clinics. In the study of Suzuki H [60], more patients with EGC were diagnosed by the private clinics (28.1%), and the contribution of the mass screening program was less than 10%. Of the asymptomatic patients, only 12.3% participated in the mass screening program; the rest were examined outside of mass screening. Thus, most of the patients with EGC were detected outside the mass screening program regardless of symptoms. In addition, univariate analysis showed that the proportion of men was higher in the asymptomatic group than the symptomatic group. The reason for this discrepancy may be due to the fact that men have greater accessibility to health checkups (including mass screening or private health assessment clinics) at the workplace than women in Japan [60]. The proportion of EGC cases among those of gastric cancer is more than 50% in Japan [46], whereas in the West the proportion is much lower [61]. In the West, it is widely believed that this difference is due to the mass screening program [62]. However, the study of Suzuki et al [60] suggests that the reason for the increased detection of EGC in Japan is not only the success of the mass screening program but also the cautious attitude of Japanese people and physicians toward gastric cancer. The awareness of the risk of gastric cancer and the importance of early detection has increased recently, and many individuals attend private health assessment clinics without symptoms [51]. Also, if individuals have symptoms, they generally seek medical consultation at outpatient clinics. Similarly, all physicians perform some kind of investigation to rule out gastric malignancy. This suggests that outpatient clinics or private clinics have a more important role in early detection than mass screening [60]. From the aspect of medical science, EGD was promising in the earlier detection of gastric cancer [54,55]. To detect gastric cancer at an earlier stage and to reduce the mortality due to gastric cancer, mass screening using EGD may be useful screening program. However, no studies have directly examined whether the screening using EGD reduced the mortality due to gastric cancer. Therefore, this endoscopic screening program should be evaluated in terms of the mortality due to gastric cancer. In addition, from the aspect of medical economics, despite its diagnostic advantages, its cost is much higher and it requires more staff and technical expertise compared to radiology [63]. In financial terms, perhaps its economic efficiency is low [60]. Therefore, at this moment mass screening using EGD with governmental support would be beneficial only in a population at high risk for gastric cancer. Measures similar to those of employed in Japan with an aim of earlier detection of gastric cancer should be considered in the areas with a high incidence of gastric cancer, such as Latin America and eastern Europe [64]. They may decrease the morbidity and mortality of this formidable disease and improve its dismal prognosis throughout the world [60].

Diagnostic accuracy in H. pylori infection is, and will be, an increasing problem in the Western populations in which the incidence rate of H. pylori is rapidly declining [28]. This presupposes that the sensitivity and specificity of the diagnostic test applied to clinical practice has to be high. This may not be the case in many serologic and other noninvasive tests, including the breath test and stool antigen tests. For example, if the sensitivity and specificity of the test is 95%, as is the case in most of the tests, the predictive value of the positive test result is only 68% to 77% if the prevalence of the infection is 15% to 20% in the study population [28].

A growing interest in non-invasive detection of Helicobacter pylori infection and its consequences has led to development of a large number of tests that have been used in different clinical situations or for different purposes. Stool antigen tests have been extensively evaluated in pre- and post-treatment settings both in adults and children, and the urea breath test has been studied as a predictor of bacterial load, severity of gastric inflammation, and response to eradication treatment. Several studies have also explored the usefulness of some serologic markers as indicators of the gastric mucosa status.

The potential indications for the use of non-invasive methods for H. pylori detection include: 1, screening of patients who do not require direct examination of gastric mucosa; 2, difficulties in obtaining biopsies (e.g., bleeding ulcers, anticoagulant therapy); 3, evaluation of eradication efficacy; and 4, epidemiologic studies [65,66]. The urea breath test (UBT) is considered to be the most accurate non-invasive method to detect H. pylori infection. Some studies revealed that the urea blood test had a similar performance to UBT both for diagnosis and assessment of H. pylori eradication [67,68]. Some authors studied the 13C-UBT value as predictor of gastric lesions severity, bacterial load, and response to eradication therapy. Zagari et al. showed a correlation between UBT values, activity of gastritis, and H. pylori colonization density [69], whereas Tseng et al. did not find significant differences in UBT values between patients with gastritis, duodenal ulcer, gastric ulcer, and gastric cancer [70]. The available studies indicate that stool antigen tests are usually inferior to the UBT, but they may represent an alternative option in patients with limited access to UBT who do not require endoscopy of the gastrointestinal tract [65].

Numerous serologic tests are currently available for H. pylori testing. Several studies investigated the usefulness of serologic markers as predictors of the gastric mucosa status. Serum anti-parietal cell antibodies were found to correlate with antral atrophy [71], and serum pepsinogen I/II ratio was inversely related to the grade of corpus atrophy [72]. One study showed that the combination of anti- H. pylori antibodies, serum pepsinogens I and II, and gastrin-17 could be used not only to identify patients with atrophic gastritis but also to localize the site of atrophy [73]. In other studies, anti-H. pylori antibodies combined with serum pepsinogens I and II [74] or the level of H. pylori IgG2 antibodies [75] appeared to be a predictive marker for the development of gastric carcinoma.

Thus, a variety of blood tests exist that indirectly measure the function of antrum and corpus mucosa. Some of these tests could be used as a panel in easy, "noninvasive" diagnosis of the status of the gastric mucosa [28]. The proposed panel consists of a noninvasive H. pylori test, an assay of serum level pepsinogen groups I and II, and a determination of a postprandial increase of serum gastrin-17 after an ingestion of a protein-rich drink or meal. The serum level of pepsinogen group I and serum level of gastrin-17 after prandial stimulus reflect the status of corpus and antral mucosa, respectively, and these test values are decreased in the presence of atrophic gastritis (i.e., in the presence of the loss [atrophy] of oxyntic or antral glands [G cells], respectively). Like endoscopy and microscopic evaluation of the antral and corpus biopsies, the panel of the proposed serologic blood tests could be used in estimation of the risk and likelihood of various gastric diseases.

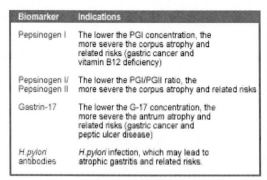
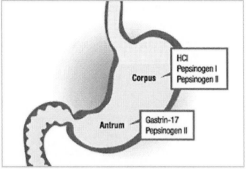

Figure 1. Physiological background and biomarkers for diagnosis of atrophic gastritis (from kind permission of Professor Osmo Suovaniemi).

The substantiation for use of such a diagnostic panel has come from gastric physiology (Figure 1).

Sipponen et al. [76, 77], Oksanen et al. [78], Samloff et al. [79], and other investigators attempted to draw practical conclusions from correlations between mucosal pathology and assessment of different markers of atrophic gastritis [80–83]. PGI is located in the chief and mucous neck cells of the fundic gland (Figure 2) [84]. Thus, if pepsinogen I leaks exclusively from peptic cells in the oxyntic gland area into the circulation and its serum level reflects the secretory activity of these cells, therefore, it was speculated and previously demonstrated that PGI reflects the atrophic condition of the whole stomach induced by H. pylori infection [85] (Figure 3). Furthermore, changing PGI value should reflect the stage of atrophic progression. It should be emphasized that another marker for screening atrophic gastritis and precancerous gastric conditions is the level of plasma pepsinogen II, which, like pepsinogen I, originates from peptic cells of the oxyntic gland areas (Figure 4) as well as those present in the pyloric glands in the antrum (Figure 5) and Brunner's glands of the upper duodenum [76, 79].

Atrophic gastritis involving the entire gastric mucosa may cause a fall in the plasma level of pepsinogen II, which usually shows directional changes similar to those of pepsinogen I [76, 86]. However, because of its partially duodenal origin, it is not considered useful in detecting fundic atrophic gastritis, as pepsinogen I and the ratio of the pepsinogen I/pepsinogen II concentrations, rather than pepsinogen II alone, is considered useful additional marker of high sensitivity and specificity as demonstrated by Sipponen et al. [76], Kitahara et al. [86], and others. The levels of serum gastrin reflects the secretory activity of G cells normally present in the antral mucosa and, in lower numbers, also in the upper duodenum. Hypergastrinemia occurs in patients treated for a long time with proton pump inhibitors, e.g., for reflux esophagitis and, most typically, in gastrinoma [87]. In patients with gastric cancer, moderate to high hypergastrinemia may be considered secondary phenomenon due to hypochlorhydria in fundic atrophic gastritis or cancerous stomach and loss of normal gastric acid-induced suppression of gastrin release from antral G cells, but it may also originate from the cancer cells themselves, which have been shown to be capable of expressing and releasing gastrin [88]. Moreover, the interpretation of changes in gastrin levels in patients with H. pylori infection may change depending on the phase of infection. In the initial, "acute phase" of infection H. pylori colonizes mostly the antral portion of the stomach, causing suppression of the G cells and gastrin release as well as achlorhydria. Later on, after the first phase, when chronic active gastritis develops and lasts for weeks to years, it may be associated with pronounced hypergastrinemia (Figure 6). Typically elevated gastrin levels are observed in the majority of patients with chronic H. pylori infection and atrophy of the oxyntic part of the mucosa such as occur typically in autoimmune metaplastic atrophic gastritis and proximal gastric cancer [23, 88, 90].

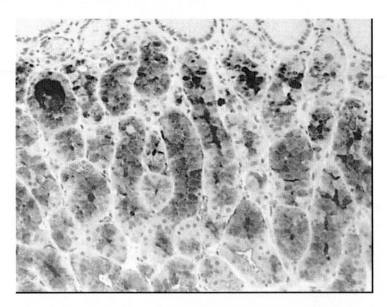

Figure 2. Positive immunohistochemistry for Pepsinogen I in the chief and mucous neck cells of the fundic glands (the preparation of Professor Pentti Sipponen).

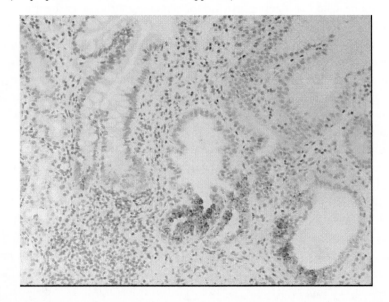

Figure 3. Pepsinogen I in severely atrophic corpus mucosa. Only some cell remnants are stained positively in the atrophic mucosa. The absence of pepsinogen secreting cells is an objective sign of severe atrophy (the preparation of Professor Pentti Sipponen).

Marked atrophy of the antral mucosa related to long-lasting H. pylori infection may, however, lead to a decline in gastrin release (Figure 7) and to decreased serum levels of this hormone as observed by Rembiasz et al. [89]. This phenomenon has been also reported by Sipponen and coworkers [77] and others. This had initiated discussion about the value of assessment of gastrin levels in patients with atrophic gastritis of the antral mucosa. The difference in gastrin concentration become more evident if postprandial levels were taken into consideration. This was observed in all study groups. In patients with atrophy of the mucosa of the antrum, serum gastrin was markedly lower than in controls [89].

In general, the more severe is the atrophic gastritis in the corpus mucosa of the stomach, the lower is the concentration of pepsinogen I and pepsinogen I/II ratio in the blood sample. Similarly, the more severe the atrophic gastritis in the antrum mucosa of the stomach, the lower the measured gastrin-17 concentration. The measured concentrations of pepsinogens (I and II) and gastrin-17 represent the overall condition of the mucosa of the stomach, its functional status and the severity of atrophy.

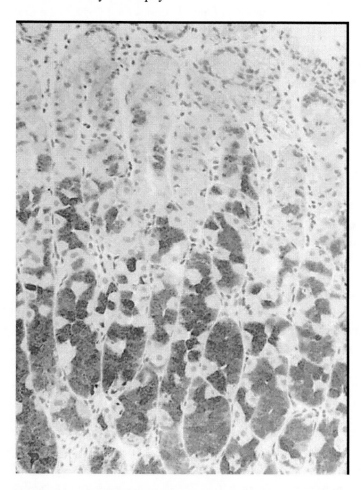

Figure 4. Positive immunohistochemistry for Pepsinogen II in the chief and mucous neck cells of the fundic glands (the preparation of Professor Pentti Sipponen).

To investigate the utility of serum PG1 and/or G-17 concentrations for the objective evaluation of atrophic gastritis, we have performed the study of 360 H. pylori-positive patients with different dyspeptic complaints were investigated. H. pylori positivity was defined by the rapid urease test during endoscopy and was verified by subsequent histologic examination of biopsies. The patients were 38 to 80 years of age and none had received treatment with proton pump inhibitors or NSAIDs (non-steroidal anti-inflammatory drugs) before endoscopy. Basal blood samples for measurement of PG1 and anti-H. pylori antibodies (HPAbs) were drawn after an overnight fast. The samples for postprandial G-17 were taken 20 min after a protein drink containing 10 g protein. The samples were centrifuged at 1500g for 10 min and the serum samples were stored at -20°C until analyzed. Serum specimens were investigated by means of enzyme immunoassay using a commercial program, Biohit GastroPanel ® (Biohit Plc.,Helsinki, Finland) with an estimation of serum G-17 and PG1 levels, and counting the HPAb titers. According to applied instructions, serum concentrations of PG1 <25 µg/l were considered as markers of corpus atrophy; serum concentrations of G-17 <5 pmol/l were considered as markers of antral atrophy, and G-17 <10 pmol/l if PG1 <50 µg/l as markers of mild corpus atrophy. Interpretation of results of HPAb detection was carried out as follows: HPAb titers <32 EIU: negative result; 32-44 EIU: doubtful result; >44 EIU: positive result. In addition, we performed diagnostic upper gastrointestinal endoscopy with biopsy. The biopsies were taken randomly from the antrum (1 from the lesser curvature and 1 from the greater curvature of the middle antrum) and from the corpus (1 from the anterior wall and 1 from the posterior wall of the middle corpus). Biopsy specimens were stained with hematoxylin and eosin, Giemsa and alcian blue (pH 2.5)/PAS stain. The degree of histologic mucosal atrophy was scored on a scale of 0 to 3 according to the updated Sydney System [42]. The histology and the serology were done blindly. The statistics were calculated by means of the computer program Primer of Biostatistics 4.03, using the Mann-Whitney criterion, Spearman's correlation coefficient (r_s), prevalence and mean values, with 95% confidence intervals (95% CI). We also defined the positive predictive value (PPV, the possibility of the presence of disease on obtaining a positive (pathological) result of the test) and negative predictive value (NPV, the possibility of the absence of disease on obtaining a negative (normal) result of the test) for an enzyme immunoassay by Biohit GastroPanel.

The results (Table 1) indicate a consecutive decrease in serum G-17 levels along with a worsening of the antral atrophy; similar decrease in serum levels of PG1 during progression of the corpus atrophy. In the multifocal atrophic gastritis, the values for PG1 and G-17 serum concentrations were significantly lower than the respective cut-off values. Conversely, HPAb titers in the atrophic gastritis were higher than the established cut-off values. Statistical analysis revealed statistically significant differences between the serum levels of PG1 and G-17 measured at different stages of stomach mucosal atrophy, whereas the dynamics of HPAb titers was statistically non-significant.

There was a strong reverse correlation between histological antral atrophy and serum G-17 levels (r_s= -0.63), and between histological corpus atrophy and serum PG1 levels (r_s= -0.86). Moreover, there was a strong reverse correlation between the antral atrophy on endoscopy and the serum G-17 levels (r_s= -0.53), and especially between the corpus atrophy on endoscopy and the serum PG1 levels (r_s= -0.79). Furthermore, the statistical analysis did not reveal any significant differences between the morphological and serological tests in the diagnosis of antral (p=0.826), corpus (p=0.278) or multifocal (p=0.595) atrophy, or in diagnosis of non-atrophic gastritis (p=0.212).

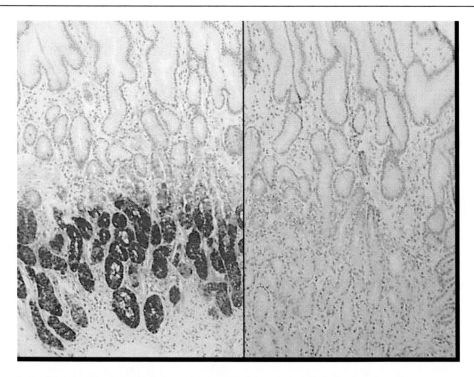

Figure 5. Positive immunohistochemistry for PG1(right) and PG2 (left) in the normal antrum (the preparation of Professor Pentti Sipponen).

Table 1. Mean values of serum PG-1, G-17 concentrations, Hp-Ab titers in the different grades of gastric mucosal atrophy

Histologic diagnosis	PG-1, µg/l	G-17, pmol/l	HPAb, EIU
Non-anrophic gastritis	98,0±10,25	6,88±0,98	62,62±5,63
Corpus-predominant atrophy			
weak	18,71±0,95*		77,21±6,13
moderate	11,91±0,49**		76,47±5,04
severe	6,92±0,45**		85,68±17,81
Antrum-predominant atrophy			
weak		8,91±0,47*	78,25±5,86
moderate		6,40±0,18**	74,08±4,39
severe		1,82±0,26**	73,38±5,38
Multifocal atrophy			
weak	18,15±3,66*	8,45±1,53*	78,45±/30,54
moderate	11,95±2,99**	6,32±1,58**	79,11±/33,40
severe	6,90±2,38**	5,26±2,36**	83,40±/30,22

* $P<0,05$ compared with corresponding non-anrophic state.

** $P<0,05$ compared with corresponding previous degree of atrophy.

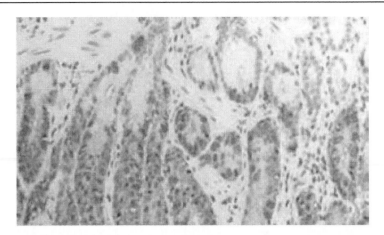

Figure 6. Gastrin-17 in antral mucosa in patients with severe atrophic gastritis in corpus and pernicious anemia. Number of G cells is increased (hyperplasia) in antrum and the cells are strongly stained (from kind permission of Professor Pentti Sipponen).

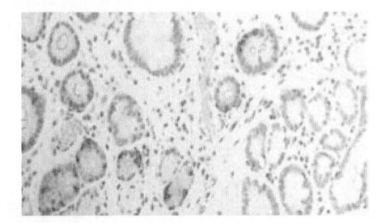

Figure 7. Gastrin-17 in mild atrophic antrum. Number of G cells has remarkably decreased (from kind permission of Professor Pentti Sipponen).

Table 2. Sensitivity (Se) and specificity (Sp), PPV and NPV of Biohit GastroPanel® in diagnosis of stomach mucosal atrophy

The degree of stomach mucosal atrophy (by histology)	Se	Sp	PPV	NPV
No antral atrophy	83%	95%	53%	99%
Mild antral atrophy	61%	84%	45%	91%
Moderate antral atrophy	67%	90%	81%	81%
Severe antral atrophy	89%	99%	98%	94%
No corpus atrophy	92%	97%	98%	91%
Mild corpus atrophy	71%	92%	48%	97%
Moderate corpus atrophy	72%	96%	81%	93%
Severe corpus atrophy	88%	97%	82%	98%

The highest sensitivity of the Biohit Gastro Panel in the diagnostics of atrophic gastritis (see Table 2) was demonstrated in cases of weak and severe antral atrophy and in cases of moderate and severe corpus atrophy. Similarly, the greatest specificity of the Biohit GastroPanel was demonstrated in cases of non-atrophic gastritis and in the presence of severe antral/corpus atrophy. The positive predictive value of the Biohit GastroPanel was maximal in the cases of moderate antral atrophy and in non-atrophic corpus gastritis. The negative predictive value of the Biohit GastroPanel was maximal in the cases of non-atrophic or severe antral atrophic gastritis, as well as in weak and severe corpus gastritis. Overall, the Biohit GastroPanel was quite sensitive and specific in the diagnostics of gastric mucosal atrophy.

In order to assess what preclinical and clinical evidence is currently available, a number of statements were formulated and discussed at a workshop with experts in the field of H. pylori research, held in 2005 in Lejondal, near Stockholm [91]. The evidence for each suggested statement was presented by one of the experts in that particular field and a vote was taken concerning the validity of the statement and the level of supportive documentary evidence. In view of the depth of information required for each statement, two parallel workshops took place, one dealing with experimental and microbiological evidence and the other with clinical evidence. These were followed by a joint plenary session with all experts present, at which they were invited to vote on all statements under discussion and to agree/disagree with the suggested level of the evidence. The statements subjected to the critical analysis are presenred in Table 3.

Table 3. Preclinical Evidence, Clinical Evidence, and Risks subjected to the state-of-the-art critique of evidence on Lejondal H. pylori–Gastric Cancer Task Force [91]

Experimental and microbiological evidence
1. Certain H. pylori characteristics are associated with an increased risk of gastric cancer, but currently genotyping cannot predict individual risk of disease.
2. Host genetic factors contribute to an increased risk of gastric cancer
3. There is strong cell biological evidence to implicate H. pylori in gastric carcinogenesis
4. Experimental studies with animal models provide evidence that eradication of H. pylori at an early time point can prevent gastric cancer development
5. There is correlation between effects of eradication and expression of molecular markers linked to gastric carcinogenesis
Clinical evidence
6a. H. pylori eradication heals chronic activation of atrophic gastritis and halts the progression to preneoplastic conditions (atrophic gastritis and intestinal metaplasia)
6b. In a subset of patients, regression of preneoplastic conditions (atrophic gastritis & intestinal metaplasia) may occur.
7. H. pylori eradication can reduce the risk of developing gastric cancer
Risks
8. The use of antimicrobials for H. pylori is a moderate risk for antimicrobial resistance in H. pylori and other bacteria
9. There is an inverse association between H. pylori infection and GERD
10. H. pylori eradication in the short term does not lead to GERD symptoms and/or erosive esophagitis
11. There is an inverse association between H. pylori infection and esophageal adenocarcinoma.

The contributors to the Lejondal H. pylori–Gastric Cancer Task Force have concluded that H. pylori infection continues to play a key role in acid-related disorders, with a general consensus that colonization with the bacterium invariably results in the outcome of chronic gastritis. Subsets of patients have a progression of the chronic gastritis to either ulcer or cancer. Several indications have proved beneficial over the years but are not as yet implemented on a large scale. Apart from the classical indications such as peptic ulcer [92], there are several other beneficial indications for H. pylori eradication and therapy strategies. In patients with uninvestigated dyspepsia who are less than 45–50 yr of age with no alarm symptoms, the key variable in determining the appropriateness and cost-effectiveness of screening for H. pylori infection versus initiation of empiric proton pump inhibitor therapy is the prevalence of the infection and peptic ulcer disease in the local population. The test and treat approach is considered cost-effective if the prevalence of H. pylori in the population is 20% or greater, while empiric proton pump inhibitor therapy is favored when prevalence is less than 20%. Epidemiological evidence indicates that the proportion of all gastric cancers attributable to H. pylori infection and hence potentially preventable upon elimination of this risk factor is somewhere in the range of 60–90%. This portends significant benefit in terms of morbidity and mortality, not least in populations with high prevalence of H. pylori infection coupled with high incidence of gastric cancer. While there is some discordance regarding who should undergo a search and treat strategy with the current available therapy, there is broad agreement that cure of the infection reduces the risk for gastric cancer development. Whether the association between H. pylori infection and gastric cancer is causal or not is no longer an issue. Largely consistent results from epidemiological studies and animal experiments all support a carcinogenic role of the microorganism, and a web of plausible mechanisms is slowly emerging. Although the true strength of the association, and the proportion of all gastric cancers that can be attributed to H. pylori, is still under debate, it is becoming increasingly evident that the early studies may have underestimated the importance of the infection. The effect of prophylactic eradication on gastric cancer incidence in humans remains unknown, though.

Results from ongoing randomized trials are eagerly awaited, but it will probably take many years before strong conclusive results from such studies will become available, if at all. Given the growing number of studies showing considerable variation in H. pylori strain type and genetic predisposition of the host, and the admittedly remote possibility that elimination of the infection might increase the risk for other adverse health outcomes, including an increase in the prevalence of antibiotic-resistant micro-organisms, there is a need for "simple" risk stratification and a targeted approach to chemoprevention. There is little scientific support for the notion that patients who seek health care for dyspeptic symptoms constitute a high-risk group that should be particularly targeted. This population will, in any case, have the opportunity for therapy with the dual aim of relieving their symptoms and preventing H. pylori-related complications. Presently, the critical question is whether it is justifiable to wait with chemoprevention for another decade or two, until the desired solid scientific data are at hand, or whether prophylactic eradication should be offered already now to some selected groups. In conclusion, a majority of this scientific panel favored a test-and-treat strategy in first-degree relatives of gastric cancer patients. The overwhelming majority also felt that a more general screen-and-treat strategy should be focused in the first instance on a population with a high incidence of H. pylori-associated diseases.

Table 4. Summary of the data provided by the GastroPanel examination and the ^{13}C-urea breath – or stool antigen test of the "test-and-treat" strategy to the doctor in charge.

At an early stage …	The GastroSoft report states:	^{13}C - urea breath test or Stool antigen test report:
The diagnosis for Functional vs. organic dyspepsia. When GastroPanel indicates the gastric mucosa is healthy, the dyspepsia complaints are often caused by functional dyspepsia or another disease not involving the gastric mucosa	YES	NO
H. pylori infection (gastritis)	YES	NOT RELIABLE (1)
Atrophic gastritis (damaged and severely dysfunctional gastric mucosa) and the probabilities of different conditions affecting the mucosa of the gastric corpus or antrum or both (normal, gastritis or atrophic gastritis)	YES	NO
The risks (related to atrophic gastritis) of		
Gastric cancer	YES	YES/NO (2)
Vitamin B12 deficiency	YES	NO
Peptic ulcer disease	YES	YES/NO (3)
The risks of the complications of Gastroesophageal reflux disease:		
Esophagitis and Barrett's esophagus	YES (4)	NO
If necessary, a recommendation for		
Gastroscopy and biopsy examination	YES	NO
Treatment of *H. pylori* infection	YES	YES/NO (5)
Determination of vitamin B12 and homocysteine	YES	NO
Follow-up examination to monitor		
the incidence of atrophic gastritis	YES	NO
the healing of the *H. pylori* infection	YES	YES
the healing of atrophic gastritis	YES	NO

The GastroSoft program supplies a patient report and in consecutive examinations the graphs on the probabilities of different conditions. The reports produced by the stochastic GastroSoft are based on clinical studies comparing the results of GastroPanel examinations with results from gastroscopy and biopsy examinations (www.biohit.com/gastrosoft).

1) The ^{13}C- urea breath - and stool antigen tests give *false negative results* if the patient has *a) atrophic gastritis* (a risk of gastric cancer and peptic ulcer disease and vitamin B12 deficiency and related diseases, such as dementia, depression and polyneuropathies as well as atherosclerosis, strokes and heart attacks), *b) MALT*

lymphoma or *c) bleeding peptic ulcer disease* or *d) if the patient is currently receiving antibiotics or PPIs* (proton pump inhibitors).

2)   The risk of gastric cancer is very low without atrophic gastritis in corpus, antrum or both. But in some cases, a *H. pylori* infection without histologically observable atrophic gastritis may be associated with gastric cancer and peptic ulcer disease.

3)   No peptic ulcer disease with corpus atrophy (no acid, no ulcer). The risk of peptic ulcer disease is very low without antrum atrophy.

4)   High pepsinogen I (over 150 μg /l) and high pepsinogen I and II ratio (over 10) and low gastrin-17 (below 2 pmol /l) indicate high acid (HCl) output (see Figure 8) and risks for the complications of esophageal reflux disease.

5)   When the incidence of *H. pylori* -related atrophic gastritis is monitored, the patient can be offered targeted, safe treatment at the right time. The need for medication and the costs and adverse effects of medication can thus be reduced. If the patient has been diagnosed with peptic ulcer disease (gastric or duodenal ulcer), the *H. pylori* infection has to be treated (6). It should also be treated if the patient has atrophic gastritis. The patient and the doctor may also agree on eradication treatment for other reasons for example when the patient's close relatives have been diagnosed with gastric cancer.

6)   Press Release: The 2005 Nobel Prize in Physiology or Medicine, 3 October 2005 jointly to Barry Marshall and J. Robin Warren for their discovery of "the bacterium *Helicobacter pylori* and its role in gastritis and peptic ulcer disease": - "An indiscriminate use of antibiotics to eradicate *Helicobacter pylori* also from healthy carriers would lead to severe problems with bacterial resistance against these important drugs. Therefore, treatment against *Helicobacter pylori* should be used restrictively in patients without documented gastric or duodenal ulcer disease." http://nobelprize.org/medicine/laureates/2005/press.html

Until now, it has only been possible to diagnose the diseases of the stomach mucosa through H. pylori tests (the "test-and-treat" strategy) and limited endoscopic resources [92]. The test-and-treat strategy is not able to diagnose atrophic gastritis and related risks, such as early gastric cancer, which could be treated successfully in most cases. In addition to this, the ^{13}C urea breath test and stool antigen tests recommended in the test-and-treat strategy give false negative results if the patient has atrophic gastritis, MALT lymphoma or bleeding peptic ulcer disease or if the patient is receiving antibiotics or PPI medication. Therefore, the current diagnosing guidelines for dyspeptic patients and for H. pylori infection do not promote evidence-based, safe treatment. In addition, diagnosis and treatment of dyspepsia-type complaints are often based exclusively on symptoms reported by the patient and good guesses made by the doctor.

Thus, the analysis of the literature data and results of our own research allow us to conclude that the serious medical and ethical problems of the "test and treat" strategy can be corrected simply and economically by replacing its ^{13}C- urea breath – or stool antigen test by the GastroPanel examination (Table 4). Talley et al. (2004) indicate that in many countries, such as Sweden and the US, the "test and treat" strategy alone is not considered sufficient [93]. The H. pylori tests of the "test and treat" strategy does not find atrophic gastirits and related risks, such as gastric cancer and precancerous lesions, which should be confirmed by gastroscopy and biopsy specimen examination and would be successfully treated.

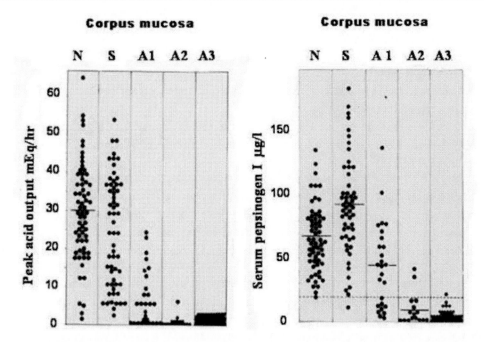

Figure 8. Peak acid (HCl) output and serum pepsinogen I in different grades of atrophic corpus gastritis. Data from the study of Varis and Isokoski [94]; data presented with permission of the authors. Abbreviations: N=normal and healthy corpus mucosa. S=non-atrophic ("superficial") gastritis, A1=mild atrophic gastritis, A2=moderate atrophic gastritis, or A3=severe atrophic gastritis in corpus, respectively.

Consequently, GastroPanel & gastroscopy and biopsy specimen examinations reveal patient with precancerous lesions and early stage gastric cancers, and, therefore, save people from unnecessary deaths because of gastric cancer.

REFERENCES

[1]   Murray CJ, Lopez AD. Mortality by cause for eight regions of the world: global burden of disease study. *Lancet.* 1997; 349: 1269-76.

[2]   Nishi M, Ishihara S, Nakajima T, Ohta K, Ohyama S, Ohta H. Chronological changes of characteristics of early gastric cancer and therapy: experience in the Cancer Institute Hospital of Tokyo, 1950–1994. *J Cancer Res Clin Oncol* 1995;121:535–41.

[3]   Gotoda T, Yanagisawa A, Sasako M, Ono H, Nakanishi Y, Shimoda T, et al. Incidence of lymph node metastasis from early gastric cancer: estimation with a large number of cases at two large centers. *Gastric Cancer* 2000; 3:219–25.

[4]   Gotoda T, Sasako M, Ono H, Katai H, Sano T, Shimoda T. Evaluation of the necessity for gastrectomy with lymph node dissection for patients with submucosal invasive gastric cancer. *Br J Surg* 2001;88:444–9

[5]   Soetikno R, Kaltenbach T, Yeh R, Gotoda T. Endoscopic mucosal resection for early cancers of the upper gastrointestinal tract. *J Clin Oncol* 2005;23:4490–8.

[6]   Tsukuma H, Mishima T, Oshima A. Prospective study of "early" gastric cancer. *Int J Cancer* 1983;31:421–6.

[7]   Look M, Tan YY, Vijayan A, Teh CH, Low CH. Management delays for early gastric cancer in a country without mass screening. *Hepatogastroenterology* 2003;50:873–6.

[8]   Sano T, Katai H, Sasako M, Maruyama K. The management of early gastric cancer. *Surg Oncol* 2000;9:17–22.

[9]   Kong SH, Park do J, Lee HJ, Jung HC, Lee KU, Choe KJ, et al. Clinicopathologic features of asymptomatic gastric adenocarcinoma patients in Korea. *Jpn J Clin Oncol* 2004;34:1–7.

[10] Oliveira FJ, Ferrao H, Furtado E, Batista H, Conceicao L. Early gastric cancer: report of 58 cases. *Gastric Cancer* 1998;1:51–6.

[11] Matsukuma A, Furusawa M, Tomoda H, Seo Y. A clinicopathological study of asymptomatic gastric cancer. *Br J Cancer* 1996;74: 1647–50.

[12] Pinto E, Roviello F, de Stefano A, Vindigni C. Early gastric cancer: report on 142 patients observed over 13 years. *Jpn J Clin Oncol* 1994;24:12–9.

[13] Boldys H, Marek TA, Wanczura P, Matusik P, Nowak A. Even young patients with no alarm symptoms should undergo endoscopy for earlier diagnosis of gastric cancer. *Endoscopy* 2003;35: 61–7.

[14] Fernandez E, Porta M, Malats N, Belloc J, Gallen M. Symptom-to-diagnosis interval and survival in cancers of the digestive tract. *Dig Dis Sci* 2002;47:2434–40.

[15] Everett SM, Axon ATR. Early gastric cancer in Europe. *Gut* 1997;41:142–50.

[16] Maruyama M, Barreto-Zuniga R, Kimura K. Misconceptions on early gastric cancer in Japan. *Hepatogastroenterology* 2001;48: 1560–4.

[17] Eckardt VF, Giessler W, Kanzler G, Remmele W, Bernhard G. Clinical and morphological characteristics of early gastric cancer: a case-control study: *Gastroenterology* 1990;98:708–14.

[18] Biasco G, Paganelli GM, Azzaroni D, Grigioni WF, Merighi SM, Stoja R, et al. Early gastric cancer in Italy: clinical and pathological observations on 80 cases. *Dig Dis Sci* 1987;32:113–20.

[19] Malcolm R. Dyspepsia: Challenges in diagnosis and selection of treatment. *Clin Therapeutics* 2001;23:1130–44.

[20] Agreus L, Talley N. Dyspepsia: current understanding and management. *Annu Rev Med* 1997;49:475–93.

[21] Correa P, Haenszel W, Cuello C, Tannenbaum S, Archer M. A model for gastric cancer epidemiology. *Lancet.* 1975; 2: 58-9.

[22] Kuipers EJ, Uyterlinde AM, Pena AS, Roosendaal R, Pals G, Nelis GF. Long term sequelae of Helicobacter pylori gastritis. *Lancet.* 1995;345: 1525-8.

[23] Sipponen P, Kekki M, Haapakoski J, Ihamaki T, Siurala M. Gastric cancer risk in chronic atrophic gastritis: statistical calculations of crosssectional data. *Int J Cancer.* 1985; 35: 173-7.

[24] Kuipers EJ. Review article: relationship between Helicobacter pylori, atrophic gastritis and gastric cancer. *Aliment Pharmacol Ther.* 1998; 12: 25-36.

[25] Correa P. A human model of gastric carcinogenesis. *Cancer Res.* 1988;48:3554–60.

[26] Correa P. Human gastric carcinogenesis: a multistep and multifactorial process. First American Cancer Society Award Lecture on Cancer Epidemiology and Prevention. *Cancer Res.* 1992;52:6735–40.

[27]   Rugge M., Russo V. M. & Guido M. Review article: what have we learnt from gastric biopsy? *Aliment Pharmacol Ther*. 2003; 17 (Suppl. 2): 68–74.

[28]   Sipponen P. Update on the Pathologic Approach to the Diagnosis of Gastritis, Gastric Atrophy, and Helicobacter pylori and its Sequelae. *J Clin Gastroenterol*. 2001;32(3):196–202.

[29]   Sipponen P, Varis K, Fraki O, et al. Cumulative 10-year risk of symptomatic duodenal and gastric ulcer in patients with or without gastritis. A clinical follow up of 454 outpatients. *Scand J Gastroenterol*. 1990;25:966–73.

[30]   Sipponen P, Hyvarinen H, Siurala M. H. pylori corpus gastritis: relation to acid output. *J Physiol Pharmacol*. 1996;47:151–9.

[31]   Yardley JH. Pathology of chronic gastritis and duodenitis. In: Goldman H, Appelman HD, Kaufman N, eds. Gastrointestinal pathology. Baltimore: William & Wilkins, 1990:69–143

[32]   Varis K. Surveillance of pernicious anemia. In: Sherlock P, Morson BC, Barbara L, et al., eds. Precancerous lesions of the gastrointestinal tract. New York: Raven Press, 1983:189–94.

[33]   Correa P. The epidemiology and pathogenesis of chronic gastritis: three etiologic entities. *Front Gastrointest Res*. 1980;6:98-108

[34]   Sipponen P, Kekki M, Siurala M. The Sydney System: Epidemiology and natural history of chronic gastritis. *J Gastroenterol Hepatol*. 1991;6:244–251.

[35]   Siurala M, Sipponen P, Kekki M. Chronic gastritis: dynamic and clinical aspects. *Scand J Gastroenterol*. 1985;20(suppl 109):69–76.

[36]   Graham DY. Helicobacter pylori: its epidemiology and its role in duodenal ulcer disease. *Gastroenterol Hepatol*. 1991;6:105–13.

[37]   Mihara M, Haruma K, Kamada T, et al. The role of endoscopic findings for the diagnosis of Helicobacter pylori infection: evaluation in a country with high prevalence of atrophic gastritis. *Helicobacter*. 1999;4:40–8.

[38]   Kokkola A, Rautelin H, Puolakkainen P, et al. Diagnosis of Helicobacter pylori infection in patients with atrophic gastritis: comparison of histology, 13C-urea breath test, and serology. *Scand J Gastroenterol*. 2000;35:138–41.

[39]   Karnes WE Jr, Samloff IM, Siurala M, et al. Positive serum antibody and negative tissue staining of Helicobacter pylori in subjects with atrophic gastritis. *Gastroenterology*. 1991;101:167–74

[40]   Andrew A, Wyatt JI, Dixon MF. Observer variation in the assessment of chronic gastritis according to the Sydney system. *Histopathology*. 1994;25:317–22

[41]   Price AB. The Sydney system: Histological division. *J Gastroenterol Hepatol*. 1991;6:209–222.

[42]   Dixon MF, Genta RM, Yardley JH, Correa P, participants in the InternationalWorkshop on the Histopathology of Gastritis, Houston 1994. Classification and grading of gastritis. The updated Sydney system. *Am J Surg Pathol*. 1996;20:1161–1181.

[43]   Wald NJ. Guidance on terminology. *J Med Screen* 1994;1:76

[44]   Wald N., Editorial. The definition of screening. *J Med Screen* 2001;8:1.

[45]   Nomura K, editor. Cancer Statistics in Japan 2005. Tokyo: Foundation for Promotion Cancer Research 2006.

[46]   Hisamichi S. Screening for gastric cancer. *World J Surg* 1989;13:31–7.

[47]   Tsubono Y, Nishino Y, Hisamichi S. Screening for gastric cancer in Miyagi, Japan: evaluation with a population-based cancer registry. *Asian Pacific J Cancer Prev* 2000;1:57–60.

[48]   Tsubono Y, Nishino Y, Hisamichi S. Screening for gastric cancer in Japan. *Gastric Cancer* 2000;3:9–18.

[49]   Shiratori Y, Nakagawa S, Kikuchi A, Ishii M, Ueno M, Miyashita T, et al. Significance of a gastric mass screening survey. *Am J Gastroenterol* 1985;80:831–4.

[50]   Han JY, Son H, Lee WC, Choi BG. The correlation between gastric cancer screening method and the clinicopathologic features of gastric cancer. *Med Oncol* 2003;20:265–9.

[51]   Kampschoer GH, Fujii A, Masuda Y. Gastric cancer detected by mass survey: comparison between mass survey and outpatient detection. *Scand J Gastroenterol* 1989;24:813–7.

[52]   Statistics and Information Department, Ministry of Health, Labour, and Welfare. National Reports on Cancer Screening Programs 2004. Tokyo: Health and Welfare Statistics Association 2006.

[53]   Hamashima C. The Japanese Guidelines for Gastric Cancer Screening. *Jpn J Clin Oncol* 2008;38(4)259–267

[54]   Hosokawa O, Watanabe K, Hattori M, Douden K, Hayashi H, Kaizaki Y. Detection of gastric cancer by repeat endoscopy within a short time after negative examination. *Endoscopy* 2001;33:301– 5

[55]   Triantafillidis JK, Cheracakis P. Diagnostic evaluation of patients with early gastric cancer — a literature review. *Hepatogastroenterology* 2004;51:618–24.

[56]   Yoshida S, Yamaguchi H, Tajiri H, Saito D, Hijikata A, Yoshimori M, et al. Diagnosis of early gastric cancer seen as less malignant endoscopically. *Jpn J Clin Oncol* 1984;14:225–41.

[57]   Yoshida S, Yoshimori M, Hirashima T, Yamaguchi H, Tajiri H, Nakamura K, et al. Nonulcerative lesion detected by endoscopy as an early expression of gastric malignancy: retrospective observation of 72 cases of gastric carcinoma. *Jpn J Clin Oncol* 1981;11:495–506.

[58]   Ono H, Kondo H, Gotoda T, Shirao K, Yamaguchi H, Saito D, et al. Endoscopic mucosal resection for treatment of early gastric cancer. *Gut* 2001; 48:225–9.

[59]   Cancer statistics in Japan — 1997. Foundation for Promotion of Cancer Research, National Cancer Center, 1997.

[60]   Suzuki H. Detection of early gastric cancer: misunderstanding the role of mass screening. *Gastric Cancer* 2006; 9: 315–319.

[61]   Sue-Ling HM, Martin I, Griffith J, Ward DC, Quirke P, Dixon MF, et al. Early gastric cancer: 46 cases treated in one surgical department. *Gut* 1992;33:1318–22.

[62]   Everett SM, Axon ATR. Early gastric cancer: disease or pseudodisease. *Lancet* 1998; 351:1350–2.

[63]   Waye JD, Aabakken L, Armengol-Miro JR, Llorens P, Williams CB, Zhang QL. Screening for GI cancer and payment mechanisms. *Gastrointest Endosc* 2002;55:453–4

[64]   Cancer statistics in Japan — 2005. Foundation for Promotion of Cancer Research, National Cancer Center, 2005.

[65] Dzierzanowska-Fangrat K., Lehours P., Megraud F., Dzierzanowska D. Diagnosis of Helicobacter pylori Infection. *Helicobacter*. 2006;11 (Suppl.1): 6–13

[66] Hirschl AM, Makristathis A. Non-invasive Helicobacter pylori diagnosis: stool or breath tests? *Dig Liver Dis*. 2005;37:732–4.

[67] Ahmed F, Murthy UK, Chey WD, Toskes PP, Wagner DA. Evaluation of the Ez-HBT Helicobacter blood test to establish Helicobacter pylori eradication. *Aliment Pharmacol Ther*. 2005;22:875–80.

[68] Fry LC, Curioso WH, Rickes S, Horton G, Hirschowitz BI, Monkemuller K. Comparison of 13C-urea blood test to 13C-breath test and rapid urease test for the diagnosis of Helicobacter pylori infection. *Acta Gastroenterol Latinoam*. 2005;35:225–9.

[69] Zagari RM, Pozzato P, Martuzzi C, et al. 13C-urea breath test to assess Helicobacter pylori bacterial load. *Helicobacter*. 2005;10:615–9.

[70] Tseng CA, Wu JY, Pan YS, Yu FJ, Fuccio L, Martinelli G, Roda E, Bazzoli F. Comparison of 13C-urea breath test values in gastric cancer, peptic ulcer, and gastritis. *Hepatogastroenterology*. 2005;52:1636–40.

[71] Lo CC, Hsu PI, Lo GH, et al. Implications of anti-parietal cell antibodies and anti-Helicobacter pylori antibodies in histological gastritis and patient outcome. *World J Gastroenterol*. 2005;11:4715–20.

[72] Graham DY, Nurgalieva ZZ, El-Zimaity HM, Opekun AR, Campos A, Guerrero L, Chavez A, Cardenas V. Non-invasive versus histologic detection of gastric atrophy in a Hispanic population in North America. *Clin Gastroenterol Hepatol*. 2006;4:306–14.

[73] Germana B, Di Mario F, Cavallaro LG, et al. Clinical usefulness of serum pepsinogens I and II, gastrin-17, and anti-Helicobacter pylori antibodies in the management of dyspeptic patients in primary care. *Dig Liver Dis*. 2005;37:501–8.

[74] Watabe H, Mitsushima T, Yamaji Y, Okamoto M, Wada R, Kokubo T, Doi H, Yoshida H, Kawabe T, Omata M. Predicting the development of gastric cancer from combining Helicobacter pylori antibodies and serum pepsinogen status: a prospective endoscopic cohort study. *Gut*. 2005;54:764–8.

[75] Ren Z, Borody T, Pang G, Li LC, Dunkley M, Clancy R. Selective reduction of anti-Helicobacter pylori IgG subclass antibody in gastric carcinoma. *J Gastroenterol Hepatol*. 2005;20:1338–43.

[76] Sipponen P, Samloff IM, Saukkonen M,Varis K. Serum pepsinogens I and II and gastric mucosal histology after partial gastrectomy. *Gut*. 1985;26:1179–1182.

[77] Sipponen P, Linnala A, Sande N, Vaananen H, Rasmussen M, Tunturi-Hihnala H, Sotka M, Turunen M, Sandstrom R, Heiskanen I, Suovaniemi O, Harkonen M. Serum levels of gastrin-17 pepsinogen I and H. pylori antibodies in nonendoscopic diagnosis of atrophic gastritis. *Gut*. 2001;49:1718.

[78] Oksanen A, Sipponen P, Karttunen R, Miettinen A, Veijola L, Sarna S, Rautelin H. Atrophic gastritis and Helicobacter pylori infection in outpatients referred for gastroscopy. *Gut*. 2000;46(4):460–463.

[79] Samloff IM, Varis K, Ihamaki T, Siurala M, Rotter JI. Relationships among serum pepsinogen I, pepsinogen II and gastric mucosal histology. A study in relatives of patients with pernicious anemia. *Gastroenterology*. 1982;83:204–209.

[80] Knight T, Wyatt J, Wilson A, Greaved S, Newell D, Hengels K, Corlett M, Webb P, Forman D, Elder J. H. pylori gastritis and serum pepsinogen levels in a healthy

population: development of a biomarker strategy for gastric atrophy in a high risk group. *Br J Cancer*. 1996;73:819–824.

[81]   Matsumoto K, Konishi N, Ohshima M, Hiasa Y, Kimura E, Samori T. Association between Helicobacter pylori infection and serum pepsinogen concentration in gastroduodenal diseases. *J Clin Pathol*. 1996;49:1005–1008.

[82]   Plebani M, Basso D, Scrigner M, Toma A, Di Mario F, Dal Bo N, Samloff IM. Serum pepsinogen C a useful marker of H. pylori eradication? *J Clin Lab Anal*. 1996;10(1):1–5.

[83]   Westerveld BD, Pals G, Lamers CB, Defize J, Pronk JC, Frants RR, Ooms EC, Kreuning J, Kostense PJ, Eriksson AW. Clinical significance of pepsinogen A isozymogens, serum pepsinogen A and C levels, and serum gastrin levels. *Cancer*. 1987;59:952–958.

[84]   Samloff IM. Cellular localization of group I pepsinogens in human gastric mucosa by immunofluorenscence. *Gastroeterology*. 1971;61:185–188.

[85]   Karita M, Noriyasu A, Kosako E, Teramukai S, Matsumoto S. Relationship between pepsinogen I&II and H. pylori infection considered with grade of atrophy and gastroduodenal diseases. *Dig Dis Sci*. 2003;48:1839–1845.

[86]   Kitahara F, Kobyashi K, Sato T, Kojima Y, Araki T, Fujimo MA. Accracy of screening of gastric cancer using serum pepsinogen concentrations. *Gut*. 1999;44:693–697.

[87]   Konturek SJ, Konturek PC, Bielanski W, Lorens K, Sito E, Konturek JW, Kwiecien S, Bobrzynski A, Pawlik T, Karcz D, Areny H. Case presentation of gastrinoma combined wih carcinoidband with longest survival record—Zollinger–Ellison syndrome. *Med Sci Monit*. 2002;8:CS43–59.

[88]   Konturek PC, Konturek SJ, Bielanski W, Kania J, Zuchowicy M, Harwich A, Rehfeld JF, Hahn EG. Influence of COX-2 inhibition by rofecoxib on serum and tumor progastrin and gastrin levels and expression of PPARgamma and apoptosis-related proteins in gastric cancer patients. *Dig Dis Sci*. 2003 Oct; 48(10):2005-17.

[89]   Rembiasz K., Konturek P. C., Karcz D., Konturek S. J., Ochmanski W., Bielanski W., Budzynski A., Stachura J. Biomarkers in Various Types of Atrophic Gastritis and Their Diagnostic Usefulness. *Dig Dis Sci*. 2005; 50(3):474–482.

[90]   Waldum HL, Fossmark, Bakke I, Martinsen TC, Qvigstad G. Hypergastrinemia in animals and man. Causes and consequences. *Scand J Gastroenterol*. 2004;39:505–509.

[91]   Malfertheiner P., Sipponen P., Naumann M., Moayyedi P., Megraud F., Xiao S.–D., Sugano K., Nyren O. Helicobacter pylori Eradication Has the Potential to Prevent Gastric Cancer: A State-of-the-Art Critique. *Am J Gastroenterol* . 2005;100: 2100–2115.

[92]   Malfertheiner P, Megraud F, O'Morain C, et al. Current concepts in the management of Helicobacter pylori infection—The Maastricht 2-2000 Consensus Report. *Aliment Pharmacol Ther*. 2002;16:167–80.

[93]   Talley NJ, Vakil N, Delaney G, et al. Management issues in dyspepsia: current consensus and controversies. *Scand J Gastroenterol*. 2004;39 (10): 913-918.

[94]   Varis K, Isokoski M. Screening of type A gastritis. *Ann Clin Res*. 1981;13(3):133-8.

In: Gastric Cancer: Diagnosis, Early Prevention, and Treatment   ISBN 978-1-61668-313-9
Editor: V. D. Pasechnikov, pp. 173-196   © 2010 Nova Science Publishers, Inc.

Chapter V

PRIMARY AND SECONDARY PREVENTION OF GASTRIC CANCER AND EARLY GASTRIC CANCER RECURRENCE AFTER ENDOSCOPIC REMOVAL

Jan Bornschein, Michael Selgrad, Peter Malfertheiner[*]

Department of Gastroenterology, Hepatology and Infectious Diseases,
Otto-von-Guericke-University of Magdeburg, Leipziger Str.44, D-39120 Magdeburg,
Germany

ABSTRACT

Detection and eradication of *H. pylori* infection appears to be the only promising preventive strategy at the moment although its effectiveness is not definitely proven yet. High risk individuals, like first degree family members of gastric cancer patients should be evaluated for the status of *H. pylori* infection and under certain criteria also for the presence of genetic alterations like mutations of the e-cadherin gene or polymorphisms of the IL1-β gene. Endoscopy is the most reliable screening modality, best for reasons of cost-effectiveness it can only be recommended for high-incidence regions where experienced examiners are available in sufficient numbers. Serological tests (*H. pylori* antibody, pepsinogen 1, gastrin 17) are not ready for routine gastric cancer screening, but can provide information to identify individuals at high risk. The identification of more robust serological markers for preselection of patients for endoscopic screening will be an important task for the next years.

Environmental and dietary factors hold some value but interventional studies have not obtained significant results for gastric cancer prevention.

---

[*] Corresponding author: Peter Malfertheiner, Department of Gastroenterology, Hepatology and Infectious Diseases, Otto-von-Guericke-University of Magdeburg, Leipziger Str. 44, D-39120 Magdeburg. Tel: 0049 391 6713100; Fax: 0049 391 6713105. Email: peter.malfertheiner@med.ovgu.de

INTRODUCTION

Gastric cancer is usually diagnosed at an advanced stage with only limited treatment options available. There is tremendous need for effective tools for prevention and early detection of gastric cancer (see also Chapter IV). In case of early gastric carcinoma treated by endoscopic mucosal resection (EMR) or limited surgical removal of parts of the stomach, recurrence rates in the stomach remnant are high for both local and metastastic disease. Therefore, research should also focus on means for the fight against recurrence.

Besides surveillance strategies after curative partial gastric resection or endoscopic treatment, prevention of recurrence relies on the elimination of the persistent risk condition.

The main impact is given by eradication of *H. pylori*. Indeed, treatment of the *H. pylori* infection has not only the potential to prevent gastric cancer, but also reduces the recurrence rate of gastric neoplasia after EMR or endoscopic submucosal dissection [1]. International guidelines so far, have not addressed the issue of secondary gastric cancer prevention whereas the role of *H. pylori* eradication is recognized in both the Western world as well as for the Asia-Pacific region [2;3]. In the Japanese guidelines *H. pylori* eradication is recommended at class B level after the EMR of early gastric cancer, and in case of atrophic gastritis [4].

Aim of this overview is to address the rationale for *H. pylori* treatment in the primary and secondary gastric cancer prevention as well as the role of non-invasive surveillance strategies.

H. PYLORI AND GASTRIC CANCER RISK

Infection with *Helicobacter pylori* (*H. pylori*) is the major risk factor for the development of gastric cancer and medical intervention represents the best option for prevention of the disease. In 1994, the WHO classified *H. pylori* as class I carcinogene based mainly on epidemiological evidence for its role in the pathogenesis of gastric adenocarcinoma [5]. The infection rate with *H. pylori* varies among the populations, but remains still high (40-50%) in people over 50 years of age in many Western countries.

Numerous studies attempted to assess the attributable risk of *H. pylori* infection for gastric carcinogenesis. An important analysis has been presented by the *Helicobacter* and Cancer Collaborative Group evaluating the combined data from all (and only) case control studies nested with prospective cohorts to assess more reliably the relative risk of gastric cancer. In this study 1228 patients were included and a clear association of *H. pylori* infection to non-cardia gastric cancer (OR 3.0; 95% CI 2.3-3.8) was reported. This association was even stronger when blood samples for *H. pylori* serology were obtained 10 years or longer before cancer diagnosis (OR 5.9; 3.4-10.3) [6]. An explanation is the loss of *H. pylori* colonization in the presence of atrophic gastritis and IM, so that gastric cancer patients have a negative serological Helicobacter result, although they have been formerly infected.

Another meta-analysis from Asia analysed 19 studies including approximately 2500 gastric cancer patients and almost 4000 matched controls. This study demonstrated an OR of 1.92 (1.32-2.78) for the development of non-cardia gastric cancer in *H. pylori* positive patients [7] which was in concordant with a previous similar analysis [8].

For a more meticulous assessment of the *H. pylori*-attributable risk for gastric carcinogenesis, bacterial virulence factors had been taken into consideration for risk analysis.

Several studies have shown, that the risk of gastric cancer is influenced by the presence of the cytotoxic antigen A (cagA), that is translocated by a type IV secretion system in the host epithelial cell leading to higher degrees of inflammation [9]. A meta-analysis by Huang and colleagues revealed a further 1.64-fold increase of GC risk for cagA-positive strains compared to cagA-negative ones (16 studies, n = 5054) [10]. Ekström reported an increase of the *H. pylori*-attributable OR for non-cardia cancer from 2.2 to 21.0 if the cagA status was co-evaluated by immunoblot analysis [11]. In this analysis, 71 to 91% of GC in the studied population was attributable to *H. pylori* infection.

H. PYLORI ERADICATION FOR GASTRIC CANCER PREVENTION

Despite the strong evidence for the pathogenetic relevance of *H. pylori* in gastric cancer development, the decisive question has not been answered yet: Has eradication of *H. pylori* the potential to prevent gastric cancer? Evidence pointing towards a positive answer is given by observational and interventional studies. A retrospective multicenter study from Japan analysed the GC incidence in patients after *H. pylori* eradication for a 5-years follow-up in 23 centers including more than 3000 patients [12]. GC developped in 1% of patients who had been successfully eradicated and 4% of patients with persistent infection (OR 0.36; 0.22-0.62). Uemura and colleagues could demonstrate in an observational study, that gastric cancer develops only in persons infected with *H. pylori*, but not in uninfected persons [13]. They performed upper gastrointestinal endoscopy on 1526 patients for dyspeptic symptoms or dyspeptic ulcer disease. During a median follow-up period of 7.8 years, 36 of the *H. pylori*-positive patients (2.9%) developed gastric cancer, in contrast to no case (0%) of gastric malignancy among the *H.pylori*-negative patients [13].

In a prospective interventional study from Japan, patients suffering from *H. pylori*-induced peptic ulcer disease have been followed up(n = 1342) for a median of 3.4 years [14]. Eradication therapy was not successful in 15%. GC occurred in 0.8% of the successfully eradicated patients in contrast to 2.3% of patients with eradication failure [14]. Unfortunately, statistical significance was not reached.

A prospective, randomized, placebo-controlled, population-based primary prevention study has been performed in China [15]. In total, 1630 healthy individuals were recruited for randomization on either *H. pylori* eradication treatment or placebo scheme. Within a follow-up period of 7.5 years, there have been 18 new cases of GC, 7 in the eradication group and 11 in the placebo group (P = 0.33). However, subgroup analysis of individuals that presented with preneoplastic mucosal alterations at baseline, revealed six patients with first diagnosis of GC in the placebo group versus no case in patients with successfull *H.pylori* eradication (P = 0.02) [15].

Table 1 gives an overview about further interventional studies that have been performed to analyse the effect of *H. pylori* eradication on GC incidence (Table 1).

Table 1. H. pylori and incidence of gastric cancer

Author	Year	Country	Number of pat.	Typ of study	Primary end point	Follow-up	Gastric cancer incidence
Uemura [16]	1997	Japan	132	prospective, placebo-controlled	Occurence of gastric cancer after endoscopic removal of early gastric cancer	3 years	Hp neg: 0/65 (0 %), Hp pos: 6/67 (9 %) (p=0.011)
Saito [17]	2000	Japan	64	prospective, placebo-controlled	Progression of an adenoma in *H. pylori*-positive patients	2 years	Hp neg: 0/32 (0 %), Hp pos: 4/32 (12,5 %) (p<0.05)
Uemura [13]	2001	Japan	1526	prospective, case-control	Occurence of gastric cancer in *H. pylori*-positive patients	7.8 years	Hp neg: 0/280 (0 %), Hp pos: 36/1246 (2.9 %) (*P*<0.001)
Wong [15]	2004	China	1630	populationbased, prospective, randomised, placebo-controlled	Occurence of gastric cancer after *H. pylori* eradication	7.5 years	Patients without precancerous lesions: Hp neg: 0 vs. Hp pos: 6 (p=0.02) No difference concerning pat. with precancerous lesions
Zhou [18]	2005	China	552	populationbased, prospective, randomised, placebo-controlled	Occurence of gastric cancer after *H. pylori* eradication	8 years	Hp neg: 1/246 (0.4 %) Hp pos: 6/306 (2.0 %) H. pylori-eradication results in significant reduction of gastric atrophy
Leung [19]	2004	China	435	randomised, double-blinded, placebo-controlled	Occurence of gastric cancer after *H. pylori* eradication	5 years	Hp pos: eradication: 4/220 (1.8%); placebo: 6/215 (2.8%)
Take [14]	2005	Japan	1120	Non-randomised, not double-blinded, not placebo-controlled	Re-infection, or further antibiotic treatment	3.4 years	After eradication: Succesfull eradication: 8/944 (0.8%) Hp-persistencacy: 4/176 (23%)
You [20]	2006	China	3365	randomised, double-blinded, placebo-controlled	Occurence of gastric cancer/premalignant lesions of defined dignity	7.3 years	Hp pos patients: eradikation: 19/1130 (1.7%) placebo: 27/1128 (2.4%)

Ogura [21]	2006	Japan	708	Non-radomised	Occurence of gastric cancer	3 years	Hp pos: 13/304 (4.3%) Hp neg: 6/404 (1.5%) Difference in incidence only for highly differenciated carcinomas.

Despite a strong tendency, pooled data of these studies could not confirm a significant impact of eradication therapy on gastric carcinogenesis [22]. For the final proof, a large scale prospective, randomized, placebo-controlled study is needed. The main problem for the design and set up of such a study is the sample size that would be necessary. Graham et al. calculated that a total of 17,625 patients in each group is needed to demonstrate a 50 % reduction of the *H. pylori* attributed GC incidence within a ten years period [23]. Due to obvious ethical and also economical reasons, such a trial cannot be undertaken, so that the final proof is not going to be delivered.

PREVENTION OF RECURRENCE

A major issue is not only the primary prevention and early detection of gastric cancer but also the prevention of GC recurrence after curative treatment. In about 80%, diagnosis is made at advanced stage, when only restricted treatment options are available. Even in case of endoscopic or surgical treatment with curative intent, general five-year survival rates remain low at about 24% [24]. Only in well selected patients, endoscopic mucosa resection (EMR) or endoscopic submucosal dissection (ESD) are real options for a curative approach in case of early gastric cancer (EGC) (See also chapter VI) [25]. The frequency of secondary GC is reported to be 3-7% [26]. In most cases, there are multilocular sites of recurrence, mainly in the same third of the stomach where the primary lesion was located and the tumor presents with the same histopahological characteristics [27].

A meticulous pre-interventional staging is arbitrative to provide the best possible outcome and minor rates of recurrence. Besides a regular follow-up regimen, strategies for prevention of recurrence can be based on *H. pylori* eradication, which represents one of the most important features of prevention. There is strong evidence, that assessment of *H. pylori* status at time of first diagnosis and prompt eradication in case of proof has an effect on recurrence rates after endoscopic treatment of EGC.

In a retrospective multicenter analysis the data of 2835 patients in 31 Japanese centers were evaluated for a median follow-up period of 2 years. In 356 cases *H. pylori* eradication was performed (13%). Metachronous GC was detected in 8/356 eradicated patients versus 129/2479 patients without *H. pylori* therapy (2.2 vs 5.2%; OR 0.42; 0.20-0.86) [28].

Uemura and colleagues conducted a non-randomized trial perfomring *H. pylori* eradication in patients after endoscopic removal of gastric cancer [16]. After a 3-years follow-up, 6 of 67 metachronous cancers developed in those not treated compared to no cancer in 65 patients who received anti-*H. pylori* therapy.

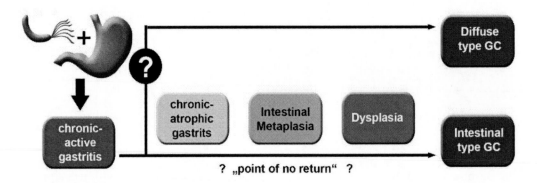

Figure 1. Schematic image of the Correa-Model.

Recently, a multi-center, randomized controlled trial from Japan confirmed the effect of *H. pylori* eradication on the incidence of metachronous GC after EMR [1]. Aim of the study was not only to verify that treatment of the infection has an inhibitory effect on recurrence of GC, but also to demonstrate that *H. pylori* is a promotor of gastric carcinogenesis [29]. Five-hundred and fourty-four patients with EGC have been included, with 272 being randomized for eradication treatment. Clinical and endoscopic follow-up have been performed at 6, 12, 24 and 36 months after allocation. At 36 months, GC has been recurred in 9/272 patients in the eradication group and 24/272 in the non-eradication group (3.3 vs 8.8%) with an OR for metachronous GC of 0.35 (0.16-0.78) [1]. Further prospective randomized trials are still ungoing to address this issue of *H. pylori* eradication for GC recurrence prevention [26].

However, while evidence supporting a preventive effect of *H. pylori* eradication on incidence and recurrence of GC is constantly growing, a major issue remains the further investigation of conditions that might influence the preventive efficacy and the pre-interventional risk-assessment. A major target is the characterization of mucosal alterations (intestinal metaplasia, glandular atrophy) in the stomach at time of eradication. When is the "point of no return", when is progression towards malignant neoplasia not stoppable any more and which are the patients that benefit from *H. pylori* eradication?

POINT OF NO RETURN/PREVENTION OF "PREMALIGNANT LESIONS"

In 1988, Correa suggested a sequence of alterations of the gastric mucosa leading from *H. pylori* driven chronic active gastritis via intestinal metaplasia and glandular atrophy (or chronic atrophic gastritis) to dyplasia and finally malignant neoplastic tissue formation (Figure 1) [30].

Model of sequential mucosal alterations in the development of intestinal type gastric cancer on the basis of *H. pylori* driven chronic active gastritis. In contrast to the adenoma-carcinoma sequence for colorectal cancer, order of appearance can be different and certain steps can be missed.

However, this model refers primarily to the intestinal and not to the diffuse type of gastric adenocarcinoma although the specific alterations can occur in both types. The multistep sequence of mucosal alterations in the stomach has been clearly demonstrated in mongolian gerbils after *Helicobacter* eradication showing the potential to interrupt further progression of pre-malignant lesions [31-33].

As mentioned above, a prospective interventional trial from China has demonstrated a preventive effect of eradication on human gastric carcinogenesis only for the subgroup of patients that presented without any pre-neoplastic lesions at baseline [15]. This gives the rational to search for the crucial step in this process, the "point of no return", when eradication of *H. pylori* will not have any protective effect on further progression of IM and atrophic gastritis [34].

A prospective observational study from Japan including 1787 patients for a 9-years follow-up period described the clinical and histopathological characteristics of patients who still develop GC after eradication [35]. All patients who developed GC presented with severe atrophic gastritis at baseline [35]. The risk for gastric carcinogenesis has been reported to be even increased in positive correlation to the degree of baseline atrophy [36]. The hazard ratio (HR) for gastric cancer development is significantly higher for patients with atrophic gastritis than for those with *H. pylori* infection alone [37]. In a prospective study from Japan, 4655 healthy, asymptomatic individuals have been followed-up endoscopically for 7.7 years presenting a HR for GC of 7.13 in case of *H. pylori* infection without glandular atrophy, 14.85 if both conditions had been detected and 61.85 if *H. pylori* infection could not be detected any more due to the atrophic changes of the gastric mucosa [37].

Compared to chronic atrophic gastritis, there is less evidence for the influence of intestinal metaplasia on gastric cancer risk. However, on multiple logistic regression analysis, degree and distribution of IM have also been demonstrated to be independent risk factors for GC development [38].

H. PYLORI ERADICATION AND MUCOSAL ALTERATIONS

Numerous studies have been published about the effect of *H. pylori* eradication on the regression of glandular atrophy and intestinal metaplasia. Uemura reported in 1997 a decrease of the degree of IM after eradication therapy in patients endoscopically treated for early gastric cancer in a three years follow-up [16]. These results have been confirmed for healthy volunteers in China without any history of malignant disease [39]. After eradication of *H. pylori,* the degree of IM decreased, whereas in individuals with persistent infection, there was an increase in the degree of IM and gastric atrophy already within one year [39].

However, the data about the actual regression of IM or glandular atrophy is controversial, since several authors report an improvement only of inflammation within one year after eradication but no changes concerning metaplasia or atrophy scores [40;41]. It was suggested, that the decisive factor whether or not there is an effect of *H. pylori* eradication is the time of follow-up. Some studies have shown, that an improvement of gastritis scores can be documented within the first six or latest the first twelve months after eradication, whereas a follow-up period of at least one year is neccessary to find an effect on IM and atrophic changes [42;43]. It was stated that the regression in histopathology scores after eradication therapy can be calculated as a function of the square of the time being *H. pylori* negative [44]. Also the side of biopsy sampling may be an important influencing factor [43].

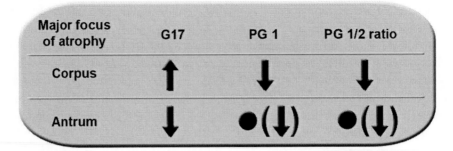

Figure 2. Pattern of a serological biopsy for the assessment of gatsric cancer.

Other risk factors for IM/atrophy progression that are crucial besides *H. pylori* infection are age, male gender, abuse of alcohol and drinking water from a well [19].

However, the issue of the necessary time of follow-up is not solved yet, since even after longer control periods there might be no change in the degree of IM or atrophic gastritis, which refers one to the unsolved question of the "point of no return" [45].

"SEROLOGICAL BIOPSY"

For prospective studies, invasive procedures like endoscopical biopsy sampling is not mandatory for the monitoring of atrophic gastritis since there are valuable serum markers available. These are mainly gastrin 17, pepsinogen 1 and pepsinogen 2 as well as the ratio of pepsinogen 1 to 2, all of them measured under standard conditions in the fasting serum (Figure 2).

The main relevant factors for diagnosis of atrophic changes of the gastric mucosa are shown with respect to main topographical location of the mucosal alterations. Gastrin 17 (G17) is expressed only in the antrum, whereas Pepsinogen 1 (PG1) is expressed in the corpus and the fundus area. Expression of Pepsinogen 2 (PG 2) is in the pre-pyloric region and the duodenum and only represented concerning the PG1 / 2 ration in this scheme. Arrow up: up-regulation; arrow down: down-regulation; dot: no change; arrow in brackets: potential change. For assessment of gastric cancer risk, *H. pylori* antibodies should be included in the analysis.

Several authors report a normalization of these parameters after *H. pylori* eradication, either completely or at least by trend [46-48]. Follow-up has been documented for one to five years and the treatment-induced decrease of gastrin 17 levels and increase in pepsinogen (pepsinogen 1) correlated with histologically proven improvement of atrophic gastritis (of the corpus predominant type). However, data concerning the necessary time of follow-up and the degree of regression of the documented changes are not congruent.

H. PYLORI AND MOLECULAR ALTERATIONS

Some of the changes in the gastric mucosa caused by *H. pylori* infection and secondly after its eradication can be followed on the molecular level. Patients with *H. pylori* infection present with higher Ki67 levels as a marker for proliferation, in addition to a shift of the Bax – Bcl2 balance towards the antiaptotic side with an overexpreison of Bcl2 and low Bax levels [49]. This is even more evident, in case of pre-neoplastic mucosal alterations resulting in a higher risk for the development of GC. Patients with *H. pylori* induced chronic atrophic gastritis have an abnormal DNA content in the epithelium with further patholgical expression of p53 and cMyc [50;51]. These genomic changes disappeared completely twelve months after eradication of *H. pylori* partially accompanied by complete regression of IM and mucosal atrophy as mentioned above. Similar results have been reported for patients with elevated p27 and decreased Cyclin D2 expression under the influence of *H. pylori* infection [52]. Even in case of GC, there was a trend to normalization of altered expression levels after eradication. *H. pylori* infection also alters the content and functionality of DNA missmatch repair proteins like hMLH1 and hMSH2 which increased to normal levels after eradication [53].

METHODS OF *H. PYLORI* DETECTION

Up to today, *H. pylori*-infection remains the major target for intervention in the fight against gastric cancer. However, there is no broad use of *H .pylori* eradication as a preventive mean on a global basis. The main arguments against are the availability of the diagnostic procedures and their costs, as well as the complexity of the consequent therapy. Also taken into account is the global increase in specific and general resistancy against antibiotics used for eradication therapy.

Invasive tests like specific histopathological staining performed on mucosa biopsies that have been obtained during gastroscopy or rapid urease test on equivalent specimens are not appropriate for a population-based screening. The laborious direct culture of the *Helicobacter* from biopsy samples is only justified in case of documented eradication failure to specify the resistance pattern of the individual strain.

For general screening, non-invasive tests should be performed. There are numerous test-kits for serological analysis commercially available, mostly based on enzyme linked immunoassays (EIA) and the detection of IgG antibodies to various *H. pylori* antigens. For most of these kits, specifity lies over 90% whereas sensitivity ranges from 60 to 90% with further possible improvement by addition of IgA analysis [54;55]. False positive results are mainly due to antibody persistence after eradication. Superior to serological assessment concerning the actual status of *H. pylori* infection is the Urea Breath Test (UBT) and the stool antigen test, with the former still representing the gold standard for non-invasive *H. pylori* diagnostics [56]. Specifity and sensitivity is in general >90% [57]. However, there are regional differences of the applied cut-off levels, so that the diagnostic report should always state the local reference values. It is controversely discussed if the results of these tests allow conclusions about density of *H. pylori* colonization, which could not yet be established [58;59].

The main factor influencing the outcome of the UBT is the intake of PPI which could lead to false negative results and should therefore be interrupted at least two weeks before testing.

In the late 1990ies, the stool antigen test for *Helicobacter* detection has been introduced to clinical practice. The most accurate results can be achieved by monoclonal antibody tests with sensitivity and specifity comparable to the UBT. Only in the post-eradication setting, the UBT is clearly superior to the stool antigen test.

Especially in regions with low incidence for *H. pylori* infection, an increase in the diagnostic value can always be achieved by combination of the mehods mentioned above.

H. PYLORI ERADICATION

Goldstandard for eradication therapy is still a triple therapy based on the use of one proton pump inhibitor (PPI), clarithromycin and amoxicillin/metronidazole in populations with less than 15-20% resistance to clarithromycin [2]. A decline of 70% in the eradication rates has been reported in case of resistance to clarithromycin [60]. Although there has been conflicting data, the Maastricht III consensus stated that a 14 days period of treatment might be more effective than the 7-days treatment [2]. However in regions with acceptable eradication rates, the one week treatment might be sufficient and a extension to two weeks should be just considered in regions where local studies show a failure of the one-week treatment.

The main risk factor for treatment failure represents the regional increase in clarihromycin resistance [61;62], so that in these areas, clarithromycin might be replaced by metronidazole. Alternatively a bismuth-based quadruple therapy can be applied, which is also often used as second-line treatment after failure of the recommended first-line options. Levofloxacin has gained importance as salvage therapy in case of eradication failure. In case of repeated failure of eradication, microbiological culture of the *H. pylori* is necessary to enable a resistance-adapted therapy [63].

A new option is the sequential therapy, consisting of dual ten-day regimen with PPI and amoxicillin for the first five days followed by a triple therapy of PPI, clarithromycin and tinidazole for the remaining five days. Zullo and colleagues presented the results of a pooled data-analysis demonstrating an overall eradication rate of 93.5% at the intention to treat analysis for this scheme [64]. The sequential therapy was also superior to traditional triple therapy in a head to head analysis (eradication rate: 91% vs 78%) [65]. Although the sequential therapy may become an alternative treatment option, it has to be considered that it is a complex scheme and most of the studies have been carried out in Italy and thus its efficacy has to be proven in other countries.

COST EFFECTIVENESS OF "SCREEN-AND-ERADICATE"

Despite the convincing data about eradication rates, the antibiotic treatment remains complex, expensive and may lead to a further increase of the global antibiotic resistance rates. If the expenses for the prior diagnostic procedures are taken into account, this result in a poor cost-effectiveness of a "screen-and-eradicate"-schedule for the prevention of gastric cancer. In 1996, Parsonnet and colleagues analysed the cost-effectiveness of *H. pylori* screening for GC prevention in the United States, assuming a 30% decrease of GC incidence by population-based *H. pylori* screening and consequent eradication [66]. Costs per life-year safed have been € 25,000 with an increase if the assumed preventive efficacy of eradication was even lower than 30%.

Several U.S.-studies supported these data, suggesting costs for *H. pylori* screening and treatment between € 6,300 to 25,000 per life-year saved [66-69]. Two U.K. models suggested that the strategy would at most cost € 8,500 per life year saved and under some assumptions the program could even save the health service money [70;71]. The model suggesting that *H. pylori* test and treat was cost saving also assessed the possibility that the strategy would reduce the dyspepsia burden in the community [71].

A further conclusion was that a population-based screening for *H. pylori* infection with the aim of GC prevention is more reasonable in high incidence regions [67;71].

Therefore, screening for *H. pylori* should be performed in individuals with a certain risk profile, including patients with peptic ulcer disease or gastric cancer, also after potentially curative treatment, and their first degree relatives. Another group are patients in whom long-term acid antisecretory therapy or long-term nonsteroidal anti-inflammatory drug therapy (including low-dose aspirin) is planned [72]. However, the definite decrease of GC incidence as a consequence of *H. pylori* eradication remains the decisive variable for these calculations [70].

Screening would be dispensable if an effective vaccine against *H. pylori* is ubiquitous available, which would furthermore lead to an improvement of cost-effectiveness mainly in developed countries. A prediction model estimates, that a ten-years vaccination program would cause a decrease of *H. pylori* prevalence in the USA down to 0.07% by the end of the 21st century [73]. This would not only have an effect on GC but also on other *H. pylori*-related diseases. Animal studies have demonstrated that vaccination against *H. pylori* can be effective, although there is no data yet about an effective vaccine for human conditions, but promising trials are ongoing [74-76].

CHEMOPREVENTION

Despite the option of *H. pylori* eradication as a tool for GC prevention, the development of cheap and easily applicable chemopreventive agents is worthwile, while considering the low cost-effectiveness of the *H. pylori* "screen and eradicate"-strategy.

COX-INHIBITION

A major focus of research has been on cyclo-oxygenase (COX) –inhibitors, especially specific inhibitors of the inducible COX-isoform 2. There are numerous studies reporting the induction of COX-2 in GC tissue and its association to invasive growth, lymph vessel invasion and nodal involvement, especially for intestinal type tumors [77-79]. Since changes in COX-2 expression can already be detected in early dyplastic lesions, induced by *H. pylori* driven inflammation, they are considered to be an early event in gastric carcinogenesis and thus a target for prevention [80]. Although there has never been a randomized controlled trial to evaluate the potential of COX-inhibitors on GC development, several case-control and cohort studies have been carried out about this issue. The largest assessment was performed by Thun and colleagues who observed more than 650 000 individuals taking aspirin for different reasons for about 10 years, supported by the American Cancer society [81]. They documented a protective effect against GC (OR 0.53; 0.34-0.81), resulting in an almost 50% reduction of GC incidence for participants who took aspirin more often than 16 times a month. Non-aspirin NSAID use was analysed from the population-based North Jutland prescription database and the Danish Cancer Registry, following more than 170 000 individuals for over nine years showing a clear tendency of GC risk reduction (OR 0.70; 0.4-1.1) [82]. Several case-control studies confirm these data and rise an association between duration of Aspirin or NSAID intake and GC risk reduction [83]. Even a positive effect on IM-regression has been reported for patients using selective COX-2 inhibitors [84]. However, these data have not been transferred into clinical practice due to the reason of cost-effectiveness and drug-induced morbidity like e.g. NSAID induced gastric ulcer bleeding, which has to be considered as a severe side-effect of those drugs causing high morbidity and mortality.

Besides these data, it has been reported that *H. pylori* eradication has the potential to reduce COX-2 overexpression, that is present in patients with atrophic gastritis [85].

GASTRIN-MODULATION

Within recent years, the importance of gastrin for an intact mucosal homeostasis in the stomach has been recognized and its complex role in gastric carcinogenesis has been revealed, including the gastrin induced mediation of proliferation, angiogenesis and tissue invasion [86]. Animal models have shown that constitutive high expression leads to development of GC in 100% [87]. In these so-called InsGas mice, the insulin promotor was used for constitutive expression of gastrin 17. Gastric carcinogenesis was even more rapidly progressive in animals that have additionally been infected by *Helicobacter felis*.

Gastrin also influences *Helicobacter*-induced mucosal alterations. Antagonism of the upregulated gastrin expression and its secretion in *H. felis* related atrophic gastritis delayed or even arrested the progression of glandular atrophy towards malignant changes in InsGas mice [88]. Konturek and colleagues suggested in 1999 for the first time a putative autocrine mechanism of stimulation of GC progression with GC cells expressing both, gastrin and its receptor [85]. Median gastrin levels were higher in GC patients compared to controls, both concerning plasma and luminal levels. Gastrin itself is reported to be expressed in 47% of GC samples and its receptor, the cholecystokinin (CCK-) B receptor in 56% [89]. Positive expression is associated with better differentiation and intestinal type GC. The potential of modulation of gastrin-dependent pathways in human conditions still needs to be evaluated [85].

ALIMENTARY FACTORS AND GASTRIC CANCER

The relevance of diet for the development of gastric cancer has been under investigation for decades. It has been suggested that dietary factors account for about 30% of cancers in Western countries and around 20% in developing countries [90;91]. For gastric cancer, the World Health Organization stated in 1982 that eating habits are the main factors involved in carcinogenesis. This was prior to the discovery of *H. pylori* by Warren and Marshall in 1983.

There are several dietary factors associated with gastric cancer development. The identification of protective dietary factors has prompted to conduct a series of studies.

Evidence from case-control, ecological and cohort studies has been gained showing that a diet high in fruit and vegetables reduces the risk for GC development whereas high intake of various salt-preserved foods increases this risk. However, prospective studies did not meet the expectations in support of a protective effect for fruit and vegetables. Thus, the International Agency for Research on Cancer (IARC) determined that higher intake of vegetables "possibly" and higher intake of fruit "probably" reduce the risk of GC [92]. On the other hand, there is substantial evidence that high intake of salt-preserved foods and salt per se increases the risk of GC and should therefore be avoided or at least reduced [93].

There are several potential mechanisms through which a diet high in fruit and vegetables may be protective against cancer.

Fruit and vegetables are rich of carotenoids, vitamin C, folates, and phytochemicals, which each by itself or in concert may protect against GC. Fruits and vegetables have a high antixodant capacity, which is related to their content of beta-carotene, alpha-tocepherol and vitamin C.

In a Cochrane analysis randomised trials comparing antioxidant supplements with placebo for prevention of cancers of the gastrointestinal tract, Bjelakovic and colleagues did not prove the preventive effect against GC by antioxidants. These data were further strengthened by a recent meta-analysis [94].

Vitamin C as a protective agent against GC has also been reported with conflicting results. This is due to the complex relationship of Vitamin C with the *H. pylori* infection. *H. pylori* infection reduces the bioavailability of this nutrient, leading subsequently to decreased Vitamin C concentrations in the plasma and gastric juice [95;96], whereas the luminal concentration of reactive oxygen species is increased in *H. pylori* infection [97]. The EPIC (European Prospective Investigation into Cancer and Nutrition) study analysed the association of plasma Vitamin C with the risk of GC, while taking into account factors like body mass index, total energy intake, smoking, and *H. pylori* status. This study did not demonstrate an association of Vitamin C levels with GC development [98].

In a randomised controlled trial carried out in Colombia, patients at high risk for GC were treated after *H. pylori* eradication with a combination of Vitamin C and beta-carotene or placebo. In the group with Vitamin C supplementation, regression of pre-malignant lesions was observed [99]. According to the biological plausibility, Vitamin C intake via dietary or supplement agents probably decreases the risk of GC [99]. In animal experiments conducted on beagles a protective effect was reported for folic acid supplementation [100]. However, these results have not been confirmed in humans.

Garlic as a member of the *Allium* family is suggested to have a protective effect in GC. Several case-control studies found a protective effect against GC by high intake of raw and/or cooked garlic. In a meta-analysis, garlic consumption led to a risk reduction of 0.53 (95% CI: 0.31, 0.92) [101]. However, results so far are conflicting. In a prospective randomized trial, 3365 inhabitants of 13 villages in China received either *H. pylori* eradication or supplementation of garlic or vitamins [20]. After a median follow-up of 7.3 years, no protective effect was reported for supplement therapy concerning the incidence of gastric cancer or even pre-neoplastic changes.

Tea as one of the most popular beverages world-wide is also proposed for cancer prevention. The anti-cancerogen ingredients catechins have a strong anti-angiogenic and anti-oxidant acitivity. They further have the potential to modulate signal transduction pathways and thereby lead to inhibition of cell proliferation and transformation. It has been reported that catechins are able to induce apoptosis and cell-cycle arrest, which may explain their protection against GC [102-104]. Five case-control studies were included in the WCRF/AICR report, investigating the relation between tea intake and GC risk. Of these five, four studies suggested a protective effect. Most of these studies showed a dose-dependent effect, but in contrast one study did not find an essential association for green tea. Thus, again the WCRF/AICR report concluded that high intake of green tea "possibly" decreases the risk of GC [105].

Animal studies have proven that ingestion of salt causes gastritis by destroying the mucosal barrier leading to inflammation and damage such as diffuse erosion and degeneration [106-108]. It is thought that chronic inflammation and degeneration is associated with an increased regeneration promoting the effect of food-derived carcinogenesis. In 1997 the World Cancer Research Fund and the American Institute for Cancer Research analysed 16 case-control studies, stating an association between salt or salted food and the risk of GC [105]. More recent case-control studies confirmed this association [109-112]. One prospective study examined GC prevalence in 2476 men and women and evaluated the salt intake by a 70-item food frequency questionnaire. In this patient population 93 cases of GC were identified and after consideration of *H. pylori* infection high salt-intake was shown to be significantly associated with GC [113]. In summary, there is an abundance of evidence that reduction of salt and salted food is protective against gastric carcinogenesis.

N-nitroso compounds (NOCs) are potent carcinogens and humans are exposed to various NOCs from general diet, tobacco consumption, and drinking water [114;115]. NOCs are formed in vivo by the nitrosation of amides or amines in the stomach by nitrites. Nitrosation is increased in chronic inflammation, as well as in GC and oesophageal cancer [114]. Nitrosamines are found mainly in cured meat products, smoked preserved food, and pickled and salt-preserved food [116]. Evidence for these associations was provided in animal experiments [117]. Epidemiological studies however, have failed to prove that nitrosamines are carcinogenic in humans [105].

ALCOHOL AND GASTRIC CANCER

Chronic alcohol abuse is a major health care problem worldwide. However, more than 40 epidemiological, mostly retrospective studies have been carried out and they did not confirm an association between chronic alcohol consumption and GC. Even intake of large amounts of alcohol (more than 200 g per day) was not significantly associated with increased risk of GC, neither was the type of alcohol nor the concentration (percentage of ethanol) [118;119].

In two prospective studies and four case-control studies, no significant correlation between alcohol consumption and cancer of the gastric cardia was reported [120].

SMOKING AND GASTRIC CANCER

About 60 different components in cigarette smoke are considered to be carcinogenic. The most important are polycyclic aromatic hydrocarbons, nitrosamines, aromatic amine, trace metals, as well as nicotine [121]. A recent systematic review analyzed the relation between cigarette smoking and GC. In this review 42 cohort, case-cohort, and case-control studies were included the study provided solid evidence that smoking was significantly associated with both gastric cardia (RR = 1.87; 95% CI: 1.31–2.67) and non-cardia cancers (RR = 1.60; 95% CI: 1.41–1.80). This is conform with a previous meta-analysis [122] and the results of a large European prospective Study (EPIC), which estimated that 17.6% (95% CI = 10.5-29.5%) of GC are related to smoking [123]. In conclusion, smoking seems to be the most important lifestyle risk factor for GC.

CONCLUSION

Eradication of *H. pylori* is the most effective tool for primary prevention of gastric cancer and moreover reduces the recurrence of the disease after endoscopic removal of early gastric cancer. In spite of a low cost-effectiveness, a general screen-and-treat strategy can currently only be recommended for high risk populations. For an adequate risk assessment besides environmental and specific host factors, the presence of pre-neoplastic mucosal alterations has to be considered since there is reasonable evidence, that beyond a certain point of mucosal alteration treatment of the infection has a limited benefit in withholding the progression to dysplastic and/or neoplastic lesions.

Adjustment of dietary habits or intake of supplemental medication like COX-inhibitors or antioxidants has a subordinate and at the best a supportive role. A significant carcinogenic influence is attributed to tobacco smoking, particularly in *H. pylori* infected subjects.

Strategies which are generally applicable, easily available and cost-effective for population based screening are in the phase of evaluation.

REFERENCES

[1]   Fukase K, Kato M, Kikuchi S, Inoue K, Uemura N, Okamoto S, Terao S, Amagai K, Hayashi S, Asaka M: Effect of eradication of Helicobacter pylori on incidence of metachronous gastric carcinoma after endoscopic resection of early gastric cancer: an open-label, randomised controlled trial. *Lancet.2008 Aug* 2;372:392-397.

[2]   Malfertheiner P, Megraud F, O'Morain C, Bazzoli F, El-Omar E, Graham D, Hunt R, Rokkas T, Vakil N, Kuipers EJ: Current concepts in the management of Helicobacter pylori infection: the Maastricht III Consensus Report. *Gut.2007 Jun* 56:772-781.

[3]   Fock KM, Talley N, Moayyedi P, Hunt R, Azuma T, Sugano K, Xiao SD, Lam SK, Goh KL, Chiba T, Uemura N, Kim JG, Kim N, Ang TL, Mahachai V, Mitchell H, Rani AA, Liou JM, Vilaichone RK, Sollano J: Asia-Pacific consensus guidelines on gastric cancer prevention. *J Gastroenterol Hepatol.2008 Mar* 23:351-365.

[4]   Fujioka T, Yoshiiwa A, Okimoto T, Kodama M, Murakami K: Guidelines for the management of Helicobacter pylori infection in Japan: current status and future prospects. *J Gastroenterol.2007 Jan* 42 Suppl;17:3-6.

[5]   Schistosomes, liver flukes and Helicobacter pylori. IARC Working Group on the Evaluation of Carcinogenic Risks to Humans. Lyon, 7-14 June 1994. *IARC Monogr Eval Carcinog Risks Hum.1994* 61:1-241.

[6]   Gastric cancer and Helicobacter pylori: a combined analysis of 12 case control studies nested within prospective cohorts. *Gut.2001 Sep* 49:347-353.

[7]   Huang JQ, Sridhar S, Chen Y, Hunt RH: Meta-analysis of the relationship between Helicobacter pylori seropositivity and gastric cancer. *Gastroenterology.1998 Jun* 114:1169-1179.

[8]   Eslick GD, Lim LL, Byles JE, Xia HH, Talley NJ: Association of Helicobacter pylori infection with gastric carcinoma: a meta-analysis. *Am J Gastroenterol.1999 Sep* 94:2373-2379.

[9]   Selgrad M, Malfertheiner P, Fini L, Goel A, Boland CR, Ricciardiello L: The role of viral and bacterial pathogens in gastrointestinal cancer. *J Cell Physiol.2008 Aug* 216:378-388.

[10]   Huang JQ, Zheng GF, Sumanac K, Irvine EJ, Hunt RH: Meta-analysis of the relationship between cagA seropositivity and gastric cancer. *Gastroenterology.2003 Dec* 125:1636-1644.

[11]   Ekstrom AM, Held M, Hansson LE, Engstrand L, Nyren O: Helicobacter pylori in gastric cancer established by CagA immunoblot as a marker of past infection. *Gastroenterology.2001 Oct* 121:784-791.

[12]   Kato M, Asaka M, Nakamura T, Azuma T, Tomita E, Kamoshida T, Sato K, Inaba T, Shirasaka D, Okamoto S, Takahashi S, Terao S, Suwaki K, Isomoto H, Yamagata H, Nomura H, Yagi K, Sone Y, Urabe T, Akamatsu T, Ohara S, Takagi A, Miwa J, Inatsuchi S: Helicobacter pylori eradication prevents the development of gastric cancer - results of a long-term retrospective study in Japan. *Aliment Pharmacol Ther* 2006, 24 (Suppl. 4):203-206.

[13]   Uemura N, Okamoto S, Yamamoto S, Matsumura N, Yamaguchi S, Yamakido M, Taniyama K, Sasaki N, Schlemper RJ: Helicobacter pylori infection and the development of gastric cancer. *N Engl J Med.2001 Sep* 13;345:784-789.

[14] Take S, Mizuno M, Ishiki K, Nagahara Y, Yoshida T, Yokota K, Oguma K, Okada H, Shiratori Y: The effect of eradicating helicobacter pylori on the development of gastric cancer in patients with peptic ulcer disease. *Am J Gastroenterol.2005 May* 100:1037-1042.

[15] Wong BC, Lam SK, Wong WM, Chen JS, Zheng TT, Feng RE, Lai KC, Hu WH, Yuen ST, Leung SY, Fong DY, Ho J, Ching CK, Chen JS: Helicobacter pylori eradication to prevent gastric cancer in a high-risk region of China: a randomized controlled trial. *JAMA.2004 Jan* 14;291:187-194.

[16] Uemura N, Mukai T, Okamoto S, Yamaguchi S, Mashiba H, Taniyama K, Sasaki N, Haruma K, Sumii K, Kajiyama G: Effect of Helicobacter pylori eradication on subsequent development of cancer after endoscopic resection of early gastric cancer. *Cancer Epidemiol Biomarkers Prev.1997 Aug* 6:639-642.

[17] Saito K, Arai K, Mori M, Kobayashi R, Ohki I: Effect of Helicobacter pylori eradication on malignant transformation of gastric adenoma. *Gastrointest Endosc.2000 Jul* 52:27-32.

[18] Zhou LY, Lin SR, Ding SG, Huang XB, Zhang L, Meng LM, Cui RL, Zhu J: The changing trends of the incidence of gastric cancer after Helicobacter pylori eradication in Shandong area. *Chin J Dig Dis.2005* 6:114-115.

[19] Leung WK, Lin SR, Ching JY, To KF, Ng EK, Chan FK, Lau JY, Sung JJ: Factors predicting progression of gastric intestinal metaplasia: results of a randomised trial on Helicobacter pylori eradication. *Gut.2004 Sep* 53:1244-1249.

[20] You WC, Brown LM, Zhang L, Li JY, Jin ML, Chang YS, Ma JL, Pan KF, Liu WD, Hu Y, Crystal-Mansour S, Pee D, Blot WJ, Fraumeni JF, Jr., Xu GW, Gail MH: Randomized double-blind factorial trial of three treatments to reduce the prevalence of precancerous gastric lesions. *J Natl Cancer Inst.2006 Jul* 19;98:974-983.

[21] Ogura K, Hirata Y, Yanai A, Shibata W, Ohmae T, Mitsuno Y, Maeda S, Watabe H, Yamaji Y, Okamoto M, Yoshida H, Kawabe T, Omata M: The Effect of Helicobacter Pylori Eradication On Incident of Gastric Cancer [abstract]. *Gastroenterology* 2006, 130 (4 Suppl. 2):A183.

[22] Fuccio L, Zagari RM, Minardi ME, Bazzoli F: Systematic review: Helicobacter pylori eradication for the prevention of gastric cancer. *Aliment Pharmacol Ther.2007 Jan* 15;25:133-141.

[23] Graham DY, Shiotani A: The time to eradicate gastric cancer is now. *Gut.2005 Jun* 54:735-738.

[24] Coleman MP, Gatta G, Verdecchia A, Esteve J, Sant M, Storm H, Allemani C, Ciccolallo L, Santaquilani M, Berrino F: EUROCARE-3 summary: cancer survival in Europe at the end of the 20th century. *Ann Oncol.2003* 14 Suppl;5:v128-v149.

[25] Ono H, Kondo H, Gotoda T, Shirao K, Yamaguchi H, Saito D, Hosokawa K, Shimoda T, Yoshida S: Endoscopic mucosal resection for treatment of early gastric cancer. *Gut.2001 Feb* 48:225-229.

[26] Kato M, Asaka M, Ono S, Nakagawa M, Nakagawa S, Shimizu Y, Chuma M, Kawakami H, Komatsu Y, Hige S, Takeda H: Eradication of Helicobacter pylori for primary gastric cancer and secondary gastric cancer after endoscopic mucosal resection. *J Gastroenterol.2007 Jan* 42 Suppl;17:16-20.

[27]   Nasu J, Doi T, Endo H, Nishina T, Hirasaki S, Hyodo I: Characteristics of metachronous multiple early gastric cancers after endoscopic mucosal resection. *Endoscopy.2005 Oct* 37:990-993.

[28]   Nakagawa S, Asaka M, Kato M, Nakamura T, Kato C, Fujioka T, Tatsuta M, Keida K, Terao S, Takahashi S, Uemura N, Kato T, Aoyama N, Saito D, Suzuki M, Imamura A, Sato K, Miwa H, Nomura H, Kaise M, Oohara S, Kawai T, Urabe N, Sakaki N, Ito S, Noda Y, Yanaka A, Kusugami K, Goto H, Furuta T, Fujino M, Kinjyou F, Ookusa T: Helicobacter pylori eradication and metachronous gastric cancer after endoscopic mucosal resection of early gastric cancer. *Aliment Pharmacol Ther* 2006, 24 (Suppl. 4):214-218.

[29]   Kikuchi S, Kato M, Katsuyama T, Tominaga S, Asaka M: Design and planned analyses of an ongoing randomized trial assessing the preventive effect of Helicobacter pylori eradication on occurrence of new gastric carcinomas after endoscopic resection. *Helicobacter.2006 Jun* 11:147-151.

[30]   Correa P: A human model of gastric carcinogenesis. *Cancer Res.1988 Jul* 1;48:3554-3560.

[31]   Watanabe T, Tada M, Nagai H, Sasaki S, Nakao M: Helicobacter pylori infection induces gastric cancer in mongolian gerbils. *Gastroenterology.1998 Sep* 115:642-648.

[32]   Honda S, Fujioka T, Tokieda M, Satoh R, Nishizono A, Nasu M: Development of Helicobacter pylori-induced gastric carcinoma in Mongolian gerbils. *Cancer Res.1998 Oct* 1;58:4255-4259.

[33]   Nozaki K, Shimizu N, Ikehara Y, Inoue M, Tsukamoto T, Inada K, Tanaka H, Kumagai T, Kaminishi M, Tatematsu M: Effect of early eradication on Helicobacter pylori-related gastric carcinogenesis in Mongolian gerbils. *Cancer Sci.2003 Mar* 94:235-239.

[34]   Domellof L: Reversal of gastric atrophy after Helicobacter pylori eradication: is it possible or not? *Am J Gastroenterol.1998 Sep* 93:1407-1408.

[35]   Kamada T, Hata J, Sugiu K, Kusunoki H, Ito M, Tanaka S, Inoue K, Kawamura Y, Chayama K, Haruma K: Clinical features of gastric cancer discovered after successful eradication of Helicobacter pylori: results from a 9-year prospective follow-up study in Japan. *Aliment Pharmacol Ther.2005 May* 1;21:1121-1126.

[36]   Take S, Mizuno M, Ishiki K, Nagahara Y, Yoshida T, Yokota K, Oguma K: Baseline gastric mucosal atrophy is a risk factor associated with the development of gastric cancer after Helicobacter pylori eradication therapy in patients with peptic ulcer diseases. *J Gastroenterol.2007 Jan* 42 Suppl;17:21-27.

[37]   Ohata H, Kitauchi S, Yoshimura N, Mugitani K, Iwane M, Nakamura H, Yoshikawa A, Yanaoka K, Arii K, Tamai H, Shimizu Y, Takeshita T, Mohara O, Ichinose M: Progression of chronic atrophic gastritis associated with Helicobacter pylori infection increases risk of gastric cancer. *Int J Cancer.2004 Mar* 109:138-143.

[38]   Cassaro M, Rugge M, Gutierrez O, Leandro G, Graham DY, Genta RM: Topographic patterns of intestinal metaplasia and gastric cancer. *Am J Gastroenterol.2000 Jun* 95:1431-1438.

[39]   Sung JJ, Lin SR, Ching JY, Zhou LY, To KF, Wang RT, Leung WK, Ng EK, Lau JY, Lee YT, Yeung CK, Chao W, Chung SC: Atrophy and intestinal metaplasia one year after cure of H. pylori infection: a prospective, randomized study. *Gastroenterology.2000 Jul* 119:7-14.

[40]   Schenk BE, Kuipers EJ, Nelis GF, Bloemena E, Thijs JC, Snel P, Luckers AE, Klinkenberg-Knol EC, Festen HP, Viergever PP, Lindeman J, Meuwissen SG: Effect of Helicobacter pylori eradication on chronic gastritis during omeprazole therapy. *Gut.2000 May* 46:615-621.

[41]   Salih BA, Abasiyanik MF, Saribasak H, Huten O, Sander E: A follow-up study on the effect of Helicobacter pylori eradication on the severity of gastric histology. *Dig Dis Sci.2005 Aug* 50:1517-1522.

[42]   Ohkusa T, Fujiki K, Takashimizu I, Kumagai J, Tanizawa T, Eishi Y, Yokoyama T, Watanabe M: Improvement in atrophic gastritis and intestinal metaplasia in patients in whom Helicobacter pylori was eradicated. *Ann Intern Med.2001 Mar* 6;134:380-386.

[43]   Sugiyama T, Sakaki N, Kozawa H, Sato R, Fujioka T, Satoh K, Sugano K, Sekine H, Takagi A, Ajioka Y, Takizawa T: Sensitivity of biopsy site in evaluating regression of gastric atrophy after Helicobacter pylori eradication treatment. *Aliment Pharmacol Ther.2002 Apr* 16 Suppl;2:187-190.

[44]   Mera R, Fontham ET, Bravo LE, Bravo JC, Piazuelo MB, Camargo MC, Correa P: Long term follow up of patients treated for Helicobacter pylori infection. *Gut.2005 Nov* 54:1536-1540.

[45]   Zhou L, Sung JJ, Lin S, Jin Z, Ding S, Huang X, Xia Z, Guo H, Liu J, Chao W: A five-year follow-up study on the pathological changes of gastric mucosa after H. pylori eradication. *Chin Med J (Engl).2003 Jan* 116:11-14.

[46]   Ohkusa T, Miwa H, Nomura T, Asaoka D, Kurosawa A, Sakamoto N, Abe S, Hojo M, Terai T, Ogihara T, Sato N: Improvement in serum pepsinogens and gastrin in long-term monitoring after eradication of Helicobacter pylori: comparison with H. pylori-negative patients. *Aliment Pharmacol Ther.2004 Jul* 20 Suppl;1:25-32.

[47]   Ito M, Haruma K, Kamada T, Mihara M, Kim S, Kitadai Y, Sumii M, Tanaka S, Yoshihara M, Chayama K: Helicobacter pylori eradication therapy improves atrophic gastritis and intestinal metaplasia: a 5-year prospective study of patients with atrophic gastritis. *Aliment Pharmacol Ther.2002 Aug* 16:1449-1456.

[48]   Annibale B, Di GE, Caruana P, Lahner E, Capurso G, Bordi C, Delle FG: The long-term effects of cure of Helicobacter pylori infection on patients with atrophic body gastritis. *Aliment Pharmacol Ther.2002 Oct* 16:1723-1731.

[49]   Xia HH, Zhang GS, Talley NJ, Wong BC, Yang Y, Henwood C, Wyatt JM, Adams S, Cheung K, Xia B, Zhu YQ, Lam SK: Topographic association of gastric epithelial expression of Ki-67, Bax, and Bcl-2 with antralization in the gastric incisura, body, and fundus. *Am J Gastroenterol.2002 Dec* 97:3023-3031.

[50]   Jones NL, Shannon PT, Cutz E, Yeger H, Sherman PM: Increase in proliferation and apoptosis of gastric epithelial cells early in the natural history of Helicobacter pylori infection. *Am J Pathol.1997 Dec* 151:1695-1703.

[51]   Nardone G, Staibano S, Rocco A, Mezza E, D'armiento FP, Insabato L, Coppola A, Salvatore G, Lucariello A, Figura N, De RG, Budillon G: Effect of Helicobacter pylori infection and its eradication on cell proliferation, DNA status, and oncogene expression in patients with chronic gastritis. *Gut.1999 Jun* 44:789-799.

[52]   Yu J, Leung WK, Ng EK, To KF, Ebert MP, Go MY, Chan WY, Chan FK, Chung SC, Malfertheiner P, Sung JJ: Effect of Helicobacter pylori eradication on expression of cyclin D2 and p27 in gastric intestinal metaplasia. *Aliment Pharmacol Ther* 2001 Sep;15:1505-1511.

[53]   Park DI, Park SH, Kim SH, Kim JW, Cho YK, Kim HJ, Sohn CI, Jeon WK, Kim BI, Cho EY, Kim EJ, Chae SW, Sohn JH, Sung IK, Sepulveda AR, Kim JJ: Effect of Helicobacter pylori infection on the expression of DNA mismatch repair protein. *Helicobacter.2005 Jun* 10:179-184.

[54]   Herbrink P, Van Doorn LJ: Serological methods for diagnosis of Helicobacter pylori infection and monitoring of eradication therapy. *Eur J Clin Microbiol Infect Dis.2000 Mar* 19:164-173.

[55]   Lim LG, Yeoh KG, Ho B, Lim SG: Validation of four Helicobacter pylori rapid blood tests in a multi-ethnic Asian population. *World J Gastroenterol.2005 Nov* 14;11:6681-6683.

[56]   Graham DY, Klein PD, Evans DJ, Jr., Evans DG, Alpert LC, Opekun AR, Boutton TW: Campylobacter pylori detected noninvasively by the 13C-urea breath test. *Lancet.1987 May* 23;1:1174-1177.

[57]   Gisbert JP, Pajares JM: Review article: C-urea breath test in the diagnosis of Helicobacter pylori infection -- a critical review. *Aliment Pharmacol Ther.2004 Nov* 15;20:1001-1017.

[58]   Zagari RM, Pozzato P, Martuzzi C, Fuccio L, Martinelli G, Roda E, Bazzoli F: 13C-urea breath test to assess Helicobacter pylori bacterial load. *Helicobacter.2005 Dec* 10:615-619.

[59]   Tummala S, Sheth SG, Goldsmith JD, Goldar-Najafi A, Murphy CK, Osburne MS, Mullin S, Buxton D, Wagner DA, Kelly CP: Quantifying gastric Helicobacter pylori infection: a comparison of quantitative culture, urease breath testing, and histology. *Dig Dis Sci.2007 Feb* 52:396-401.

[60]   Houben MH, van de BD, Hensen EF, Craen AJ, Rauws EA, Tytgat GN: A systematic review of Helicobacter pylori eradication therapy--the impact of antimicrobial resistance on eradication rates. *Aliment Pharmacol Ther.1999 Aug* 13:1047-1055.

[61]   Megraud F, Lamouliatte H: Review article: the treatment of refractory Helicobacter pylori infection. *Aliment Pharmacol Ther.2003 Jun* 1;17:1333-1343.

[62]   McMahon BJ, Hennessy TW, Bensler JM, Bruden DL, Parkinson AJ, Morris JM, Reasonover AL, Hurlburt DA, Bruce MG, Sacco F, Butler JC: The relationship among previous antimicrobial use, antimicrobial resistance, and treatment outcomes for Helicobacter pylori infections. *Ann Intern Med.2003 Sep* 16;139:463-469.

[63]   Selgrad M, Malfertheiner P: New strategies for Helicobacter pylori eradication. *Curr Opin Pharmacol.2008 Oct* 8:593-597.

[64]   Zullo A, De F, V, Hassan C, Morini S, Vaira D: The sequential therapy regimen for Helicobacter pylori eradication: a pooled-data analysis. *Gut.2007 Oct* 56:1353-1357.

[65]   Vaira D, Zullo A, Vakil N, Gatta L, Ricci C, Perna F, Hassan C, Bernabucci V, Tampieri A, Morini S: Sequential therapy versus standard triple-drug therapy for Helicobacter pylori eradication: a randomized trial. *Ann Intern Med.2007 Apr* 17;146:556-563.

[66]   Parsonnet J, Harris RA, Hack HM, Owens DK: Modelling cost-effectiveness of Helicobacter pylori screening to prevent gastric cancer: a mandate for clinical trials. *Lancet.1996 Jul* 20;348:150-154.

[67]   Fendrick AM, Chernew ME, Hirth RA, Bloom BS, Bandekar RR, Scheiman JM: Clinical and economic effects of population-based Helicobacter pylori screening to prevent gastric cancer. *Arch Intern Med.1999 Jan* 25;159:142-148.

[68]   Harris RA, Owens DK, Witherell H, Parsonnet J: Helicobacter pylori and gastric cancer: what are the benefits of screening only for the CagA phenotype of H. pylori? *Helicobacter.1999 Jun* 4:69-76.

[69]   Sonnenberg A, Inadomi JM: Review article: Medical decision models of Helicobacter pylori therapy to prevent gastric cancer. *Aliment Pharmacol Ther.1998 Feb* 12 Suppl;1:111-121.

[70]   Roderick P, Davies R, Raftery J, Crabbe D, Pearce R, Patel P, Bhandari P: Cost-effectiveness of population screening for Helicobacter pylori in preventing gastric cancer and peptic ulcer disease, using simulation. *J Med Screen.2003* 10:148-156.

[71]   Mason J, Axon AT, Forman D, Duffett S, Drummond M, Crocombe W, Feltbower R, Mason S, Brown J, Moayyedi P: The cost-effectiveness of population Helicobacter pylori screening and treatment: a Markov model using economic data from a randomized controlled trial. *Aliment Pharmacol Ther.2002 Mar* 16:559-568.

[72]   Forman D, Graham DY: Review article: impact of Helicobacter pylori on society-role for a strategy of 'search and eradicate'. *Aliment Pharmacol Ther.2004 Feb* 19 Suppl;1:17-21.

[73]   Rupnow MF, Shachter RD, Owens DK, Parsonnet J: Quantifying the population impact of a prophylactic Helicobacter pylori vaccine. *Vaccine.2001 Dec* 12;20:879-885.

[74]   Marchetti M, Rossi M, Giannelli V, Giuliani MM, Pizza M, Censini S, Covacci A, Massari P, Pagliaccia C, Manetti R, Telford JL, Douce G, Dougan G, Rappuoli R, Ghiara P: Protection against Helicobacter pylori infection in mice by intragastric vaccination with H. pylori antigens is achieved using a non-toxic mutant of E. coli heat-labile enterotoxin (LT) as adjuvant. *Vaccine.1998 Jan* 16:33-37.

[75]   Del GG, Covacci A, Telford JL, Montecucco C, Rappuoli R: The design of vaccines against Helicobacter pylori and their development. *Annu Rev Immunol.2001* 19:523-563.

[76]   Malfertheiner P, Schultze V, Rosenkranz B, Kaufmann SH, Ulrichs T, Novicki D, Norelli F, Contorni M, Peppoloni S, Berti D, Tornese D, Ganju J, Palla E, Rappuoli R, Scharschmidt BF, Del GG: Safety and immunogenicity of an intramuscular Helicobacter pylori vaccine in noninfected volunteers: a phase I study. *Gastroenterology.2008 Sep* 135:787-795.

[77]   Murata H, Kawano S, Tsuji S, Tsuji M, Sawaoka H, Kimura Y, Shiozaki H, Hori M: Cyclooxygenase-2 overexpression enhances lymphatic invasion and metastasis in human gastric carcinoma. *Am J Gastroenterol.1999 Feb* 94:451-455.

[78]   Joo YE, Oh WT, Rew JS, Park CS, Choi SK, Kim SJ: Cyclooxygenase-2 expression is associated with well-differentiated and intestinal-type pathways in gastric carcinogenesis. *Digestion.2002* 66:222-229.

[79]   Yamac D, Ayyildiz T, Coskun U, Akyurek N, Dursun A, Seckin S, Koybasioglu F: Cyclooxygenase-2 expression and its association with angiogenesis, Helicobacter pylori, and clinicopathologic characteristics of gastric carcinoma. *Pathol Res Pract.2008* 204:527-536.

[80]   van Rees BP, Saukkonen K, Ristimaki A, Polkowski W, Tytgat GN, Drillenburg P, Offerhaus GJ: Cyclooxygenase-2 expression during carcinogenesis in the human stomach. *J Pathol.2002 Feb* 196:171-179.

[81]   Thun MJ, Namboodiri MM, Calle EE, Flanders WD, Heath CW, Jr.: Aspirin use and risk of fatal cancer. *Cancer Res.1993 Mar* 15;53:1322-1327.

[82]   Sorensen HT, Friis S, Norgard B, Mellemkjaer L, Blot WJ, McLaughlin JK, Ekbom A, Baron JA: Risk of cancer in a large cohort of nonaspirin NSAID users: a population-based study. *Br J Cancer.2003 Jun* 2;88:1687-1692.

[83]   Nardone G, Rocco A, Malfertheiner P: Review article: helicobacter pylori and molecular events in precancerous gastric lesions. *Aliment Pharmacol Ther* 2004 Aug;1;20:261-270.

[84]   Yang HB, Cheng HC, Sheu BS, Hung KH, Liou MF, Wu JJ: Chronic celecoxib users more often show regression of gastric intestinal metaplasia after Helicobacter pylori eradication. *Aliment Pharmacol Ther.2007 Feb* 15;25:455-461.

[85]   Konturek PC, Konturek SJ, Bielanski W, Karczewska E, Pierzchalski P, Duda A, Starzynska T, Marlicz K, Popiela T, Hartwich A, Hahn EG: Role of gastrin in gastric cancerogenesis in Helicobacter pylori infected humans. *J Physiol Pharmacol.1999 Dec* 50:857-873.

[86]   Watson SA, Grabowska AM, El-Zaatari M, Takhar A: Gastrin - active participant or bystander in gastric carcinogenesis? *Nat Rev Cancer.2006 Dec* 6:936-946.

[87]   Wang TC, Dangler CA, Chen D, Goldenring J, Koh T, Raychowdhury R, Coffey RJ, Ito S, Varro A, Dockray GJ, Fox JG: Synergistic interaction between hypergastrinemia and Helicobacter infection in a mouse model of gastric cancer. *Gastroenterology.2000 Jan* 118:36-47.

[88]   Takaishi S, Cui G, Frederick DM, Carlson JE, Houghton J, Varro A, Dockray GJ, Ge Z, Whary MT, Rogers AB, Fox JG, Wang TC: Synergistic inhibitory effects of gastrin and histamine receptor antagonists on Helicobacter-induced gastric cancer. *Gastroenterology.2005 Jun* 128:1965-1983.

[89]   Hur K, Kwak MK, Lee HJ, Park DJ, Lee HK, Lee HS, Kim WH, Michaeli D, Yang HK: Expression of gastrin and its receptor in human gastric cancer tissues. *J Cancer Res Clin Oncol.2006 Feb* 132:85-91.

[90]   Doll R, Peto R: The causes of cancer: quantitative estimates of avoidable risks of cancer in the United States today. *J Natl Cancer Inst.1981 Jun* 66:1191-1308.

[91]   Miller AB: Diet and cancer. A review. *Acta Oncol.1990* 29:87-95.

[92]   *IARC Handbooks of Cancer Prevention: Fruit and Vegetables*. Edited by IARC. Lyon: 2003.

[93]   Palli D: Epidemiology of gastric cancer: an evaluation of available evidence. *J Gastroenterol.2000* 35 Suppl;12:84-89.

[94]   Bjelakovic G, Nikolova D, Simonetti RG, Gluud C: Systematic review: primary and secondary prevention of gastrointestinal cancers with antioxidant supplements. *Aliment Pharmacol Ther.2008 Sep* 15;28:689-703.

[95]   Woodward M, Tunstall-Pedoe H, McColl K: Helicobacter pylori infection reduces systemic availability of dietary vitamin C. *Eur J Gastroenterol Hepatol.2001 Mar* 13:233-237.

[96]   Banerjee S, Hawksby C, Miller S, Dahill S, Beattie AD, Mccoll KE: Effect of Helicobacter pylori and its eradication on gastric juice ascorbic acid. *Gut.1994 Mar* 35:317-322.

[97]   Drake IM, Mapstone NP, Schorah CJ, White KL, Chalmers DM, Dixon MF, Axon AT: Reactive oxygen species activity and lipid peroxidation in Helicobacter pylori

associated gastritis: relation to gastric mucosal ascorbic acid concentrations and effect of H pylori eradication. *Gut.1998 Jun* 42:768-771.

[98] Jenab M, Riboli E, Ferrari P, Sabate J, Slimani N, Norat T, Friesen M, Tjonneland A, Olsen A, Overvad K, Boutron-Ruault MC, Clavel-Chapelon F, Touvier M, Boeing H, Schulz M, Linseisen J, Nagel G, Trichopoulou A, Naska A, Oikonomou E, Krogh V, Panico S, Masala G, Sacerdote C, Tumino R, Peeters PH, Numans ME, Bueno-de-Mesquita HB, Buchner FL, Lund E, Pera G, Sanchez CN, Sanchez MJ, Arriola L, Barricarte A, Quiros J, Hallmans G, Stenling R, Berglund G, Bingham S, Khaw KT, Key T, Allen N, Carneiro F, Mahlke U, Del GG, Palli D, Kaaks R, Gonzalez CA: Plasma and dietary vitamin C levels and risk of gastric cancer in the European Prospective Investigation into Cancer and Nutrition (EPIC-EURGAST). *Carcinogenesis.2006 Nov* 27:2250-2257.

[99] Correa P, Fontham ET, Bravo JC, Bravo LE, Ruiz B, Zarama G, Realpe JL, Malcom GT, Li D, Johnson WD, Mera R: Chemoprevention of gastric dysplasia: randomized trial of antioxidant supplements and anti-helicobacter pylori therapy. *J Natl Cancer Inst.2000 Dec* 6;92:1881-1888.

[100] Xiao F, Crissey MA, Lynch JP, Kaestner KH, Silberg DG, Suh E: Intestinal Metaplasia with a High Salt Diet Induces Epithelial Proliferation and Alters Cell Composition in the Gastric Mucosa of Mice. *Cancer Biol Ther* 2005 Jun;11;4.

[101] Fleischauer AT, Poole C, Arab L: Garlic consumption and cancer prevention: meta-analyses of colorectal and stomach cancers. *Am J Clin Nutr.2000 Oct* 72:1047-1052.

[102] Wang ZY, Cheng SJ, Zhou ZC, Athar M, Khan WA, Bickers DR, Mukhtar H: Antimutagenic activity of green tea polyphenols. *Mutat Res.1989 Jul* 223:273-285.

[103] Xu Y, Ho CT, Amin SG, Han C, Chung FL: Inhibition of tobacco-specific nitrosamine-induced lung tumorigenesis in A/J mice by green tea and its major polyphenol as antioxidants. *Cancer Res.1992 Jul* 15;52:3875-3879.

[104] Wang ZY, Hong JY, Huang MT, Reuhl KR, Conney AH, Yang CS: Inhibition of N-nitrosodiethylamine- and 4-(methylnitrosamino)-1-(3-pyridyl)-1-butanone-induced tumorigenesis in A/J mice by green tea and black tea. *Cancer Res.1992 Apr* 1;52:1943-1947.

[105] Glade MJ: Food, nutrition, and the prevention of cancer: a global perspective. American Institute for Cancer Research/World Cancer Research Fund, American Institute for Cancer Research, 1997. *Nutrition.1999 Jun* 15:523-526.

[106] Tatematsu M, Takahashi M, Hananouchi M, Shirai T, Hirose M: Protective effect of mucin on experimental gastric cancer induced by N-methyl-N'-nitro-N-nitrosoguanidine plus sodium chloride in rats. *Gann.1976 Apr* 67:223-229.

[107] Takahashi M, Hasegawa R: Enhancing effects of dietary salt on both initiation and promotion stages of rat gastric carcinogenesis. *Princess Takamatsu Symp.1985* 16:169-182.

[108] Liu C, Russell RM: Nutrition and gastric cancer risk: an update. *Nutr Rev.2008 May* 66:237-249.

[109] Ye WM, Yi YN, Luo RX, Zhou TS, Lin RT, Chen GD: Diet and gastric cancer: a casecontrol study in Fujian Province, China. *World J Gastroenterol.1998 Dec* 4:516-518.

[110] Ward MH, Lopez-Carrillo L: Dietary factors and the risk of gastric cancer in Mexico City. *Am J Epidemiol.1999 May* 15;149:925-932.

[111] Lee SA, Kang D, Shim KN, Choe JW, Hong WS, Choi H: Effect of diet and Helicobacter pylori infection to the risk of early gastric cancer. *J Epidemiol.2003 May* 13:162-168.

[112] Kim HJ, Chang WK, Kim MK, Lee SS, Choi BY: Dietary factors and gastric cancer in Korea: a case-control study. *Int J Cancer.2002 Feb* 1;97:531-535.

[113] Shikata K, Kiyohara Y, Kubo M, Yonemoto K, Ninomiya T, Shirota T, Tanizaki Y, Doi Y, Tanaka K, Oishi Y, Matsumoto T, Iida M: A prospective study of dietary salt intake and gastric cancer incidence in a defined Japanese population: the Hisayama study. *Int J Cancer.2006 Jul* 1;119:196-201.

[114] Bartsch H, Spiegelhalder B: Environmental exposure to N-nitroso compounds (NNOC) and precursors: an overview. *Eur J Cancer Prev.1996 Sep* 5 Suppl;1:11-17.

[115] Tricker AR, Preussmann R: Carcinogenic N-nitrosamines in the diet: occurrence, formation, mechanisms and carcinogenic potential. *Mutat Res.1991 Mar-Apr* 259:277-289.

[116] Jakszyn P, Gonzalez CA: Nitrosamine and related food intake and gastric and oesophageal cancer risk: a systematic review of the epidemiological evidence. *World J Gastroenterol.2006 Jul* 21;12:4296-4303.

[117] Shuker DE, Bartsch H: DNA adducts of nitrosamines. *IARC Sci Publ.1994*73-89.

[118] Franke A, Teyssen S, Singer MV: Alcohol-related diseases of the esophagus and stomach. *Dig Dis.2005* 23:204-213.

[119] Boeing H: Epidemiological research in stomach cancer: progress over the last ten years. *J Cancer Res Clin Oncol.1991* 117:133-143.

[120] Pollack ES, Nomura AM, Heilbrun LK, Stemmermann GN, Green SB: Prospective study of alcohol consumption and cancer. *N Engl J Med.1984 Mar* 8;310:617-621.

[121] Gonzalez CA, Pera G, Agudo A, Palli D, Krogh V, Vineis P, Tumino R, Panico S, Berglund G, Siman H, Nyren O, Agren A, Martinez C, Dorronsoro M, Barricarte A, Tormo MJ, Quiros J, Allen N, Bingham S, Day N, Miller A, Nagel G, Boeing H, Overvad K, Tjonneland A, Bueno-de-Mesquita HB, Boshuizen HC, Peeters P, Numans M, Clavel-Chapelon F, Helen I, Agapitos E, Lund E, Fahey M, Saracci R, Kaaks R, Riboli E: Smoking and the risk of gastric cancer in the European Prospective Investigation Into Cancer and Nutrition (EPIC). *Int J Cancer.2003 Nov* 20;107:629-634.

[122] Tredaniel J, Boffetta P, Buiatti E, Saracci R, Hirsch A: Tobacco smoking and gastric cancer: review and meta-analysis. *Int J Cancer.1997 Aug* 7;72:565-573.

[123] Ladeiras-Lopes R, Pereira AK, Nogueira A, Pinheiro-Torres T, Pinto I, Santos-Pereira R, Lunet N: Smoking and gastric cancer: systematic review and meta-analysis of cohort studies. *Cancer Causes Control.2008 Sep* 19:689-701.

In: Gastric Cancer: Diagnosis, Early Prevention, and Treatment   ISBN 978-1-61668-313-9
Editor: V. D. Pasechnikov, pp. 197-233   © 2010 Nova Science Publishers, Inc.

Chapter VI

ENDOSCOPIC DIAGNOSIS OF EARLY GASTRIC CANCER AND GASTRIC PRECANCEROUS LESIONS

Sergey Kashin[*,1], *Alexey Pavlov*[2], *Kazuhiro Gono*[3], *Alexander Nadezhin*[4]

[1]Department of Endoscopy, Yaroslavl Regional Cancer Hospital, Yaroslavl, Russia
[2]Department of Histology, Yaroslavl State Medical Academy, Yaroslavl, Russia
[3]Research Department, Olympus Medical Systems Corp., Tokyo, Japan
[4]Department of Pathology, Yaroslavl Regional Cancer Hospital, Yaroslavl, Russia

ABSTRACT

Gastric cancer is the leading cause of cancer death worldwide. Early detection of cancer or their precursors may be the only chance to reduce this high mortality. Treatment results are dependent on the stage of the disease, which is related to the extent of the tumor. Endoscopic technology has simplified the diagnosis of precancerous lesions and gastric malignancies. The commercial introduction of the first flexible fiber endoscope in 1961 marked the beginning of a revolution in the diagnosis and management of gastrointestinal disease. Since then, ongoing development has taken place in the area of endoscopy design and presently, fiberoptic (video) endoscopes are largely replaced by electronic videoendoscopes. Recent advances in biomedical optics are illuminating new ways to detect premalignant lesions and early gastric cancers with endoscopy. Relying on the interaction of light with tissue, these 'state-of-the-art' techniques potentially offer an improved strategy for diagnosis of early mucosal lesions by facilitating targeted excisional biopsies. Furthermore, the prospects of real-time 'optical biopsy' and improved staging of lesions may significantly enhance the endoscopist's ability to detect subtle neoplastic mucosal changes and lead to curative endoscopic ablation of these lesions. However, the differentiation of lesions and the diagnosis of early neoplastic changes remain difficult despite the existing recommended

---

[*] Corresponding Author: Sergey Kashin, MD, Dept of Endoscopy, Yaroslavl Regional Cancer Hospital, Chkalova streen 4a, Yaroslavl, Russia, 150054. Tel/Fax 7 4852 721294, e-mail: s_kashin@mail.ru

classifications for various mucosal surface details. Together with recent interest in new imaging techniques should be considered to represent a simple, safe and inexpensive technique that may be useful in identifying premalignant conditions and minute cancerous lesions, estimating their superficial extent and determining the histological type and submucosal invasion.

INTRODUCTION

Gastric cancer is the leading cause of cancer death worldwide. Early detection of cancer or their precursors may be the only chance to reduce this high mortality. Treatment results are dependent on the stage of the disease, which is related to the extent of the tumor. In the pursuit of a cure, gastric cancer must be diagnosed in its early stage. Gastric cancer confined to the mucosa and submucosa is regarded as defining the early stage of the disease (early gastric cancer, EGC), due to its overall favorable prognosis: the 5-year survival rate is greater than 90-95%. Most cases of ECG are asymptomatic and difficult to diagnose by X-ray examination tools such as the upper gastrointestinal series and computed tomography. Endoscopy is the gold standard procedure in early detection of precancerous conditions and neoplasia (either confirmed cancer or high-grade and low-grade dysplasia) [1].

However, poor sensitivity associated with frequent surveillance programs incorporating conventional screening tools, such as white light endoscopy and multiple random biopsies, is a significant limitation. Conventional endoscopy sometimes is limited to detecting lesions based on gross morphological changes, while new optically based devices offer the potential of detecting the very earliest mucosal changes at the microstructural level by detecting the relative changes in the way light interacts with tissue along the disease transformation pathway. Recent advances in biomedical optics are illuminating new ways to detect premalignant lesions and early cancers of the GI tract with endoscopy. Relying on the interaction of light with tissue, these 'state-of-the-art' techniques potentially offer an improved strategy for diagnosis of early mucosal lesions by facilitating targeted excisional biopsies. Furthermore, the prospects of real-time 'optical biopsy' and improved staging of lesions may significantly enhance the endoscopist's ability to detect subtle neoplastic mucosal changes and lead to curative endoscopic ablation of these lesions[2].

The detailed diagnostic procedure sometimes needed to assess the range of infiltration and depth of invasion of the carcinoma, which is always required before the appropriate therapy can be selected. Accurate staging of gastric wall invasion and lymph node involvement is important for determining prognosis and appropriate treatment. Endoscopic ultrasonography may be involved in staging the tumor.

BASICS OF EARLY GASTRIC CANCER (EGC)

Definition

ECG is defined as carcinoma confined to the mucosa and submucosa irrespective of lymph node involvement, and corresponds to a T1 tumor in the TNM classification[3]. The definition of EGC is slightly different in the West and in Japan due to the different terminological conceptions of the limit of the neoplasm in the gastric mucosa.

Despite such efforts as the Vienna classification differences still exist in the criteria used to distinguish high-grade dysplasia from intramucosal cancer by Western pathologists (who rely on invasion of the lamina propria) and those used by Japanese pathologists (who use cytological and architectural features)[4]. Endoscopic examination is the only method by which EGC can be detected, and even then careful observation is needed supported by accurate knowledge of the characteristics of EGC lesions.

Endoscopic Classification

In 1962 the Japanese Endoscopic Society introduced a definition of EGC and an endoscopic classification for an early stage of the disease. Recently, it has been recorded by the Japanese Gastric Cancer Association as a T stage of TNM classification (Figure 1)[5]. The classification of EGC into types: I (elevated), IIa (superficially elevated), IIb (flat), IIc (superficially depressed), and III (excavated), remains valid. In combined superficial types, the type occupying the largest area is described first, followed by the next most dominant type: e.g. IIc + III [1]. This classification is the result of meticulous work by Japanese endoscopists.

The Paris Endoscopic Classification of Superficial Neoplastic Lesions: Esophagus, Stomach, and Colon

Correct diagnosis of EGC is becoming more and more important not only in Japan but also internationally. There is a trend that early cancers are integrated and classified as superficial carcinomas, since they exist on or in the superficial layer. In "The Paris classification" published recently, the Japanese criteria for the classification of EGC were applied to the classification of early cancers in the esophagus and colon[6].

In "The Paris classification" like in Japan, neoplastic lesions of the stomach with a "superficial" endoscopic appearance are classified as subtypes of "type 0". The term "type 0" was chosen to distinguish the classification of "superficial" lesions from the Borrmann classification proposed in 1926 for "advanced" gastric tumors, which included types 1 to 4[7]. The Japanese Gastric Cancer Association (JGCA) also added type 5 for unclassifiable advanced tumors. Within type 0 there are polypoid and non-polypoid subtypes. The non-polypoid subtypes include lesions with a small variation of the surface (slightly elevated, flat, and slightly depressed) and excavated lesions.

The complete modification for gastric tumors is represented in the following way:

type 0 - superficial polypoid, flat/depressed, or excavated tumors
type 1 - polypoid carcinomas, usually attached on a wide base
type 2 - ulcerated carcinomas with sharply demarcated and raised margins
type 3 - ulcerated, infiltrating carcinomas without definite limits
type 4 - nonulcerated, diffusely infiltrating carcinomas
type 5 - unclassifiable advanced carcinomas

Type 0 with its subtypes adapted to endoscopic appearance of EGC. In a pragmatic and simple approach, it is mandatory to classify superficial lesions routinely in at least one of the 5 major types: 0-I, 0-IIa, 0- IIb, 0-IIc, 0-III shown in Figure 2. Polypoid 0-I lesions can be divided (mainly in colon) into type 0-Ip and type 0-Is (pedunculated and sessile)[8].

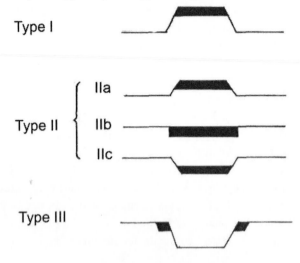

Figure 1. Japanese classification of early gastric cancer. Adopted from: Japanese Gastric Cancer Association: Japanese classification of gastric cancer. 2nd English edition. Gastric Cancer 1998 [5].

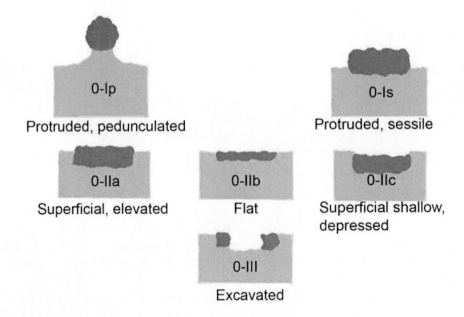

Figure 2. Schematic representation of the major variants of type 0 neoplastic lesions of the digestive tract: protruded (types 0- Ip and Is), superficial (three subtypes 0- IIa, IIb, and II c) and excavated (type 0- III). Adopted from: The macroscopic classification of early neoplasia of the digestive tract. Endoscopy 2002;34 [9].

Endoscopic Characteristics of Early Gastric Cancer

Because the criteria for the classification are subjective, there are surely individual variations in the classification of each lesion among examiners. The following points are used to detect and classify lesions.

Type 0-I, Protruded or Polypoid

A polypoid neoplastic lesion protrudes above the surrounding surface at endoscopy. In the operative specimen, the height of the lesion is more than double the thickness of the adjacent mucosa. In pedunculated polyps, the base is narrow; in sessile polyps, the base and the top of the lesion have the same diameter. Protruded lesions can be diagnosed correctly if biopsy of the lesion is made without exception [6]. Almost all type 0-I early cancers are confined to the mucosa and are a good indication for endoscopic resection including the surrounding area.

Type 0-IIa, Superficial Elevated

This type of the lesion is often detected as a sessile elevated lesion. Sometimes 0-IIa type (slightly elevated type) is difficult to differentiate from protruded lesion (type 0-I). The respective classification of these two types is made easier by placing a biopsy forceps next to the lesion as a calibrating gauge. This standard is applied to the height of the lesion and not to its diameter. Lesions protruding above the level of the closed jaws of the biopsy forceps (approximately 2.5 mm) are classified as 0-I; lesions protruding below this level are classified as 0-IIa. In general, type 0-IIa is identified as flat elevation (sometimes reddish) with a comparatively uneven surface. Submucosal invasion can be suspected on the basis of a central depression in the protrusion, which is described as type 0-IIa+IIc. Chromoendoscopy is very useful for diagnosis of superficial elevated lesions.

Type 0-IIb, Flat

Definite cases of type 0-IIb EGC are very rare, except for minute cancers discovered by a detailed histopathological search. In these cases, endoscopic assessment of the cancerous area is very difficult. Conventional endoscopy sometimes is limited to detect flat lesions based on gross morphological changes, while new optically based devices (high-magnification endoscopy and narrow band imaging) offer the potential of detecting the very earliest mucosal changes at the microstructural level. In the histology of the accompanying IIb area, most of the cases showed diffuse-type carcinoma.

Type 0-IIc, Superficial Depressed

Type 0-IIc lesions, characterized by a well-demarcated shallow depression with an irregular margin, are easy to diagnose by endoscopic findings alone. A reddish shallow depression with flat cancerous mucosa surrounded by a saw-edged border is the characteristic form of intestinal-type carcinoma, while typical diffuse-type carcinoma shows a discolored uneven depression with a sharp margin. Chromoendoscopy is most effective for diagnosing the type 0-IIc cancer [1].

Table 1. Incidence and types of early gastric cancer

Types of EGC	Proportion of patients with EGC N = 4,029
0-I	2.9%
0-IIa	14.1%
0-IIb	8.3%
0-IIc	74.2%
0-III	0.5%
Total	100%

Type 0-III, Excavated

The distinction between a depressed (0-IIc) and ulcerated lesion (0-III) during endoscopy is based upon the depth of the depression and the analysis of the epithelial surface in the depressed area. Superficial erosions in a depressed lesion involve only the most superficial layers. In the ulcerated lesion, there is loss of the mucosa and often of the submucosa. In excavated lesions (types 0-III, 0-IIc+III) and slightly depressed lesions (type 0-IIc) convergence of folds or abnormal folds are frequently found. A benign peptic ulcer occasionally occurs within a cancerous area. Depending on the healing process of a peptic ulcer surrounded by cancerous mucosa, macroscopic types can change from 0-III, to 0-IIc+III, to 0-IIc (+ ulcer scar), serially. If an active peptic ulcer covers almost the entire cancerous area (0-III), the diagnosis is difficult. For this reason, a follow-up examination is very important for accurate diagnosis of a type 0-IIc EGC with an ulcer or a scar [1].

The relative proportions of each type of EGC differ in various institutions. According to the data of Cancer Institute Hospital (Tokyo, Japan) patients with type 0-IIc and its combined types account for 75% of all patients suffering from EGC. With regard to the classification of EGC, the proportion of patients which were diagnosed in this hospital from 1973 to 2003 is shown in Table 1[6].

Endoscopic technology has simplified the diagnosis of precancerous lesions and gastric malignancies. EGC can be detected and diagnosed with the help of chromoendoscopy, high-magnification endoscopy and narrow band imaging.

CHROMOENDOSCOPY

Chromoendoscopy, *(chrom-, chromo- [Gk.Chroma] meaning color or pigment)*, synonymous with chromoscopy, is an "old" endoscopic tissue-staining technique that has been practiced in Japan since early days of fiber-endoscopy.[10]. Dye spraying allows improved visualization of a subtle mucosal lesion that is not possible with conventional examination. The most popular method - contrast method is a simple technique in which a blue pigment, such as 0.2%-0.5% indigo carmine solution, is sprayed onto the mucosal surface. Indigo carmine is a contrast stain, which accumulates in the mucosal pits and thus improves the visualization of the pit pattern and details of the mucosal surface architecture It is inexpensive, non-toxic, and does not require prior washing with a mucolytic agent. After conventional endoscopic observation gastric mucosa is sprayed with simethicone to eliminate froth and bubbles followed by dye solution through a spraying catheter or a biopsy channel. Although chromoendoscopy cannot make all invisible sites visible, it is a convenient method to differentiate a target point from surrounding tissue easily. Particularly, it facilitates to determine a site for biopsy and provides a clear border between pathological and normal sites[11]. Figure 3 shows how EGC suspected on the basis of color change in a localized area of abnormality (Figure 3a) is diagnosed as type 0-IIa+IIc EGC on the basis of typical chromoscopic findings with indigo carmine (Figure 3b).

Methylene blue is taken up by absorbing tissues such as small intestinal and colonic cells Gastric carcinogenesis is generally considered to be a multistep progression from chronic gastritis to glandular atrophy, intestinal metaplasia, dysplasia, and ultimately cancer[12]. In a prospective study from Japan, H. pylori–infected subjects with gastric intestinal metaplasia were found to have a >6-fold increase in risk of gastric cancer. Changes in gastric atrophy and intestinal metaplasia are therefore widely used as a surrogate end point in cancer chemoprevention trials [13,14]. Therefore, methylene blue chromoendoscopy has been used to screen for intestinal metaplasia, areas of dysplasia and carcinoma located in metaplasia. Areas of intestinal metaplasia in the stomach will highlight because these areas stain positively while gastric mucosa do not. Usually a concentration of 0.2-0.5% of methylene blue is used. Chromoendoscopy using methylene blue allows to estimate not only the areas of intestinal metaplasia but also the degree of metaplasia as a "field". The study of Ito et al showed a good correlation between the histological features and status of methylene blue staining[15]. In our study the grade of intestinal metaplasia was also evaluated by dye-endoscopy using methylene blue. The results of the study suggest the reversibility of intestinal metaplasia in patients with successful H. pylori eradication therapy in the gastric antrum during the follow-up period, which was confirmed by methylene blue staining (Figure 4)[16].

Safety of pigments. Indigo carmine is a safe pigment that is used as a food additive and as an injectable dye for kidney function testing[17]. However, care is needed when using methylene blue, which is absorbed during chromoendoscopy and may have adverse effects. Methylene blue can induce oxidative damage of DNA in Barrett's mucosa after chromoendoscopy when photosensitised by white light[18].

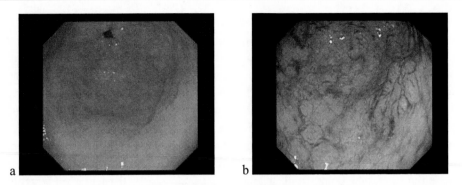

Figure 3. Type 0-IIa+IIc early gastric cancer in antrum: a. Ordinary observation; b. View with indigo carmine contrast method. Indigo carmine 0,2% solution clearly demonstrates the contour of the lesion.

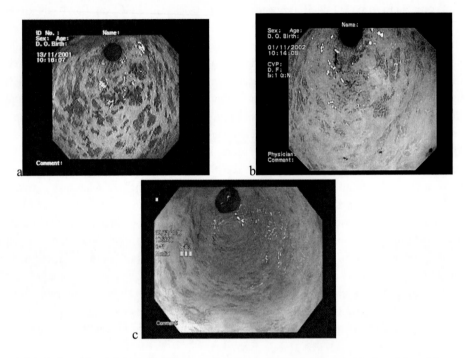

Figure 4. Methylene blue solution (0.5%) was spread over the gastric antrum before (a) and 1-year after (b) and 4-years after (c) eradication therapy. The patient was a 60-year-old female.

HIGH-RESOLUTION AND HIGH-MAGNIFICATION ENDOSCOPY

The commercial introduction of the first flexible fiber endoscope in 1961 marked the beginning of a revolution in the diagnosis and management of gastrointestinal disease. Since then, ongoing development has taken place in the area of endoscopy design and presently, fiberoptic (video) endoscopes are largely replaced by electronic videoendoscopes. Conventional videoendoscopes are equipped with CCD chips of 100K to 300K pixels, meaning that each image is built up from 100 000 to 300 000 individual pixels. This technical feature, also referred to as pixel density, is important because it relates to the image resolution and hence to the ability to discriminate two closely approximated points. The higher the pixel density, the higher the image resolution, the more likely minute lesions will be discriminated and detected. The second generation of electronic videoendoscopes is equipped with CCD chips of 400K and recently endoscopes (both gastroscopes and colonoscopes) were introduced with 850K pixel density. Endoscopes with such a high resolution are referred to as high resolution endoscopes. This terminology can be confusing at times because the adjunct high resolution is sometimes also used to refer to magnifying endoscopes. In this article the adjunct high resolution relates to pixel density of the CCD chip.

Endoscopic detection of gastrointestinal pathology currently depends on the recognition of visible mucosal lesions, but these findings on standard endoscopy have a poor correlation with histopathological diagnosis. Some endoscopes, including high resolution endoscopes, are equipped with an optical zooming facility comprising of a movable lens in the tip of the scope. By controlling the focal distance, the scope can move very close to the mucosal surface providing the magnified image. These scopes are referred to as magnifying endoscopes. Magnifying endoscopic observation of the gastrointestinal tract was first reported in 1967 by Okuyama[19]. Since then, intensive efforts have been made to analyze the characteristics of the surface structure of the gastrointestinal tract, and these attempts have succeeded in distinguishing between neoplastic and non-neoplastic lesions. Magnification endoscopy with or without chromoendoscopy is unique in that it provides a more precise evaluation of the detail of the mucosal surface, a high yield for targeted biopsy specimens and, consequently, an improvement in diagnostic accuracy[20]. There are two types of magnification available in endoscopy: electronic and optical. The electronic enlarged image provides the endoscopist with an image of bigger size with no improvements of resolution, while the optical magnification, with a zoom objective placed at the tip of the endoscope, just distal to the CCD, gives additional details of the tissue features. The endoscope with optical zoom utilizes a moveable lens, so that the endoscope can move very close to the mucosal surface to provide a magnified or enlarged image. This endoscope is comparable to the dissecting microscope. The magnifying power of the optical zoom can reach up to ´150, but ´80 is enough for the most applications. When the zoom is activated, the focal distance between the objective and the mucosal surface decreases in proportion to the power of magnification, therefore the tip of the instrument is placed at a few millimeters (~3 mm) from the target and a small area of the mucosa is explored. A transparent hood, fixed at the tip of the endoscope, helps to maintain the adequate distance, particularly in the cardiac region [21,22,23]. The gastric mucosal surface and the superficial microvasculature have been observed in detail on magnification endoscopy and named as a fine gastric mucosal pattern [24]. Magnified view shows whitish pits and sulci surrounded by reddish interstitial parts. Gastric pits and sulci are histologically identical to gastric glands. Dark spots are the center of the gastric gland (Figure 6c, Figure 11a). Two decades ago, a classification for magnified endoscopic findings of gastric pits was proposed to detect the gastric histological changes [25]. Sakaki's classification indicated successfully the progression of atrophic changes and intestinal metaplasia (Figure 5) [26].

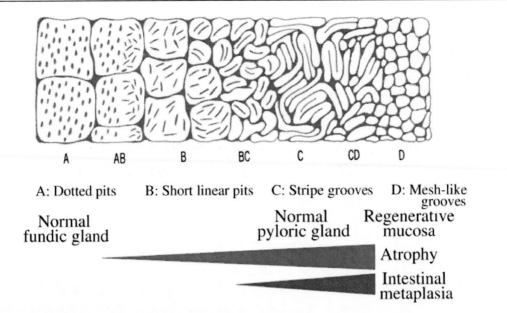

Figure 5. Classification of gastric pits (Sakaki's Classification). It indicates not only the normal microstructure of gastric mucosa but also the progression of atrophic changes and intestinal metaplasia. Adopted from reference 26: Digestive Endoscopy, 2005, Vol.17, Issue s1, P: S5-S10.

Magnification endoscopy was used to evaluate the surface mucosal architecture to distinguish between benign and malignant lesions and for improving detection of early flat and depressed cancer. Most of the differentiated intramucosal gastric carcinomas of a superficial type were observed on magnification endoscopy as well demarcated areas [27]. These areas were associated with disappearance of the subepithelial capillary-network (SECN) pattern, and were accompanied by proliferation of tumorous microvessels, which showed irregularity in size, shape, and distribution. Our studies show that magnified observation of the microvascular architecture of gastric carcinoma may be useful for characterizing flat carcinomas, the degree of differentiation, and may also be useful for determining the lateral extent of spread (Figure 6).

NARROW-BAND IMAGING (NBI)[1]

The application of opto-electronic in video-endoscopes aims to improve accuracy in diagnosis, through image processing and digital technology. Narrow band imaging, one of the most recent techniques, consists of using interference filters for the illumination of the target in narrowed red, green, and blue (R/G/B) bands of the spectrum.

---

[1] "NBI" and "Narrow Band Imaging" are registered trademarks of Olympus Corporation.

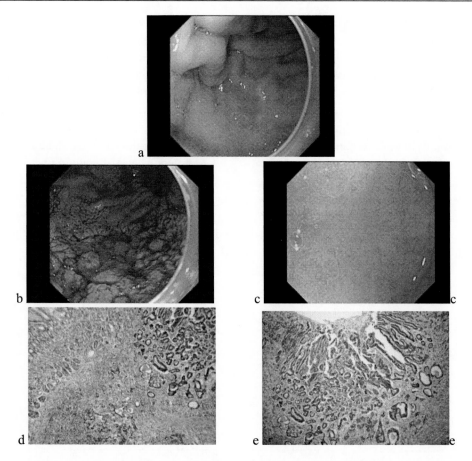

Figure 6. Diagnosis of early gastric cancer: a) conventional observation; b) indigo carmine chromoendoscopy; c) high-magnification endoscopy - presence of demarcation areas (white arrows) and capillary network (corkscrew vessels); magnified endoscopic findings of the noncarcinomatous surrounding mucosa - a regular honeycomblike subepithelial capillary network (SECN) pattern can be observed; d) Carcinoma glands surrounded with marked lymphocytic infiltrate are seen to be invading deep mucosa layer but not deeper than superficial submucosa (lamina propria is destroyed only focally). Intact neighboring gastric glands are seen at the left; e) The same case. It is clearly seen that tumor length is not more than a centimeter. At margins normal glands and just superficially spreading isolated cancer cells are seen.

Technical Explanation of Narrow Band Imaging

The chromoendoscopy is a well known method for capturing fine structures of the mucosal surface. However it still has some problems for daily clinical use, such as difficulty in achieving complete and even coating of the mucosal surface with the dye and the extra time required to perform the procedure. And the chromoendoscopy is often not effective in enhancing the capillary patterns. To resolve them, the narrow band technology (NBI) was proposed in 2005. At this time, two systems which NBI work exist - Olympus EVIS EXERA II (EXERA II) and Olympus EVIS LUCERA SPECTRUM (SPECTRUM). The EXERA II is based on a color CCD chip in which color imaging is done by several tiny color filters in each pixel. Creating color information on the SPECTRUM is a black and white CCD and the use of RGB color filter wheel equipped within the light source unit. Although both systems are based on how a color image is produced, the principle of NBI on each system is the same and activating NBI provides improved image contrast when viewing micro-vessel patterns within the superficial mucosa. A schematic diagram of the interaction between light and tissue component is shown in Figure 7. When light irradiates tissue, other than surface reflection, absorption by the blood content and scattering from cellar component occur. The fact of the wavelength dependency of both interactions is well known. That is, hemoglobin as a blood content highly absorbs light in 415 nm and 540 nm, and light is more scattered in shorter wavelength (blue range) than in longer wavelength (more reddish color). This wavelength-dependency affects light penetration depth in different wavelength. That is, the penetration depth of shorter wavelength light is highly limited within a superficial layer, and on the other hand the longer wavelength light is able to be diffused in a deeper layer of tissue.

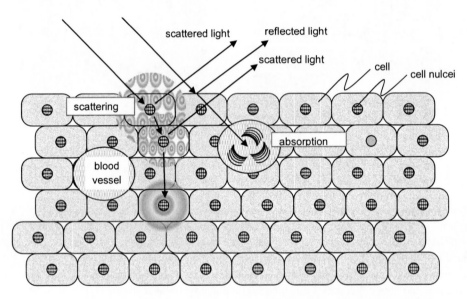

Figure 7. Schematic diagram of the interaction between light and tissue components.

Figure 8 (lower figures) shows a schematic diagram of blood vessels in tissue. Generally, diameters of blood vessels in tissue get thinner closer to the surface of mucosa. Therefore, the use of shorter wavelength light of which penetration depth is highly limited helps improve the image contrast of the capillary pattern in a superficial layer. Figure 8 (upper figures) provides images of the backside mucosa of the human tongue exposed to different center wavelengths of narrow band light. We can see the vessel images change greatly according to the center wavelength. The fine vessels presented on the 415 nm image were identified as vessels near the superficial layer of the mucosa based on a comparison with the pathological configuration of the tongue mucosa. Unlike 415 nm images, no fine vessels are presented on the images of 540 nm, one of the hemoglobin absorption. On the other hand, the vessels presented on the 540nm images are not displayed on the 415 nm images. We believe this is because 415nm light is unable to reach the depth where the vessels presented on the 540nm light are located owning to multiple scattering effect within the living tissue. The fine vessels presented on the 415 nm image are not seen on the 540 nm because the two bands have different absorption coefficient of hemoglobin. From presented images, the 415 nm image can present the structure of fine vessels at the superficial layer and the 540 nm narrow band image can display the vessel structure in the relatively deep part of the mucosa if the living tissue is observed under narrow band light of 415 nm and 540 nm which are wavelengths used in NBI systems.

In order to display NBI images in colors, the video processor of the EXERA II and the SPECTRUM is designed so that the 415 nm image can be assigned to blue and green plane and the 540 nm image can be assigned to red plane of the final image. This assignment makes fine vessels look brownish-red and thicker vessels in the deep layer look cyan as shown in Figure 9.

The NBI system uses blue narrow band light to image capillaries in the surface layers of mucosal membranes, and green narrow band light to image thick blood vessels located inside membranes while enhancing the contrast of surface capillaries. This approach also has the potential to improve the efficiency of clinical examinations by reducing examination times and unnecessary biopsies. A priority to the demonstration of the epithelial crests of the surface and the distribution of the superficial capillaries is ensured by a higher radiance obtained in the blue band. NBI creates enhanced images of capillaries in the surface layers of mucosal membranes and minute patterns on mucosal membranes by irradiating target areas with light in two narrow wave bands that are strongly absorbed by circulating hemoglobin (Figure 10). Especially in gastric mucosa, capillary and pit patterns are fundamentals for early diagnosis. We strongly believe that NBI will be a useful tool for the most physicians who have to do precise observation in daily procedures.

NBI associates two groups of technological advance: image processing and magnifying endoscopy. In the instrument developed by the Olympus Corporation the incident light is distributed in discontinuous narrow bands of photons in the Blue, Green, and Red (R/G/B), which have distinct depth of penetration into mucosa. This gives access to an improved analysis of the architecture in surface and of the capillary network just under the surface.

The classification and understanding of chronic inflammatory processes in the digestive mucosa (gastritis) become more reliable. With respect to the treatment decision, NBI technique confers an increased reliability for the classification of the lesions in four groups:

Benign without malignant potential;
Benign with a malignant potential;
Malignant with invasion limited to the mucosa and/or the submucosa;
Malignant with in-depth invasion of the digestive wall [28].

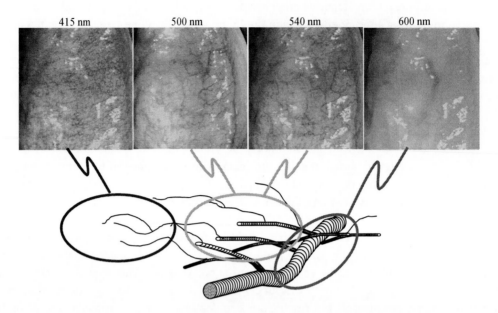

Figure 8. Images of the backside mucosa of the human tongue (upper figures) and a schematic diagram of blood vessels (lower figures).

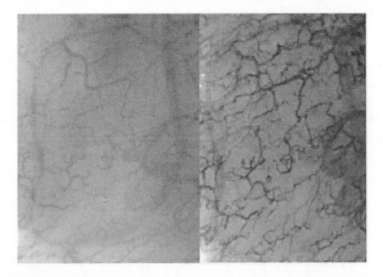

Figure 9. Color images of backside mucosa of human tongue. The left and right images were obtained by the use of WLI and NBI with magnifying endoscope respectively. The NBI image provides enhanced contrast of micro vessel pattern as brownish appearance and cyan color pattern for blood vessels in the deeper layer.

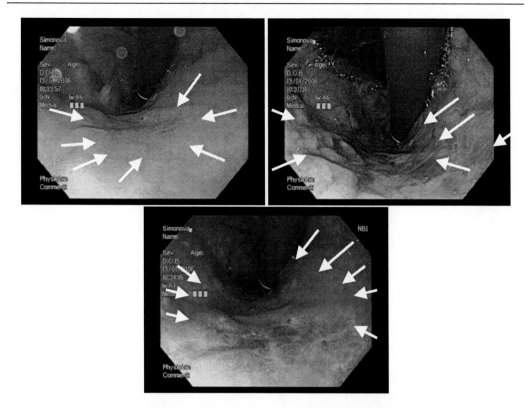

Figure 10. NBI may enhance the mucosal surface contrast without the use of dyes in cases of EGC. Demarcation areas (white arrows) of type IIc EGC are clearly diagnosed using NBI.

It is imperative for the endoscopist to make a differential diagnosis between benign and malignant lesions. For such purposes, NBI in combination with magnification endoscopy is a powerful tool for making a correct diagnosis of gastric superficial neoplasia. K. Yao unveiled NBI potential in diagnosis of benign gastric lesions and early cancer based on clearly visualization of both the microvascular architecture and the microsurface structure. He described the new optical sign for discriminating between adenoma and carcinoma - white opaque substance (WOS). The assessment of WOS regular or irregular patterns could be useful in cases when vessels are not clearly seen [29,30] (Figure 11).

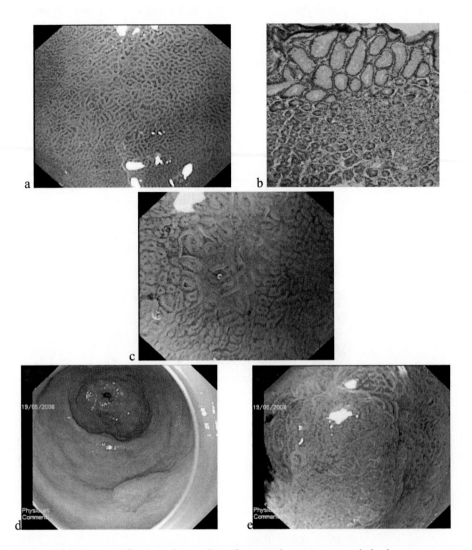

Figure 11. a). NBI high-magnification observation of noncarcinomatous gastric body mucosa - a regular honeycomblike subepithelial capillary network (SECN) pattern in correlation with histology (b), NBI enhances the contrast of surface capillaries; c). NBI observation of intestinal metaplasia in the antrum; d), e). early gastric cancer, type IIa: NBI with optical magnification helps to detect pathological vessels at the center of the tumor and WOS with an irregular distribution is present along the edges of the lesion where vessels pattern cannot be clearly visualized.

Principles of Detection of the Lesions

Characterization of a Lesion after Detection

Once an abnormal area has been detected using a video endoscope equipped with these recently developed technical facilities, the lesion should be characterized using the following steps (Figure 12):

1. Assessment of the gross morphology in standard vision with the help of NBI and chromoendoscopy.
2. Analysis of the magnification endoscopy findings should be based on two distinctive microanatomies:
    A) Microvascular (MV) architecture with two patterns: regular microvascular pattern (RMVP) with regular microvessels (in shape and arrangement) and irregular microvascular pattern (IMVP) with irregular in shape and arrangement microvessels (tortuous or irregularly branched microvessels with abnormal caliber and with various sizes). Slight vascular alterations suggest either non-neoplastic lesion or low-grade neoplasia; severe vascular alterations with numerous corkscrew vessels of irregular caliber suggest high-grade noninvasive or invasive neoplasia.
    B) Microsurface (MS) structure with three microsurface patterns:
        *   Regular microsurface pattern (RMSP),
        *   Irregular microsurface pattern (IMSP),
        *   Absent microsurface pattern (AMSP).

If we apply these categories to early gastric carcinoma, an IMVP or IMSP with the presence of a demarcation line between the lesion and the surrounding mucosa is characteristic for adenocarcinoma.

Gross morphology of the lesion. The limits and the relief of the target lesion are assessed under standard endoscopic vision. The diameter of the lesion is estimated by comparison with a guide (a graduated probe or biopsy forceps). The gross macroscopic appearance, enhanced by chromoscopy with indigo carmine for detecting depressions and ridges, is classified into subtypes of type 0 superficial neoplastic lesions. Many flat (nonpolypoid) lesions remain superficial as they increase in diameter in a transverse-type growth pattern; other flat lesions progress to invasive carcinoma in spite of their small size in a vertical-type growth pattern and these lesions usually correspond to the depressed type of superficial neoplastic lesion (0-IIc).

The microvascular network. The superficial vascular network in the suspect area is best explored without chromoscopy and with the help of magnification. Small vessels are clearly contrasted in dark green by using the NBI technique. The subepithelial capillaries reproduce the microarchitecture (crests and pits) of the normal epithelium: a honeycomb network around the neck of gastric pits in the gastric oxyntic mucosa and transverse collecting venules visible more deeply; coiled subepithelial capillaries in the gastric antral mucosa.

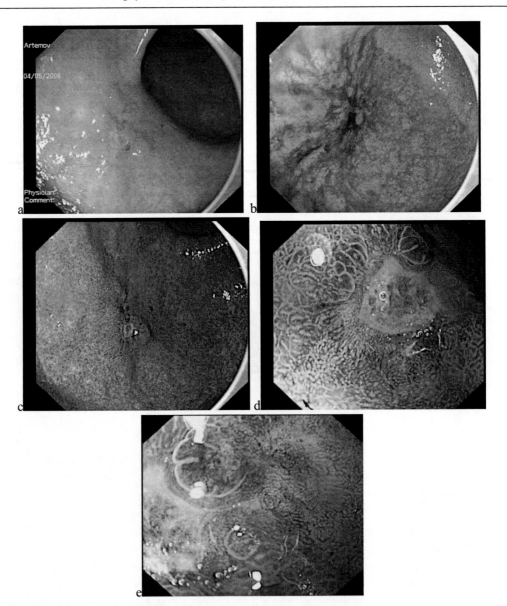

Figure 12. EGC type IIC detected and characterized using conventional observation (a), indigo carmine chromoendoscopy (b), NBI (c) and high-magnification combined with NBI (d, e) for better visualization of irregular microsurface pattern (IMSP), absent microsurface pattern (AMSP) and irregular microvascular pattern (IMVP) with pathological vessels.

In areas with chronic inflammation, various degrees of alterations are seen: in the stomach, *H. pylori* infection causes a diffuse reddening of the surface of the oxyntic mucosa with regression of the honeycomb pattern and of collecting venules.

In areas with neoplasia, various degrees of change are observed: in the stomach, intramucosal cancer is shown by abnormal superficial vessels (mesh, coil, or corkscrew), their appearance depending on the degree of tumor differentiation.

The microsurface structure of the epithelium. When using NBI or chromoscopy with the optical zoom or the macro objective lens, pits and ridges are enhanced at the surface of the mucosal depressions [31]. Magnification is particularly helpful for identifying areas with intestinal metaplasia or with a disorganized structure, suggesting low- or high-grade intraepithelial neoplasia. Magnification is also helpful for classification of neoplastic lesions.

We examined 156 lesions detected in 116 patients using high-magnification endoscopy and NBI. The results of histological examination of detected lesions are summarized in Table 2.

Table 2. The number of neoplastic and benign lesions confirmed by histology

	№ of patients	№ of lesions	Early gastric cancer	Adenoma/ dysplasia	Hyperplastic polyp	Gastric ulcer	Erosion
High-magnification endoscopy	56	80	14	15	18	12	21
Narrow band imaging	60	76	10	13	17	16	20
Total	116	156	24	28	35	28	41

The results of our study helped us create the criteria of benign and neoplastic gastric lesions.

Benign Gastric Lesions

In the margins of gastric ulcers and erosions high-magnification endoscopy and NBI detected various types of regular patterns: membranous, spindle-like, palisade-like or cobblestone-like, typical for regenerated epithelium during the healing process. Though the density of capillary vessels increased, in almost all cases there were neither dilation nor tortuous changes. These areas appeared dark brown on NBI observation. Inside the fine reddish granules of regenerated epithelium of the healing ulcer, slightly dilated and tortuous capillary vessels, without irregularity, were observed. Hyperplastic polyps showed a reddish, coarse pattern on magnifying endoscopy and also a dark brown colored pattern on NBI, caused by congestion and edema of the interstitium.

Neoplastic Gastric Lesions

Gastric adenomas with dysplasia showed a whitish, minute and regular mucosal pattern on magnifying endoscopy, which reflected the flat surface structure composed of compact and regular pits. In 5 cases of adenomas with high-grade epithelial dysplasia we detected a regular pattern and in some cases local areas with irregular or disturbed patterns at the surface of the lesion. Elevated-type early cancers of tubular papillary adenocarcinoma had an irregular mucosal pattern on magnifying endoscopy and an irregular pit pattern on microscopy. The capillary vessels observed by magnifying and NBI endoscopy were irregular and relatively thick or short with a corkscrew shape compared with those observed in hyperplastic polyps or adenomas (Figure 13). These results indicated a close relationship between the magnifying endoscopy findings and the histological features. Almost all the depressed-type early cancers had irregular tubular structures and were diagnosed by a characteristic pit pattern which was finer than that of the surrounding mucosa. In depressed-type early cancers of well to moderately differentiated adenocarcinoma, the finer pit pattern compared with the surrounding mucosa, the disappearance of a pit pattern and abnormal capillary vessels could be observed by magnifying endoscopy. On the other hand, in depressed-type early cancers of poorly differentiated adenocarcinoma or signet-ring cell carcinoma the loss of a clear pattern with depression was observed and abnormal capillary vessels, either in fine networks or corkscrew vessels, were seen when using NBI. In five cases of minute cancers of less than 7mm in size, however, it was difficult to recognize characteristic malignant indices such as the abovementioned features. Regarding depressed-type early gastric cancer, the criteria for malignancy when using conventional endoscopy are as follows: the irregular shape of the depression, the abrupt interruption of converging folds, or the demarcation line in the margin of the depression. With regard to elevated-type early gastric cancer, the indices of malignancy with conventional endoscopy are like an irregularly shaped uneven granular elevation with areas of erythematous changes and discoloration, diagnosed by NBI as dark and light spots [32,33]. The typical findings for intestinal-type gastric cancer are the disappearance of a regular capillary network pattern, the presence of an irregular microvascular pattern, and the presence of a demarcation line between the cancerous and non-cancerous mucosa. Diffuse-type gastric cancers reveal only a reduced or absent regular capillary network pattern. In contrast, coarse and irregular mucosal patterns are observed in elevated-type gastric cancers by magnifying endoscopy. Magnified features of depressed type gastric cancers are a fine pit pattern, destruction or disappearance of the mucosal microsurface structure, and abnormal capillary vessels. In the case of intestinal-type early gastric cancer, of which the extent is unclear by using conventional endoscopy, magnifying endoscopy is able to determine the lateral extent of gastric cancer by a demarcation line and tumor vessels. But NBI was superior to conventional and magnifying endoscopy in delineation of an "irregular microvascular pattern" and "demarcation line" – important signs of early gastric cancer.

Magnifying observation of the stomach is based on the analysis of the pit pattern. However, the mucosa of the stomach is much more complicated than the columnar epithelium of the colon because the pit pattern varies among the atrophic mucosa, fundic gland mucosa etc.

NBI is a novel endoscopic imaging technique that may enhance the mucosal surface contrast without the use of dyes. Preliminary studies using NBI in early gastric cancer have shown that mucosal and vascular patterns can be better observed with NBI [34].

Both techniques are operator-dependent, depend on correct interpretation of images with promising results mainly obtained in expert centers [2], further research is needed before these methods can be recommended for routine use in this setting.

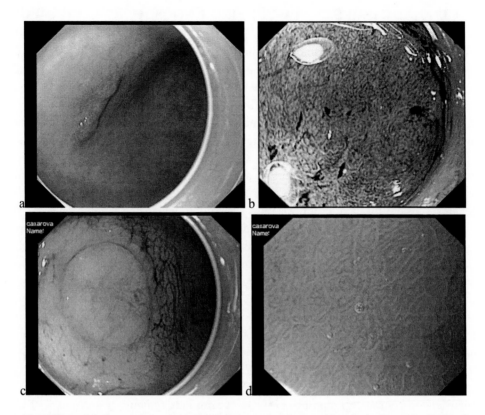

Figure 13. Differential diagnosis between EGC and gastric adenoma/dysplasia. Type II a EGC of tubular papillary adenocarcinoma (a, b) had an irregular mucosal pattern, the capillary vessels observed by magnifying and NBI endoscopy were irregular and relatively thick or short with a corkscrew shape compared with a regular mucosal and capillary pattern observed in adenoma (c, d).

Taken together, the results of high-magnification chromoendoscopy and NBI suggest that new optical techniques may enhance the detection of various neoplastic and preneoplastic lesions. Magnification with NBI confers a further strength to the clinical utility of magnification. The improved morphologic analysis of epithelial crests on the surface of the mucosa increases the reliability of the detection of intestinal metaplasia, dysplasia and early gastric cancer. The more precise analysis of the abnormal surface architecture (pit pattern) of neoplastic lesions should be relevant for treatment decision. The clear vision of the vascular network of the mucosa is probably the most important contribution of the new technique. This will stimulate the study of neo-angiogenesis in superficial digestive cancer and increase our knowledge on the pathophysiology of inflammatory conditions. Noteworthy, chromoscopy is not helpful when the exploration aims to study the vessels. Finally, there is a great potential for further developments by modifying the characteristics of the interference filters. This concerns the depth of penetration of the light and the morphology of the image as well as the color rendering.

RECENT ADVANCES IN MAGNIFYING ENDOSCOPIC TECHNOLOGY

As the next step, a new technology making it possible to obtain direct histological images of tissues in vivo was desired (virtual histology). Recent advances in technology have allowed observations using ultra-high magnifying endoscopy with a higher magnifying capability. These technologies make it possible to visualize the configuration of a cell in vivo.

Confocal endomicroscopy is a well known laboratory technique. Recent advances in technology have yielded clinically applicable tools for both ex vivo tissue analysis and potentially endoscopic applications [35]. Confocal endomicroscopy enables subsurface microscopic imaging of living tissue during ongoing endoscopy. This technique is performed by using two different contrast stains, intravenously applied - fluorescent that enhances the deeper imaging into the lamina propria, and acriflavine, which is scattered onto the surface mucosa and strongly labels the superficial epithelial cells, especially the nuclei. There have been several recent reports on the use of this confocal endomicroscop [36]. Kiesslich et al. reported the endoscopic criteria for hyperplastic and adenomatous polyps, and the presence of neoplastic changes could be predicted with high accuracy [37]. Inoue et al. studied fresh, untreated mucosal specimens from the esophagus, stomach, and colon obtained at endoscopy which used a laser scanning confocal microscope. 28 Images were obtained with a scanning time of, on average, less than two seconds and the images compared favorably with those obtained by standard haematoxylin and eosin stained light microscopy [38]. By using the nucleus to cytoplasm ratio as diagnostic criteria for cancer, light scanning confocal microscopy had a diagnostic accuracy of 89.7%. The new unique endoscopic imaging system Cellvizio® with confocal miniprobes provides the smooth dynamic observations of GI tract with the resolution ranging from 2.5 to 5 microns enabling direct and live visualization of cellular and/or vascular structures. Video sequences are immediately obtained and displayed 12 frames per second video acquisition and on-the-fly image processing (Figure 14).

The endo-cytoscopy system developed by Olympus (prototype; Olympus, Tokyo, Japan) consists of two flexible endoscopes, 380 cm long and 3.2 mm in diameter. The low-magnification type (XEC300) provides $450 \times$ magnification and a field of view of 300×300 μm tissue. The second endoscope is a higher-magnification type (XEC120) that provided $1125 \times$ magnification and a field of view of 120×120 μm tissue. These endoscopes could be passed through the instrument channel of the scope. For magnified observation vital staining using methylene blue or toluidine blue is necessary. These dyes are scattered into the digestive tract; 10–20 sec is needed for vital cell staining. The most evident feature of the observation using this endo-cytoscopy system should be the real-time, high-resolution diagnosis of abnormalities of the nuclei. In the non-neoplastic gastric mucosa, regular arranged tubules and nuclei could be observed. In cases of chronic atrophic gastritis with intestinal metaplasia Kumagai et al. detected goblet cells (Figure 15 a,b) and in gastric cancer, irregular, branched or destroyed tubules were observed by using endo-cytoscopy system. The cells show a loss of polarity, swelling and plemorphism of the nucleus (Figure 15 c). However, it is not possible to diagnose the type of histology by observation of the pit and cell structure from the surface, because only a limited area can be stained with methylene blue [36].

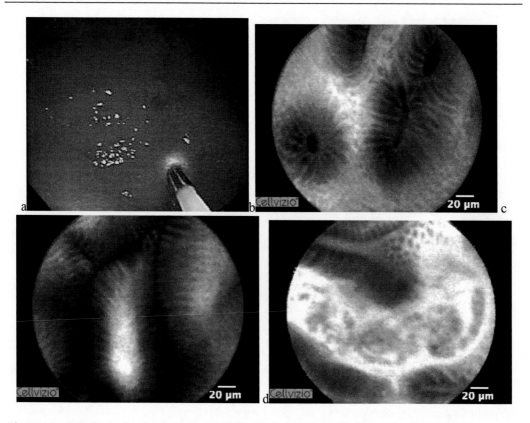

Figure 14. a). Endoscopic view remains available while imaging with the confocal microprobe Cellvizio® . Placed in contact with the mucosa, microprobe deliver real-time video sequences of the tissue microarchitecture; b). Regular gastric openings of the normal fundus mucosa; c). Normal antrum mucosa; d). Low grade epithelial dysplasia (Courtesy of Professor Chuttani, Professor Pleskow, Beth Israel Deaconness, Boston, USA and Mauna Kea Technologies, Paris, France).

OTHER PROMISING FORMS OF IMAGE ENHANCEMENT

One remarkable achievement was the application to the digestive tract of optical coherence tomography (EOCT), autofluorescence endoscopy and Raman spectroscopy. This technology provides a more detailed cross-sectional view of a lesion than endoscopic ultrasonography. Further, EOCT does not require the gastrointestinal tract to be filled with water, making the simplicity of the technique superior to EUS. However, the light penetration depth of EOCT is only about 1.5 mm from the mucosal surface, so it is not sufficient to diagnose the depth of tumor invasion. Further improvements are expected.

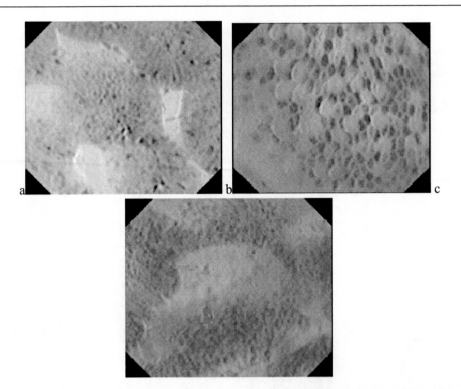

Figure 15. (a) Non-neoplastic gastric mucosa observed with XEC300 (Olympus Co., Tokyo, Japan). Regular arranged tubules could be observed. (b) Non-neoplastic gastric mucosa (intestinal metaplasia) observed with the XEC120 (Olympus Co., Tokyo, Japan) cytoscope. Regular arranged cells and goblet cells could be observed. (c) Well-differentiated adenocarcinoma observed by the XEC300 cytoscope. Irregular and branched tubules and loss of polarity of the nuclei can be observed. From reference 36: Digestive Endoscopy 2006; 18 (3), 165–172. Courtesy of Youichi Kumagai, Department of Surgery, Ohta Nishinouchi Hospital (Fukushima, Japan).

Endoscopic optical coherence tomography (EOCT) is a recently developed technique for demonstrating cross-sectional images in the GI tract using infrared light. It bears similarity to B mode ultrasound, in that incident energy is applied to target tissue, and a cross-sectional image is constructed based on the reflection of this energy from the tissue and back to a detector. Specifically, with B mode ultrasound, the echoes returning from the target tissue are visualized in the form of a gray scale map. OCT differs from B mode ultrasound in that OCT uses light rather than sound to image tissue. It has over 10 times higher resolution than currently available ultrasonography The various depths in sample tissue are discriminated as layers, and are determined by the time it takes for the incident light to contact various layers of the GI wall and reflect back to the detector. The layers of GI wall can be distinguished because of their different optical reflection. For ultrasound waves, this "time-of-flight" difference can be measured electronically using pulse-echo technology. Because OCT uses light, electronic measurement is impractical, as light travels more than 105 times faster than sound. Instead, this measurement is performed by means of optical interferometry [39]. OCT probe, can be used through the working channel of a standard endoscope, so this method is called endoscopic optical coherence tomography (EOCT). For EOCT scanning, water injection or balloon contact methods are not required because air does not interfere with the illumination beam [40].

The OCT device uses low coherent radiation with 1270-μm wavelength and 0.5-mW power and has a resolution of 15μm. Additionally, a red visible (635 nm, 0.1 mW) light emitted from the probe visualized the imaging beam position at the tissue surface. The gastric wall is observed as a layered structure with low and high reflective layers: glandular epithelium, muscularis mucosa, submucosa, and muscularis propria. Though the resolution was much higher than that of the 30-MHz US scanner, penetration of EOCT was too poor (1-1,5 mm) to use this method for assessing the depth of tumor invasion. However, by using this sophisticated instrument, the histological nature of tissues can be evaluated. EOCT if perfected might be used as a method for optical biopsy in fixture endoscopic examinations. Figure 16 presents an OCT image (a) and parallel histology (b) of the normal stomach. Three layers can be visualized: upper mucosa (UM – glandular epithelium and lamina propria), submucosa, and muscularis propria. The gastric antrum has an upper, fairly thick layer of glandular mucosa, which is less transparent then squamous epithelium because of the connective tissue interlayers lamina propria between glands. The horizontal stratified structure of the normal stomach is preserved. The submucosa is weakly contrasted from muscularis propria. Images c and d are typical for the tubulovillous adenoma of gastric antrum. The thickness of the upper mucosa is more than normal. Dark adenomatous glands can be seen.

Although EOCT has advantages over currently available imaging modalities, in its current form, it still has several limitations. The time required to obtain images is long, and the image resolution, currently 10–20 mm, is not sufficient to replace histological diagnosis. Newer, ultra-short pulsed light sources for EOCT have the potential to improve axial resolution to 2–4 mm. Just as endoscopic ultrasonography requires the endoscopist to become familiar with radiological techniques, ultrasound imaging artefacts, and three dimensional anatomy. EOCT will require the endoscopist to become more knowledgeable regarding histopathology [40].

Autofluorescence Videoendoscopy for Diagnosis of Gastric Cancer

An autofluorescence (AF) endoscopy system produces real-time pseudocolor images from computation of detecting natural tissue fluorescence from endogenous fluorophores that is emitted by excitation light. The system could specify lesions including malignancies by difference in tissue fluorescence properties and reveal early stage neoplasia not detectable by conventional white light (WL) endoscopy. Image quality of the prior autofluorescence imaging systems including fiber-optic endoscope was not feasible for general clinical use. AFI represented early stage cancers in the digestive tract as purple or magenta areas in a green background. The undifferentiated type of early gastric cancers in the fundic mucosa showed a unique pattern - green areas in a purple background. Ulcerations or inflammation caused over-diagnosis in the AF observation. AFI could reveal flat or isochromatic extensions that were not evident in the WL images. Detection of abnormal lesions with AF depends on changes in the concentration or depth distribution of endogenous fluorophores, changes in the

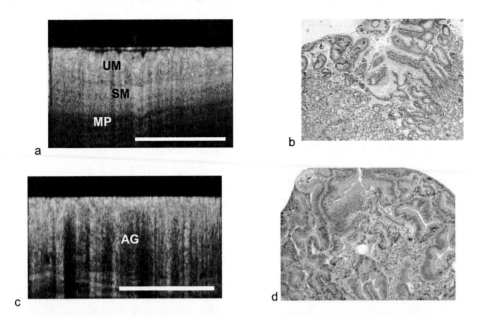

Figure 16. 1. OCT image of the stomach (gastric antrum, endoscopically normal) (a) with corresponding histology (b). Upper mucosa (UM – glandular epithelium and lamina propria) and submucosa (SM) are highly scattering. Muscularis propria (MP) are poorly scattering (bar – 1 mm). OCT image of the tubulovillous adenoma with focal high grade dysplasia. Sessile polyp of gastric antrum (d – 2 cm) (c) with corresponding histology (d). Adenomatous glands (AG) are poorly scattering (bar – 1 mm). Study presented here was performed in the Department of Gastroenterology at the Cleveland Clinic Foundation, Cleveland, Ohio, USA. These images are from data base of Professor Natalia Gladkova and Elena Zagaynova (Institute of Applied Physics and Nizhny Novgorod Medical Academy).

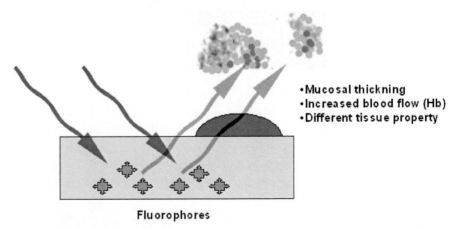

Figure17. Possible mechanisms of color difference at a tumor in the autofluorescence image. Adopted from: Novel autofluorescence videoendoscopy imaging system for diagnosis of cancers in the digestive tract. Digestive Endoscopy, 2006 Vol.18 [41].

tissue microarchitecture, or both, including altered mucosal thickness or blood (hemoglobin) concentration that affects the fluorescence intensity or spectrum. AF is basically reduced at tumors compared with normal mucosa and possible mechanisms are shown in Figure 17, 18. The difference of the fluorescence features, mainly determined by the intensity, is represented as color difference in the AF images [41].

Early gastric cancer type 0-IIa+I with retraction due to previous ulceration imaged in the antegrade view with white light endoscopy (b), autofluorescence imaging (c) - both tumor and vessels appeared dark in the AF image, narrow band imaging (d), indigo carmine chromoscopy (e). Courtesy of Jacques Bergman, MD PhD and Frederike van Vilsteren, MD, Department of Gastroenterology and Hepatology, Academic Medical Centre, Amsterdam.

Raman spectroscopy is another form of image enhancement based on the principle that incident light can cause molecules within a tissue to vibrate and rotate. The charged molecules can resonate emitting energy that can be measured spectrally. In this form of spectroscopy, light with wavelengths in the ultraviolet or infrared region of the spectrum is used to excite a target tissue. The resulting resonance spectrum represents the tissue's content of specific components such as distinct nucleic acids and proteins [42]. Thus Raman spectroscopy provides the opportunity to obtain a molecular profile or "fingerprint" of a tissue. An in vivo method of Raman spectroscopy has been developed using near infrared wavelengths for excitation. This system uses an optical fiber probe passed through the accessory channel of an endoscope. Reproducible spectra can be obtained even in the presence of blood overlying the tissue being studied. While still in their early stages, clinical studies using Raman spectroscopy to detect gastrointestinal dysplasia are currently in progress [35].

ENDOSCOPIC ULTRASONOGRAPHY (EUS)

EUS plays an important role in diagnosis and therapy of gastric lesions. The first use of the ultrasonic endoscope was reported in 1980, and the use of endoscopic ultrasonography has become widespread for examination of the gastrointestinal tract [43]. In the field of stomach diseases, the importance of tumor staging of gastric cancer has been increasing with the development of the endoscopic resection technique. Recently reported studies suggest that EUS is a more accurate diagnostic tool for staging the T aspects of gastric cancer than computerized tomography. EUS can be used to determine the depth of involvement of a lesion and makes a valuable contribution to the efficacy of endoscopic therapy. This is important information when it comes to deciding whether a tumor can be resected endoscopically or whether surgery is needed. Studies evaluating EUS staging of gastric cancers have predominantly used radial sector scanning echoendoscopes at frequencies of 7,5 and 12 MHz. A frequency of 7,5 MHz allows for a maximal depth of penetration of about 10 cm, whereas 12 MHz allows for 3 cm maximal penetration. Although 12 MHz does not allow deep penetration, it has the advantage of providing greater resolution images that may help in

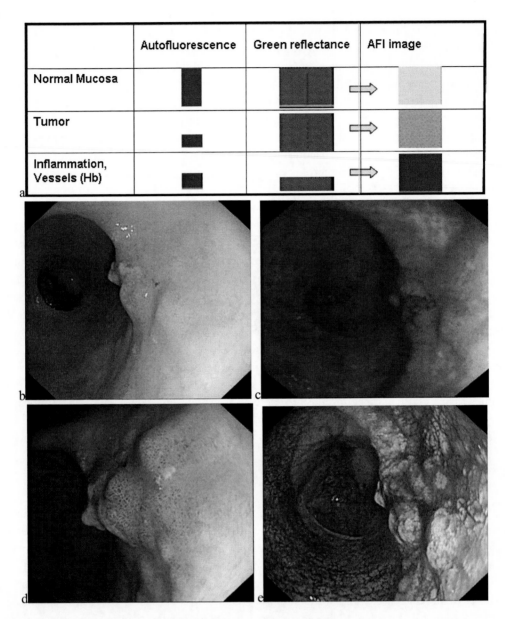

	Autofluorescence	Green reflectance		AFI image
Normal Mucosa			⇨	
Tumor			⇨	
Inflammation, Vessels (Hb)			⇨	

Figure 18. Schematic diagram of the autofluorescence (AF) and green reflection in case of early gastric cancer (a). Adopted from: Novel autofluorescence videoendoscopy imaging system for diagnosis of cancers in the digestive tract. Digestive Endoscopy 2006, Vol.18 [41].

evaluating more superficial, early gastric cancer lesions. High frequency thin endoscopic ultrasound probes have enabled us to perform target scanning with high resolution of even very small gastric cancer lesions under endoscopic control. Before evaluating a lesion deairated water is instilled into the stomach to fully cover the lesion. This provides for greater transmission of the ultrasound waves in a distended stomach, thereby enabling a larger surface of gastric lumen to be visualized. It also allows for ultrasonographic evaluation of the lesion without direct apposition of the endoscope balloon or tip of the probe over the lesion, which could result in compression of tissue planes leading to inaccuracy in determining T category. Ultrasonic evaluation of the normal stomach reveals five distinct layers, three hyperechoic and two hypoechoic, visible as an alternating bright-dark pattern. For practical purposes the first two echolayers are considered to correspond histologically with the mucosa, the third with the submucosa and the fourth with the muscularis propria and the fifth with the serosa. The layers of EUS are in good correspondence with histologic wall layers. When the muscularis mucosae and intermuscular interface of the muscularis propria are visualised, the normal gastric wall is observed as a nine layered structureUsing 30-MHz probe. The muscularis mucosae is expected to be visualized in almost 30% of cases in the stomach and the esophagus [44,45].

Gastric cancer appears as hypoechoic lesions arising in the mucosal layer which disrupts the normal layered appearance of gastric mucosa (Figure 19, 20) [46].

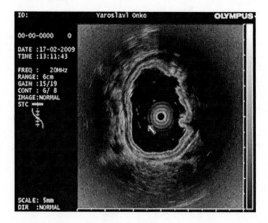

Figure 19. EUS evaluation of the normal stomach reveals five distinct layers, three hyperechoic and two hypoechoic.

Gastric Cancer EUS Staging

According to the Japanese Gastric Cancer Association classification system T1 lesions (early cancer) invade either the mucosa or submucosa (first three EUS layers), T2 lesions invade the muscularis propria (fourth EUS layer) or subserosa (not defined on EUS), T3 lesions penetrate serosa (fifth EUS layer), and T4 lesions invade adjacent organs.

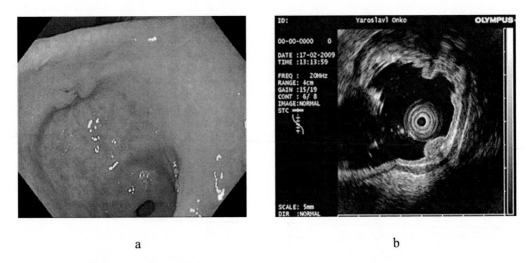

a   b

Figure 20. A case of type IIa+IIc EGC at the anterior wall of the gastric antrum. a. Conventional endoscopic image, b. EUS image shows submucosal invasion of the lesion. EUS evaluation of the stomach wall aside the tumor reveals five distinct layers, three hyperechoic and two hypoechoic, visible as an alternating bright-dark pattern. EGC appears as hypoechoic lesions arising in the mucosal and submucosal layers that disrupt the normal layered appearance of gastric wall.

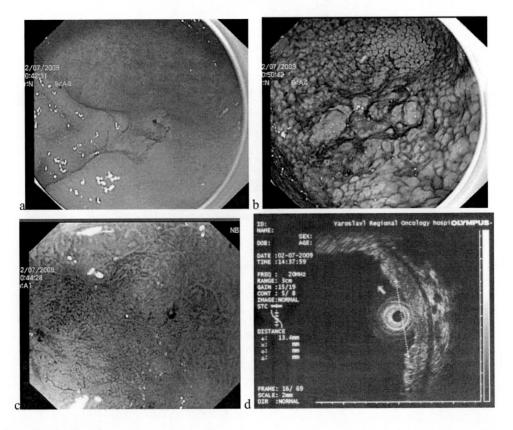

Figure 21. Continued

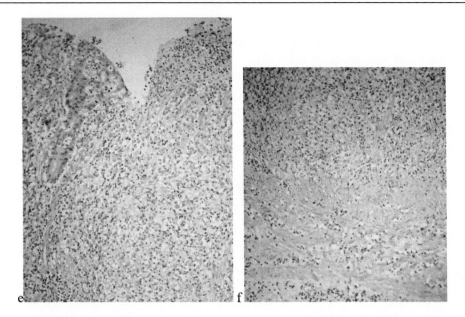

Figure 21. Early gastric cancer in antrum type 0- IIa+c: a) white light endoscopy, b) Chromoendoscopy, c) NBI with optical magnification – pathological corkscrew vessels in the center of the tumor, d) EUS – cancer with submucosal invasion – indication for surgical treatment, e) and f) histology after gastrectomy - gastric mucosa with marked signet-ring cell cancer infiltration and ulceration is seen. At the left gastric glands are seen with marked peritumorous lymphocytic infiltration (e); tumor growth extends to muscular layer of mucous. Deeper layers demonstrate no tumor cells but only lymphocytic infiltration (f), H&E stain.

EUS is a useful study for accurate staging of gastric carcinoma. Willis et al reported that overall accuracy of EUS for T staging was 78 % (T1, T2, T3, and T4 - 80 %, 63 %, 95 %, and 83 %, respectively). Regional lymph node staging was correctly conducted in 77 % [47]. Yasuda reported the diagnostic accuracy of depth of carcinoma invasion is approximately 80%, when lesions are divided into mucosal (m) carcinoma, submucosal (sm) carcinoma, carcinoma invading to the muscularis propria (pm), and carcinoma deeper than the subserosal layer (ss). The EUS diagnosis of a mucosal lesion, which is a good indication for endoscopic mucosal resection or submucosal dissection, is about 90% [40]. To determine reliable indications for endoscopic treatment suggesting submucosal tumor invasion, Matsumoto et al. retrospectively analyzed EUS images of the hyperechoic third layer which corresponds to the submucosa. The subjects enrolled in this study were 75 patients with 78 gastric cancers (diagnosed as mucosal cancer without ulcerous changes on endoscopy and as histologically differentiated adenocarcinoma on biopsy), who were also examined by EUS. EUS features of the third layer (submucosa) were classified into five groups: (1) irregular narrowing, (2) budding sign, (3) multiple echo-free spots, (4) unclear, and (5) no changes. In endoscopically diagnosed gastric mucosal cancer, 16 of the 78 lesions were associated with histologic submucosal invasion. EUS features that were associated with a high incidence of histological submucosal tumor invasion were irregular narrowing (submucosal invasion, 60.0%) and the budding sign (85.7%), and 90.9% of lesions with either of these features had submucosal invasion of tumors when tumorous changes in the third layer exceeded 1 mm in depth [48]. Further large-scale clinical trails and carefully planned investigations should be conducted to clarify those questions about the ability of EUS to differentiate tumor infiltration from fibrosis or inflammatory tissues, to detect microscopic invasions, and to discriminate the benign from malignant nodes.

The role of EUS is to evaluate the alteration of the gastrointestinal (GI) wall by carcinoma based on the ultrasonic layered structure of GI wall. That means EUS cannot be used to find a lesion, except in the rare case of gastric scirrhous carcinoma, but is used rather to evaluate the changes beneath the mucosa in order to diagnose the depth of carcinoma invasion. This assessment is an important factor in choosing a preferable treatment, such as endoscopic mucosal resection (EMR), laparoscopic surgery or laparotomy (Figure 21).

One of the most important diagnostic values of EUS is to identify indications for the endoscopic treatment of EGC. Although EUS can detect the regional metastatic lymph nodes, the rate of detection is unsatisfactory in cases of early gastric carcinoma [49].

Discussion

Considerable attention is given to the clinical diagnosis of gastrointestinal malignancies as they remain the second leading cause of cancer-associated deaths in the world. Detection and intervention at an early stage of neoplastic development significantly improve patient survival. High-risk assessment of asymptomatic patients is currently performed by strict endoscopic surveillance biopsy protocols aimed at early detection of dysplasia and malignancy. However, poor sensitivity associated with frequent surveillance programs incorporating conventional screening tools, such as white light endoscopy and multiple random biopsies, is a significant limitation. Conventional endoscopy sometimes is limited to detecting lesions based on gross morphological changes, while new optically based devices offer the potential of detecting the very earliest mucosal changes at the microstructural level by detecting the relative changes in the way light interacts with tissue along the disease transformation pathway. Recent advances in biomedical optics are illuminating new ways to detect premalignant lesions and early gastric cancers with endoscopy. Relying on the interaction of light with tissue, these 'state-of-the-art' techniques potentially offer an improved strategy for diagnosis of early mucosal lesions by facilitating targeted excisional biopsies. Furthermore, the prospects of real-time 'optical biopsy' and improved staging of lesions may significantly enhance the endoscopist's ability to detect subtle neoplastic mucosal changes and lead to curative endoscopic ablation of these lesions. However, the differentiation of lesions and the diagnosis of early neoplastic changes remain difficult despite the existing recommended classifications for various mucosal surface details.

Should we use these new optical techniques routinely? At any rate, the routine introduction of high-magnification and high-resolution endoscopy must be encouraged; this is not just a new trick. Magnification endoscopy introduces a new perspective in the mind of the endoscopist. Using these methods we must determine which lesions can be neglected, which can be treated at endoscopy, and which should be referred for surgery. However all of these techniques are operator-dependent, depend on correct interpretation of images with promising results mainly obtained in expert centers [6].

Such advancements within this specialty will be rewarded in the long term with improved patient survival and quality of life. Early diagnosis represents the most important measure to decrease gastric cancer mortality.

CONCLUSION

It is imperative for the endoscopist to detect gastrointestinal neoplasia in its early stage to ensure that the patient can receive less invasive treatment and have a good quality of life and an excellent prognosis. To make a correct diagnosis of early neoplasia in stomach, we first need to detect any lesions with subtle morphologic change and we then need to characterize such subtle mucosal lesions [29].

Observation of the stomach using modern imaging techniques provides additional detailed information to be obtained over that obtained by conventional endoscopic observation. This information includes the prediction of neoplastic changes in the lesion, depth of tumor invasion etc. Novel endoscopic microscopic imaging makes it possible to receive cellular level imaging of the tissue. This technology also offers the means of aiding our fundamental understanding of disease processes in the GI tract on a molecular level. 'Optical biopsy' refers to tissue diagnosis based on *in situ* optical measurements, which would eliminate the need for tissue removal. The above-mentioned optical techniques are striving towards this goal, but none are likely to replace conventional biopsy and histopathological interpretation in the near future. They demonstrate potential for better diagnosis with future technological refinement and large-scale clinical trials needed to assess their utility and limitation [50]. All of these new technologies may reduce the incidence of unnecessary biopsies. Further, we expect that these observations will join with the field of the molecular biology in the future.

However, endoscopists should be trained to perform standardized extremely rigorous observation with a low threshold of suspicion for neoplasia. Such property is a key requirement of a screening tool: before a suspicious small lesion can be scrutinized and discriminated (by combination of magnification endoscopy, chromoscopy and NBI) it must first be detected! Together with recent interest in new imaging techniques should be considered to represent a simple, safe and inexpensive technique that may be useful in identifying premalignant conditions and minute cancerous lesions, estimating their superficial extent and determining the histological type and submucosal invasion [51].

ACKNOWLEDGEMENTS

The authors thank Dr. Alexander Nadezhin and Dr. Artem Borbat (Department of Pathology, Yaroslavl Regional Cancer Hospital, Yaroslavl, Russia) for their contribution to the pathological and clinical material presented, Victor Kapranov (Demidov's Yaroslavl State University) for technical support and Tatyana Kasatkina (Yaroslavl State Pedagogical University, Yaroslavl, Russia) for correcting the English used in this article.

REFERENCES

[1]   Sakaki N. *How I do it: Detection of early gastric cancer using chromoendoscopy and other techniques*. OMED publications& Guidelines (http://www.omed.org/index.php/ public_guides/pu_how).

[2]   Pasechnikov V., Chukov S., Kashin S. Advances in Early Diagnosis of Gastric Cancer // in Book "Research Focus on Gastric Cancer" *Nova Science Publishers* 2008; P.21-55.

[3]   American Joint Committee on Cancer: *AJCC Cancer Staging Manual*. Philadelphia, Pa: Lippincott-Raven Publishers, 5th ed., 1997, pp 71–76.

[4]   Schlemper RJ, Riddell RH, Kato Y et al: The Vienna classification of gastrointestinal epithelial neoplasia. *Gut* 2000; 47: 251–255.

[5]   Japanese Gastric Cancer Association: Japanese classification of gastric cancer – 2nd English edition. *Gastric Cancer* 1998; 1:10–24.

[6]   Fujita R., Jass J.R., Kaminishi M., Schlemper R.J. *Early Cancer of the Gastrointestinal Tract/ Endoscopy, Pathology and Treatment*. Springer-Verlag Tokyo 2006; P 159-164.

[7]   Borrmann R. Geschwulste des Magens und Duodenums. In: Henke F, Lubarch O, editors. *Handbuch der speziellen pathologischen anatomie und histologie*. Berlin: Springer Verlag; 1926.

[8]   The Paris endoscopic classification of superficial neoplastic lesions: esophagus, stomach, and colon. *Gastrointestinal Endoscopy VOL* 58, NO. 6 (SUPPL), 2003; p 3-37.

[9]   Schlemper RJ, Hirata I, Dixon MF. The macroscopic classification of early neoplasia of the digestive tract. *Endoscopy* 2002;34:163-8.

[10]   Ida K, Hashimoto Y, Takeda S, Murakami K, Kawai K. Endoscopic diagnosis of gastric cancer with dye scattering. *Am J Gastroenterol* 1975; 63 (4): 316-20.

[11]   Okabayashi T, Gotoda T, Kondo H, Ono H, Oda I, Fujishiro M, Yachida S. Usefulness of indigocarmine chromoendoscopy and endoscopic clipping for accurate preoperative assessment of proximal gastric cancer. *Endoscopy* 2000; 32(10): S62.

[12]   Correa P. Human gastric carcinogenesis: a multistep and multifactorial process. First American Cancer Society Award Lecture on Cancer Epidemiology and Prevention. *Cancer Res* 1992;52:6735 – 40.

[13]   Leung WK, Sung JJ. Review article: intestinal metaplasia and gastric carcinogenesis. *Aliment Pharmacol Ther* 2002;16:1209–16.

[14]   Leung W., Enders K.W. Chan W., et al. Risk Factors Associated with the Development of Intestinal Metaplasia in First-Degree Relatives of Gastric Cancer Patients. *Cancer Epidemiol Biomarkers Prevention* 2005;14(12): 2982-86.

[15]   Ito M. , Haruma K., Kamada T., et al. Helicobacter pylori eradication therapy improves atrophic gastritis and intestinal metaplasia: a 5-year prospective study of patients with atrophic gastritis. *Aliment Pharmacol Ther* 2002;16: 1449–1456.

[16]   Kashin S., Nadezhin A., Kislova I., Agamov A. First Results of Regression of Atrophy and Intestinal Metaplasia (IM) after H. pylori Eradication. Abstracts XVIth International Workshop on Gastrointestinal Pathology and Helicobacter, *Helicobacter,* Vol 8, № 4, p. 406, 2003.

[17] Ida K, Hashimoto Y, Takeda S et al: Endoscopic diagnosis of gastric cancer with dye scattering. *Am J Gastroenterol* 1975; 63: 316–320.

[18] Olliver JR, Wild CP, Sahay P et al: Chromoendoscopy with methylene blue and associated DNA damage in Barrett's oesophagus. *Lancet* 2003; 362: 373–3746.

[19] Okuyama Y, Takemoto T, Tsuneoka K et al. Specially designed gastroscope for magnified observation. *Gastroenterol. Endosc.* 1967; 9: 42–3 (in Japanese).

[20] Singh S., Sharma P. Magnification endoscopy in the upper GI tract. *Digestive Endoscopy,* 2005;17 (Suppl.): S17–S19.

[21] Yao K, Oishi T. Microgastroscopic findings of mucosal microvascular architecture as visualized by magnifying endoscopy. *Digestive Endoscopy* 2001;13: S27-33.

[22] Yao K. Gastric microvascular architecture as visualized by magnifying endoscopy: Body and antrum without pathologic change demonstrate two different patterns of microvascular architecture. *Gastrointestinal Endoscopy* 2004;59:596-7.

[23] Yao K, Oishi T, Matsui T, Yao T, Iwashita A. Novel magnified endoscopic findings of microvascular architecture in intramucosal gastric cancer. *Gastrointestinal Endoscopy* 2002;56:279-84.

[24] Sakaki N, Iida Y, Saito M et al. New magnifying endoscopic classification of the fine gastric mucosa pattern. *Gastroenterol. Endosc.* 1980; 22: 377–83.

[25] Sakaki N, Iida Y, Okazaki Y et al. Magnifying endoscopic observation of gastric mucosa, particularly in patients with atrophic gastritis. *Endscopy* 1978; 10: 269–74.

[26] Kato M, Shimizu Y., Nakagawa S., et al. Usefulness of magnifying endoscopy in upper gastrointestinal tract: history and recent studies. *Digestive Endoscopy,* 2005, Vol.17, Issue s1, P: S5-S10.

[27] Otsuka Y, Niwa Y, Ohmiya N et al. Usefulness of magnifying endoscopy in the diagnosis of early gastric cancer. *Endoscopy* 2004; 36: 165–9.

[28] Rey JF, Kuznetsov K, Lambert R. Narrow band imaging: A wide field of possibilities. *Saudi J Gastroenterol* 2007;13:1-10.

[29] Yao K., Takaki Y., Matsui T., et al. Clinical Application of Magnification Endoscopy and Narrow-Bandm Imaging in the Upper Gastrointestinal Tract: New Imaging Techniques for Detecting and Characterizing Gastrointestinal Neoplasia *Gastrointest Endoscopy Clin N Am* 18 (2008): 415–433.

[30] Yao K., Iwashita A., Tanabe H., et al. White opaque substance within superficial elevated gastric neoplasia as visualized by magnification endoscopy with narrow-band imaging: a new optical sign for differentiating between adenoma and carcinoma. *Gastrointestinal Endoscopy* 2008; 68, 3: 574-579.

[31] Yao K, Iwashita A, Kikuchi Y. Novel zoom endoscopy technique for visualizing the microvascular architecture in gastric mucosa. *Clin Gastroenterol Hepatol* 2005;3(Suppl 1):S23–6.

[32] Tajiri H, Doi T, Endo H et al. Routine endoscopy using a magnifying endoscope for gastric cancer diagnosis. *Endoscopy* 2002; 34: 772–776.

[33] Kiesslich R., Jung M Magnification Endoscopy: Does It Improve Mucosal Surface Analysis for the Diagnosis of Gastrointestinal Neoplasias? *Endoscopy* 2002; 34 (10): 819–822.

[34] Gono K, Obi T, YamaguchiMet al. Appearance of enhanced tissue features in narrow-band endoscopic imaging. *J Biomed Optics* 2004; 9:568-577.

[35] Van Dam J. Novel methods of enhanced endoscopic imaging. *Gut* 2003;52 (Suppl IV): p12–16.

[36] Kumagai Y., Iida M., Yamazaki S, Magnifying endoscopic observation of the upper gastrointestinal tract. *Digestive Endoscopy* 2006;18 (3), 165–172.

[37] Kiesslich R, Goetz M, Burg J et al. Diagnosing Helicobacter pylori in vivo by confocal laser endoscopy. *Gastroenterology* 2005; 128: 2119–23.

[38] Inoue H, Igari T, Nishikage T, et al. A novel method of virtual histopathology using laser-scanning confocal microscopy in vitro with untreated fresh specimens from the gastrointestinal mucosa. *Endoscopy* 2000; 32: 439–43.

[39] Zuccaro G., Gladkova N., Zagaynova E., et al. Optical Coherence Tomography of the Esophagus and Proximal Stomach in Health and Disease. *American Journal of Gastroenterology* 2001; 96, No. 9: 2633-39.

[40] Yasuda K. EUS in the detection of early gastric cancer. *Gastrointestinal Endoscopy* 2002;56 № 4 (Suppl):68-75.

[41] Uedo N., Iishi H., Ishihara R., et al. Novel autofluorescence videoendoscopy imaging system for diagnosis of cancers in the digestive tract. *Digestive Endoscopy* 2006 Vol.18, Issue s1: S131-S136.

[42] Shim M, Song L, Marcon N, et al. In vivo near-infrared Raman spectroscopy: demonstration of feasibility during clinical gastrointestinal endoscopy. *Photochem Photobiol* 2000;72:146–50.

[43] DiMagno EP, Regan PT, Clain JE, et al. Human endoscopic ultrasonography. *Gastroenterology* 1982; 83:824–829.

[44] Yanai H., Noguchi T., Mizumachi S. A blind comparison of the effectiveness of endoscopic ultrasonography and endoscopy in staging early gastric cancer *Gut* 1999;44:361–365.

[45] Yamanaka T. JGES consensus meeting report in DDW-Japan 2000, Kobe: Interpretation of the layered structure of GI wall with endoscopic Ultrasonography. *Digestive Endoscopy* 2002; 14: 39–40.

[46] Olds G., Chak A. Endoscopic Ultrasound for Staging Gastric Cancer. In book Endoscopic Oncology Gastrointestinal Endoscopy and Cancer Management. *Humana Press* 2006; p121-128.

[47] Willis S., Truong S., Gribnitz S., Fass J., Schumpelick V. Endoscopic ultrasonography in the preoperative staging of gastric cancer: accuracy and impact on surgical therapy. *Surg Endosc* 2000; 14: 951-954.

[48] Matsumoto Y., Yanai H., Tokiyama H., et al. Endoscopic ultrasonography for diagnosis of submucosal invasion in early gastric cancer. *J Gastroenterol.* 2000;35(5):402-3.

[49] Kashin S.V., Politov I.V., Agamov A.G., Goncharov V.I., Kislova I.V., Nadezhin A.S., Velikanova E.A. The results of endoscopic treatment of early esophagogastric cancer and high grade epithelial dysplasia. Abstracts 11th UEGW, *Gut/Endoscopy, suppl.* № VI, Vol 52, A2, 2003.

[50] DaCosta R.S., Wilson B. C., Marcon N.E. New technologies for endoscopic diagnosis. *Journal of Gastroenterology and Hepatology* (2002; 17 (Suppl.) S85–S104.

[51] Dinis-Ribeiro, M. Chromoendoscopy for early diagnosis of gastric cancer. European *Journal of Gastroenterology & Hepatology:* 2006 - Volume 18 - Issue 8 - pp 831-838.

In: Gastric Cancer: Diagnosis, Early Prevention, and Treatment   ISBN 978-1-61668-313-9
Editor: V. D. Pasechnikov, pp. 235-266   © 2010 Nova Science Publishers, Inc.

Chapter VII

ENDOSCOPIC TREATMENT FOR EARLY GASTRIC CANCER

E. D. Fedorov

Department of Abdominal Surgery & Endoscopy (head - S.G.Shapovalyanz), Russia
State Medical University n.a. N.I.Pirogov, Moscow University Hospital N31
(chief – G.N.Goluchov), Russian Federation

ABSTRACT

This chapter contains review on endoscopic approaches for early gastric cancer (EGC), indications and contraindications for endoscopic resection, patient's care and complications, short- and long-term results after endoscopic resection for EGC. Endoscopic resection is indicated for EGC with no risk of lymph node metastasis. The incidence of lymph node metastasis of mucosal and submucosal gastric cancers has been reported as approximately 3% and 20% respectively. However, we cannot accurately enough predict the lymph node metastasis using CT scan or PET scan, because the lymph node metastasis from EGC is too small to detect it. Endoscopic prediction between mucosal and submucosal invasion before treatment is correctly made in only 80% to 90% of tumour even using EUS. So the indication for endoscopic resection is determined from clinicipathological finding that is considered to be as having no risk of lymph node metastasis. Endoscopic excision of cancer in many respects is comparable to conventional surgery, with the advantages of being less invasive and more economical. Endoscopic resection provides precise pathological staging without precluding future surgical therapy. This chapter also describes the methods of endoscopic treatment for early gastric cancer, with the special emphasis on the different techniques of endoscopic resection: strip biopsy, endoscopic mucosal resection (EMR) and endoscopic submucosal dissection (ESD). ESD offers the advantage to achieve one-piece resection and reduce local recurrence tumor, however, it also has several limitations. It requires a significantly longer procedure time (the median time is about 1 hour) and a considerably higher level of technical expertise in addition to there being a slightly greater risk of complications.

Anyway, after the developing ESD, the total number of patients with EGC, successfully and curatively treated with endoscopic resection is rapidly increasing.

EARLY GASTRIC CANCER: WHY ENDOSCOPIC RESECTION INSTEAD OF SURGERY OR ABLATION?

Early gastric cancer is defined when tumor invasion is limited to the mucosa or submucosa (T1 cancer), independent of the presence of lymph node metastases [41]. Endoscopic mucosal resection, also known as endoscopic resection, is defined as the resection of a fragment of the digestive wall including the mucosal membrane and the muscularis mucosae. This resection most frequently removes a part or even all of the submucosa.

Endoscopic resection mainly has been developed in Japan because the incidence of gastric cancer and the tumor description are different between East and West [82]. Although decreasing in number, the incidence of gastric cancer was approximately 80 patients per 100 000 population in Japan and more than half the patients have T1 tumors. The mortality rate of gastric cancer is seven times higher in Japan than in the United States and three times higher than in the UK and Russia. At the same time many Western pathologists diagnose the lesions without definite invasion as dysplasia, whereas they are diagnosed as well-differentiated adenocarcinoma in Japan if they have cellular and structural atypia compatible with adenocarcinoma [83]. As biopsy specimens are usually taken from the surface of the lesions, they cannot prove deeper invasion of the lesions. Therefore, many of these "dysplasia" actually invade into the submucosal layer or even deeper when they are resected and histologically examined.

Gastrectomy with lymph node dissection had been the gold standard treatment in Japan for all patients with operable gastric cancer, including early gastric cancer [55, 79, 103], considering the adverse impact of lymph node metastases on a patient's prognosis [39, 67]. This policy of radical surgery for all such cases carries significant risks of morbidity and mortality and is associated with a long-term reduction in patients' quality of life [8, 81].

Large histopathological series of specimen after gastrectomy in patients with gastric cancer showed that the incidence of lymph node metastases mainly depends on the differentiation and the depth of cancer infiltration and is just 2%–3% in T1 mucosal cancer and 15%–20% in T1 submucosal cancer [77]. Using these databases, it was possible to select patients with T1 tumors who have negligible risk of lymph node metastasis [97]. Together with the development of the instruments and technique of endoscopic mucosal resection, many of these mucosal cancers with a low risk of lymph node metastases are now treated by local endoscopic treatment.

Endoscopic excision of cancer in many respects is comparable to conventional surgery, with the advantages of being less invasive and more economical. Endoscopic mucosal resection in Japan has been widely accepted as a potentially curative treatment for early gastric cancer and it is increasingly gaining acceptance worldwide [73, 86]. The increasing ratio of early gastric cancers accelerates the development of various novel endoscopic resection techniques and, now, early gastric cancer of large size or with ulcer findings, in any location, can be resected endoscopically using advanced techniques.

Endoscopic mucosal resection is required to achieve an accurate and possibly complete local tumor staging and grading, which is critical, as this allows stratification and refinement of further treatment [35]. Other endoscopic techniques, such as laser irradiation (photodynamic therapy), microwave coagulation, or local injection of anticancer agents may also cure early gastric cancer by ablation / fulgurating it, but they do not provide any pathological specimen [46]. Without a specimen, tumor stage cannot be assessed. Thus, the patient's prognosis cannot be estimated and potential needs for additional therapy, which may be curative, cannot be assessed [58 106].

In opposite major advantage of endoscopic resection is its ability to provide pathological staging without precluding future surgical therapy [17, 104]. After endoscopic resection, pathological assessment of depth of cancer invasion, degree of differentiation of the cancer, and extent of lymphovascular invasion allows the risk of lymph node metastasis to be predicted, using published data of patients with similar findings [27]. The risk of developing lymph node metastasis or distant metastasis is then weighed against the risk of surgery [16]. Goto O. et al., based on the histology of endoscopic submucosal dissection specimens showed, that preceding endoscopic submucosal dissection itself had no negative influence on a patient's prognosis when additional gastrectomy was performed. So, it may be permissible to resect some early gastric cancers by endoscopic submucosal dissection as a first step to prevent unnecessary gastrectomy, if technically resectable [24].

Such precise staging, unfortunately, cannot be achieved as accurately with conventional biopsy studies and any imaging technique currently available, even new [105]. For example, while endoscopic ultrasound is accurate for tumor depth staging, this is only possible in 80% to 90% of cases [78]. Hence, any treatment plan based on EUS recommendations potentially means that, in 10% to 20% of cases, patients may be subjected to unnecessary surgery [6, 65, 76]. The final staging can only be done through formal histological analysis, which endoscopic excision can achieve [5, 44].

INDICATIONS FOR ENDOSCOPIC RESECTION OF EARLY GASTRIC CANCER

Patients with early gastric cancer who are identified to have no risk or a low risk of developing lymph node metastasis, relative to the perioperative risks associated with surgery, are ideal candidates for endoscopic resection [54]. Patients who have lesions suspected to contain early gastric cancer are also ideal candidates to undergo endoscopic resection.

The Japanese Gastric Cancer Association, based on extensive preliminary work, issued the first version of their gastric cancer treatment guidelines in 2001, which showed that endoscopic resection was indicated for intestinal type mucosal cancers without ulcerative findings, less or equal 20 mm in size, regardless of tumor morphology [97, 102].

At present [40], *the accepted indications* for endoscopic mucosal resection of early gastric cancer are (Table.1 and Figure 1):

1) Cancers of differentiated histological type, equal or less than 20 mm in diameter, with elevated macroscopic type, without ulceration, confined to the mucosa and have no lymphatic or vascular involvement.

(2) Cancers of differentiated histological type, equal or less than 10 mm in diameter, with depressed macroscopic type, without ulceration, confined to the mucosa and have no lymphatic or vascular involvement.

Table 1. Guideline criteria for endoscopic mucosal resection of early gastric cancer

Histological type	Size	Macroscopic type	Ulceration	Depth of tumor invasion	Lymphovascular invasion
Differentiated	≤ 20 mm	*O-I, O-IIa*	UL(-)	M	ly0, v0
Differentiated	≤ 10 mm	*O-IIc*	UL(-)	M	ly0, v0

These criteria were determined by considering two aspects: being free of lymph node metastasis and the probability of successful en bloc resection. The rationale for this recommendation is based upon the knowledge that larger-size lesions or lesions with diffuse histology type are more likely to extend into the submucosal layer and thus have a higher risk of lymph node metastasis. In addition, resection of large lesion has not been technically feasible until the development of new endoscopic mucosal resection methods using cutting devices, which is classified as endoscopic submucosal dissection (ESD) techniques.

Clinical observations have noted, however, that the accepted indications for endoscopic resection can be too strict and can lead to unnecessary surgery [40]. Therefore, extended criteria for endoscopic resection have been proposed. The upper limit of the 95% confidence interval (CI) calculated from these early studies, however, was too broad for clinical use because of their small sample size [18, 32, 66, 68, 107]. More recently, however, using a large database involving more than 5000 patients who underwent gastrectomy with meticulous R2 level lymph node dissection, Gotoda and colleagues [28] were able to define further the risk of lymph node metastasis in additional groups of patients with early gastric cancer with increased certainty (Table 2). These groups of patients were shown to have no or lower risks of lymph node metastasis than the risks of mortality from surgery. The results of this study have allowed the development of an expanded list of candidates suitable for endoscopic resection [87].

Table 2. Early gastric cancer with no risk of lymph node metastasis

Criteria	Incidence	95% CI
Intramucosal cancer Differentiated adenocarcinoma No lymphovascular invasion Irrespective of ulcer findings Tumor less than 3 cm in size	0/1230; 0%	0–0.3%
Intramucosal cancer Differentiated adenocarcinoma No lymphovascular invasion Without ulcer findings Irrespective of tumor size	0/929; 0%	0–0.4%

Table 2. Continued

Criteria	Incidence	95% CI
Undifferentiated intramucosal cancer No lymphovascular invasion Without ulcer findings Tumor less than 2 cm in size	0/141; 0%	0–2.6%
Minute submucosal penetration (SM 1) Differentiated adenocarcinoma No lymphovascular invasion Tumor less than 3 cm in size	0/145; 0%	0–2.5%

The proposed extended indications for endoscopic resection of early gastric cancer, using technique of endoscopic submucosal dissection are (Table 3 and Figure 1):

1) Cancers of differentiated histological type, more than 20 mm in diameter, elevated or depressed type, without ulceration, confined to the mucosa and has no lymphatic or vascular involvement.

2) Cancers of differentiated histological type, equal or less than 30 mm in diameter, any type, with ulceration, confined to the mucosa and have no lymphatic or vascular involvement.

3) Cancers of undifferentiated histological type, equal or less than 20 mm in diameter, elevated or depressed type, without ulceration, confined to the mucosa and have no lymphatic or vascular involvement.

4) Cancers of differentiated histological type, equal or less than 30 mm in diameter, any macroscopic type, with or without ulceration, depth of tumor invasion is SM1, and have no lymphatic or vascular involvement.

Table 3. Proposed extended criteria for endoscopic resection of early gastric cancer

Histological type	Size	Macroscopic type	Ulceration	Depth of tumor invasion	Lymphovascular invasion
Differentiated	Any size	*O-I, IIa, IIc*	UL(-)	M	ly0, v0
Differentiated	≤ 30 mm	*O-I, IIa,IIc; III*	UL(+)(-)	M	ly0, v0
Undifferentiated	≤ 20 mm	*O-I, IIa, IIc*	UL(-)	M	ly0, v0
Differentiated	≤ 30 mm	*O-I, IIa,IIc; III*	UL(+)(-)	SM1	ly0, v0

Unfortunately, there are no comparable series from Western countries, including Russia, which provide appropriate data on the correlation between cancer staging and the rate of lymph node metastases as important parameters which may justify endoscopic resection instead of surgical. But we agree with S.Ishikawa et al. [37], that treatment based on these extended indications still has to be performed as a clinical trial, especially when we are trying to perform endoscopic submucosal dissection for differentiated type mucosal cancer larger than 20 mm with ulcer, and for differentiated type cancer, when the depth of tumor invasion is SM1. Particularly these extended indications need to be thoroughly investigated in large scale prospective clinical trials.

Depth and size	Mucosal cancer				Submucosal cancer	
	Ulceration (-)		Ulceration (+)		SM1	SM2
Histology	≤20mm	>20mm	≤ 30mm	>30mm	≤ 30mm	Any size
Differentiated type	■■■	✦✦✦	✦✦✦	⁄⁄⁄	✦✦✦	⁄⁄⁄
Undifferentiated type	|||||	⁄⁄⁄	⁄⁄⁄	⁄⁄⁄	⁄⁄⁄	⁄⁄⁄

Guideline criteria for endoscopic mucosal resection.

Extended criteria for endoscopic submucosal dissection.

Consider surgery (although the possibility of metastasis is very low in this category, surgery is considered because endoscopic en-bloc removal is sometimes difficult in undifferentiated-type tumors)

Surgery.

Figure 1. Guideline criteria and proposed extended criteria for endoscopic resection of early gastric cancer.

TECHNIQUES OF ENDOSCOPIC RESECTION FOR CURE IN EARLY GASTRIC CANCER

Endoscopic procedures for the excision of early gastric cancer need to be safe, effective, and applicable to a wide range of clinical situations [84]. Several endoscopic techniques have been developed and advocated for mucosal resection for the last 40 years. Major techniques are described in Table 4 as follows: 1) the just cut, or lift and cut technique; 2) the inject, lift (or incise), and cut technique; 3) the inject, suck, and cut technique; and 4) inject, incise the mucosa, and dissect the submucosa, that is different types of endoscopic submucosal dissection.

Table 4. Techniques of endoscopic resection

7. **Just cut, or lift and cut**
   - Polypectomy (Tsuneoka K.,Uchida T., 1969)
   - Endoscopic double-snare polypectomy (EDSP) (Takekoshi T. et al., 1988)
8. **Inject, lift (or incise the mucosa), and cut**
   - Strip biopsy (Tada M, et al., 1984) [88]
   - Endoscopic resection with hypertonic saline-epinephrine solution (ERHSE) (Hirao M. et al., 1988) [33]
   - Four-point fixation endoscopic mucosal resection (Tanaka M. et al., 1997)
9. **Inject, suck, and cut [cap-assisted endoscopic mucosal resection (EMR)]**
   - EMR with cap (EMRC) (Inoue H. et al., 1993) [36]
   - Endoscopic aspiration mucosectomy (EAM) (Torii A., et al., 1995)
   - EMR with ligation (EMRL) (Masuda K., et al., 1993); [87]
10. **Inject, incise the mucosa, dissect the submucosa [endoscopic submucosal dissection (ESD)]**

- EMR with an insulation-tipped (IT) electrosurgical knife (IT-EMR) (Gotoda T. et al., 2002) [29]
- EMR with sodium hyaluronate solution (EMRSH) (Yamamoto H, 2002) [102]
- Endoscopic resection with a hook knife (Oyama T., et al., 2002) [71]
- Endoscopic resection with the tip of an electrosurgical snare (thin type)/a flex knife (Yahagi N. et al., 2004) [100]
- Endoscopic resection with a triangle-tipped knife (Inoue et al., 2003)

1. Just Cut, or Lift and Cut Technique

Endoscopic resection of early gastric cancers originated from the development of a polypectomy technique using high-frequency current to gastric polyps in 1968. Learning from the successful application of polypectomy used to remove early colon cancer [13], *endoscopic polypectomy* to treat pedunculated or semipedunculated early gastric cancer was first described in Japan in 1974. Polypectomy is usually applied to the resection of protruded tumors with a narrow base or a stalk.

2. The Inject, Lift (or Incise), and Cut Technique

The technique of endoscopic snare polypectomy became popular as endoscopic mucosal resection after the birth of a *strip biopsy method* in 1984 [88]. In this method, a double-channel endoscope is used (Figure 2a-2e). After submucosal injection of saline under the lesion, the lesion is lifted using a grasper, while a snare, inserted through the second working channel, is used to remove the lesion (Figure 3a-3g). This technique is applied to the resection of small tumors without ulcer findings regardless of morphology. The disadvantages of this technique are requirement of two assistants and existence of locations impossible for resection due to short working range of the endoscope, angulation of the gastric wall, etc.

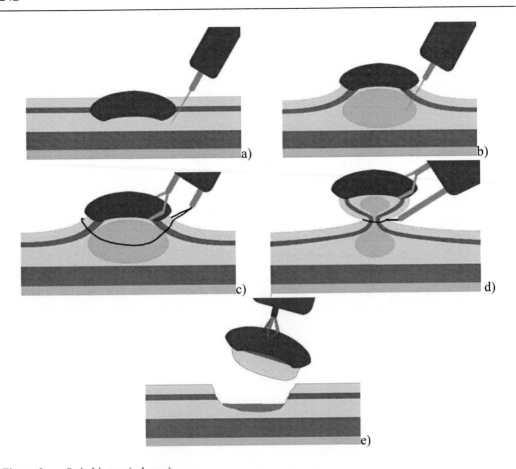

Figure 2a-e. Strip biopsy (scheme).

a) The tip of injection needle is introduced to the submucosal layer, beneath the tumor.
b) Submucosal fluid injection beneath the tumor.
c) The tumor is grasped with a pair of forceps above the snare.
d) The tumor is lifted with a pair of grasping forceps and the snare is closed snugly.
e) The tumor is resected by the snare and retrieved by the grasping forceps.

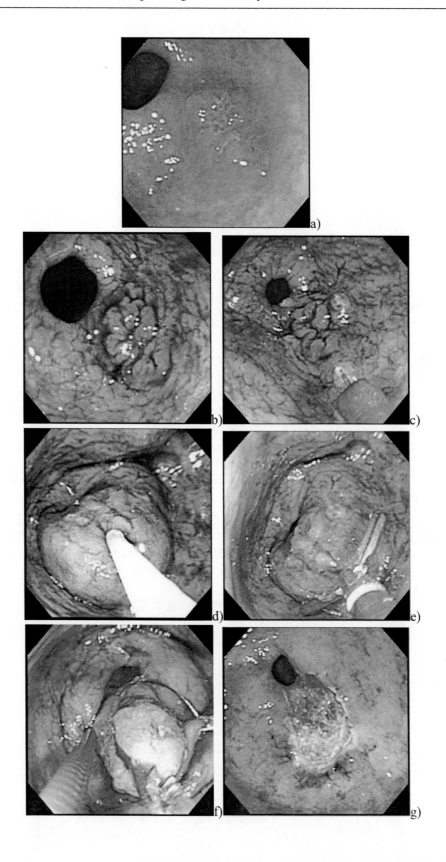

Figure 3a-g. (Continued)

Figure 3a-g. Strip biopsy (clinical application).
a) Reddish, slightly elevated tumor, on the prepyloric antrum.
b) Chromoendoscopy reveals margins of the lesion clearly.
c) Marking dots are made on the circumference of the lesion.
d) Submucosal fluid injection.
e) The lesion is grasped on the top with a pair of forceps above the polypectomy snare, placed to the base.
f) The tumor is lifted with a pair of grasping forceps, the snare is closed and the tumor is resected.
g) The resected tumor has been retrieved. Postoperative ulcer with the clean base.

In 1988, another technique, *endoscopic mucosal resection with the local injection of hypertonic saline/diluted epinephrine solution* was described [33]. In this technique, after the injection of hypertonic saline and diluted epinephrine, the periphery of the lesion is cut using a needle knife. The lesion is then removed using a snare. Endoscopic mucosal resection allowed increased precision to be applied, thus permitting the entire lesion to be removed en bloc. However, the technique also requires considerable skills, and the use of the needle knife has higher risks for perforation.

3. The Inject, Suck, and Cut Technique

A method of *endoscopic mucosal resection with a cap-fitted panendoscope* (EMR-C) developed in 1992 for the resection of early esophageal cancer, was directly applicable for the resection of early gastric cancer [36]. The technique requires a specialized transparent plastic cap that is fitted to the tip of a standard single-channel endoscope (Figure 4). Different sized caps are available according to the diameter of the endoscope and the size of the target lesions [56]. After the submucosal injection of the lesion, a specialized crescent-shaped snare is deployed in the groove of the rim of the cap. The lesion is then sucked into the cap while the snare is closed. Thus, resection can be safely performed through the submucosal layer under the lesion (Figure 5a-5c) [52]. This technique is also applied to the resection of small tumors without ulcer findings regardless of morphology. The advantages of this technique over the inject, lift, and cut technique are requirement of only one assistant, applicability even in a narrow and angular space, convenience for beginners, etc.

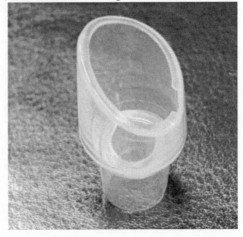

Figure 4. Wide opening oblique cap with rim (soft type) for achieving an EMR-C procedure.

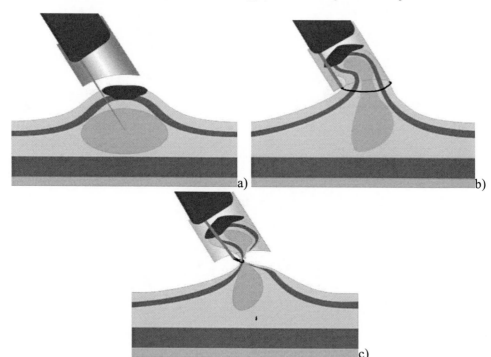

Figure 5a-c. Endoscopic mucosal resection with cap (scheme).
a) Submucosal fluid injection beneath the tumor.
b) The tumor and surrounding mucosa is drawn into the preloaded cap by suction and the snare is closing.
c) The base of the snared mucosa is released from the cap and the tumor is resected.

The technique of *endoscopic mucosal resection with ligation* (EMR-L) (Figure 6a-6c) uses a standard endoscopic variceal ligation device to capture the lesion and make it into a polypoid lesion by deploying the band underneath it [7]. The lesion above or below the band is then excised.

EMR-C and EMR-L have the advantage of being relatively simple, with the use of a standard endoscope and no requirement for an additional assistant. These methods however, due to the technique itself and the size of the accessories, do usually not allow resecting lesions larger than 15-20 mm in diameter in one piece [15, 51]. Piecemeal resection is possible, but does not allow histopathological confirmation of complete removal of gastric cancer. Specimens obtained following piecemeal resections are difficult for the pathologist to analyze, and they render pathological staging inadequate. Residual neoplastic tissue may initially not be detected by endoscopy and this is a major factor leading to the high risk of local tumor recurrence when these techniques are used [94].

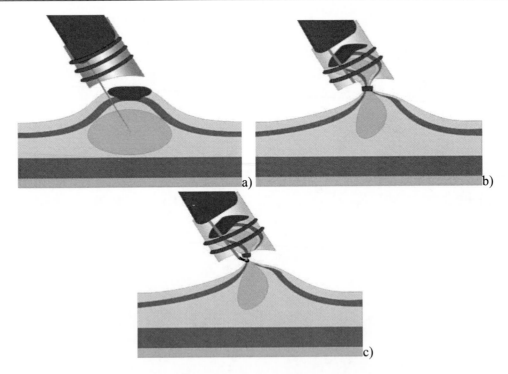

Figure 6a-c. Endoscopic mucosal resection with ligation (scheme).

a) Submucosal fluid injection beneath the tumor.

b) Endoscopic variceal ligation device is used to capture the tumor and make it into a polypoid lesion by deploying the band underneath it.

c) The lesion below the band is excised.

4. Endoscopic Submucosal Dissection (ESD)

In order to overcome these drawbacks, a new method of en-bloc resection with a standard single-channel gastroscope was developed [14]. Endoscopic techniques that involve direct dissection of the submucosa using modified needle knives have been termed **endoscopic submucosal dissection** [70]. Endoscopic submucosal dissection using an insulation-tipped diathermy knife (IT knife) (Figure 7a), was first developed at the National Cancer Center Hospital [26, 34]. Other devices used for **endoscopic submucosal dissection** have also been implemented [43], such as the flex knife [99] (Figure 7b), hook knife [71] (Figure 7c), triangle knife (Figure 7d), flash-knife and a knife in a small-caliber-tip transparent hood [100].

Standard endoscopic submucosal dissection (Figure 8a-8r) consists of 3 main steps. First, fluids are injected into the submucosal layer to separate it from the muscular layer. Second, circumferential cutting is made around the lesion. Then, the connective tissue of the submucosa is dissected under the lesion. To accurately remove the lesion, the periphery of the lesion is marked. This marking is usually performed with a standard needle knife (Figure 8e). Argon plasma coagulation is also available for peripheral marking. After marking the lesion, the fluid is injected to elevate the lesion and create a space between the submucosal and muscular layers (Figure 8f-8g). To promote elevation, several fluids such as saline, glycerol and hyaluronic acid are usually combined with diluted epinephrine, which is used for the prevention of active bleeding. With a needle knife, a small incision is made to insert the tip of the IT knife into the submucosal layer before starting circumferential mucosal incision. At the periphery of the lesion marking, the mucosa is circumferentially cut with the IT knife (Figure 8h-8i). After completion of circumferential incision, an additional solution is injected into the submucosal layer (Figure 8j) to start dissection of the submucosa (Figure 8k-8l).

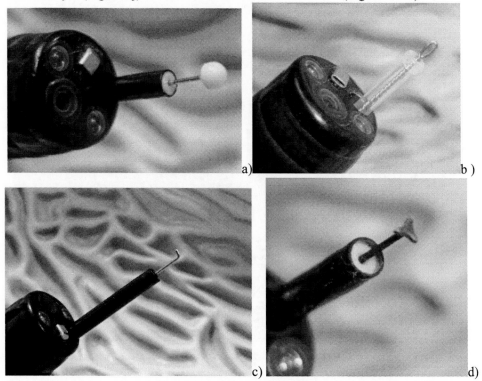

Figure 7a-d. Different types of endoscopic knives for ESD.
a) Insulation-tipped diathermic electrosurgical knife (IT knife) (Gotoda T.).
b) Flex knife (Yahagi N.).
c) Hook knife (Oyama T.).
d) Triangle knife (Inoue H.).

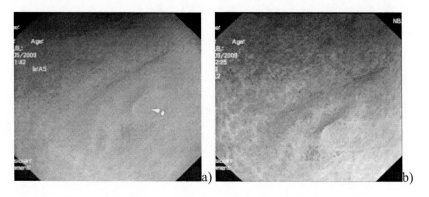

Figure 8 a-r. (Continued)

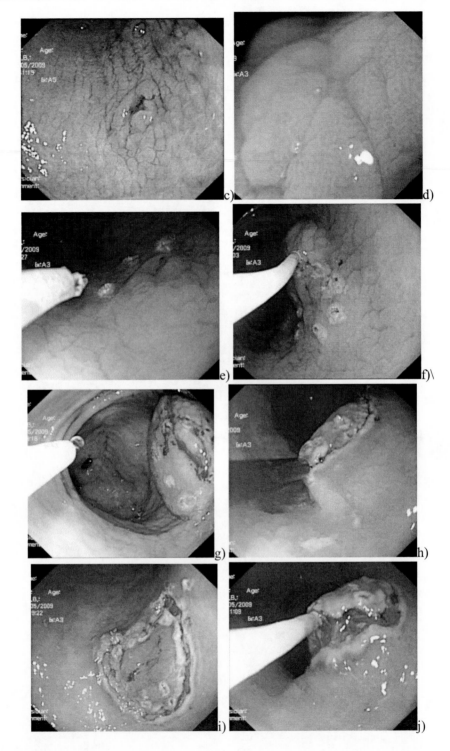

Figure 8 a-r. (Continued)

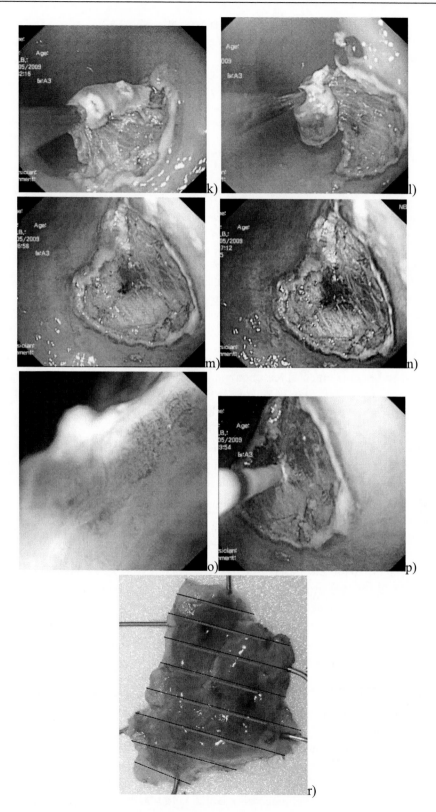

Figure 8 a-r. (Continued)

Figure 8a-r. Endoscopic submucosal dissection (ESD).

a) Reddish elevated neoplasia with central depression on the greater curvature - posterior wall of the proximal antrum.

b, c, d) NBI, chromoendoscopy and zoom reveal margins of the tumor clearly.

e) Marking dots are made on the circumference of the tumor.

f) Submucosal fluid injection is done to the distal margins of the tumor.

g) After submucosal injection of the proximal margins of the lesion, it is raised sufficiently and ready for circumferential mucosal cutting.

h) The mucosa around the marking dots is incised with flex-knife and then with IT knife in ENDO CUT mode.

i) Circumferential mucosal incision is completed and the lesion is separated from the surrounding nonneoplastic area.

j) Additional injection of diluted epinephrine to prevent perforation and facilitate dissection.

k) Submucosal dissection using an IT knife is started from the proximal edges.

l) The tumor is almost completely detached from the muscle layer.

m) No signs of bleeding or perforation in the artificial ulcer base.

n) Observation in NBI mode is made to better visualize blood vessels.

o) Zoom is applied for confirmation of free lateral margins.

p) Preventive hemostasis with argon plasma coagulation is applied.

r) The resected specimen (including all the marking dots) shows en bloc resection of the lesion.

In cases of recurrent tumor fibrosis, which makes en bloc resection difficult for conventional endoscopic mucosal resection methods, in endoscopic submucosal dissection we can cut the submucosal layer while looking at the dissected target directly, so the lesion with strong fibrosis can be resected en bloc regardless of the size and location [48], as well as stomach neoplasms after unsuccessful endoscopic resection [22]

Despite requiring significant additional technical skills and a longer procedure time [10,75], these endoscopic submucosal dissection techniques are rapidly gaining popularity in Japan and overseas, primarily because of their ability to remove even large neoplastic lesions in a single piece with a higher chance of tumor free resection margins and a lower risk of recurrences [25, 99]. The major advantages of this novel and promising technique in comparison with the other endoscopic methods in the treatment of early gastric cancer are that the resected size and shape can be controlled; en bloc resection is possible even in a large tumor and tumors with ulcerative findings are also resectable. Endoscopic submucosal dissection could be performed under the guidance of magnifying endoscopy with a combination of NBI and acetic acid installation [95]. Also, it allows precise histological staging and may prevent disease recurrence. Thus, this technique can be applied to the resection of complex tumors such as large tumors, ulcerative nonlifting tumors, and recurrent tumors. Endoscopic submucosal dissection using the IT knife is perhaps the most commonly performed endoscopic submucosal dissection today in Japan [29, 92].

The disadvantages of this new technique are the requirement of two or more assistants; also, it is technically challenging, operator-dependent and time-consuming. The bleeding and perforation, major complications of endoscopic submucosal dissection, are seems to be a little higher than in the other methods. To prevent bleeding, specially designed haemostatic forceps are used [93]. It is preferable to use a special endoscope that can splash water from the tip by a foot-switch for identification of bleeding vessels and to remove blood. To prevent perforation, investigations of submucosal injection solutions have been actively done [72]. In an attempt to minimize the chance of gastric perforation, polyethylene glycol or hyaluronic acid has been used as the injection agent; this has been reported to help make endoscopic submucosal dissection easier and safer, as these agents stay longer in the submucosa and produce clearer dissection planes [12, 20, 21, 101]. As a further improvement of hyaluronic acid solution, the usefulness of a mixture of a high molecular weight hyaluronic acid and a glycerin plus sugar solution is reported [21]. Considering the tissue damage that can occur after injection of the solution during endoscopic resection, an efficient one should be used [20].

Although several endoscopic devices have been developed solely to make endoscopic submucosal dissection easier and safer, this technique still requires an experienced endoscopist with a high level of skill, because the procedure is performed through only one gastroscope, thus requiring single-handed procedure, not a two-handed, like surgical approach [38]. In other words ESD doesn't have surgeon's left hand to obtain counter-traction for easier dissection.

In 2004 a procedure involving counter-traction of lesions for gastric endoscopic submucosal dissection has been described, but it is still under development. In brief, this process involves *percutaneous traction-assisted endoscopic mucosal resection (PTAEMR)* [50]. This invasive procedure is extremely complicated. Chen P-J. et al. [9] implemented endoscopic submucosal dissection with internal traction.

In 2006 H.Neuhaus et. al. presented first European experience with new specifically designed operative endoscope in a small series of patients. This *R−scope* has a second flexible section for improved positioning, and two instrumentation channels: one with an elevator for lifting the targeted mucosal area with rat−tooth forceps and a second one that allows knives to be moved horizontally, in order to cut the submucosal layer without moving the R−scope (Figure 9). The R−scope facilitated endoscopic submucosal dissection of large gastric areas; however the procedure is technically demanding and time−consuming. Surprisingly it was also associated with a high risk of perforation (20% in this first series). Authors think, that this may be related to an insufficient volume of solution being injected submucosally, excessively forceful lifting of the specimen or the short learning period.

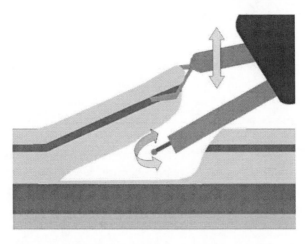

Figure 9. Endoscopic submucosal dissection with R−scope (scheme). Forceps is lifting the mucosa vertically, while the knife is moving horizontally in attempt to cut the submucosal layer.

A two-handed technique, as in conventional surgery - *magnetic-anchor-guided endoscopic submucosal dissection* for large early gastric cancers have been presented in 2008 [31, 47]. To obtain counter-traction, authors have developed a system using magnetic anchor. The magnetic anchor consists of magnetic weight, connecting thread and end-clip. After completion of mucosal incision, a magnetic anchor is transferred to the stomach. The magnetic anchor is placed on the lesion using endoclip. The lesion attached by the magnetic anchor is lifted by an electromagnet control forces from the outside of abdomen. En bloc resection rate was excellent - 100% and there was no complication such as perforations. However, median procedure time was not shortened, still 80 min, because it is a little complicated technique to obtain counter-traction for proper direction. Authors conclude that they need more improvement for simplifying this technique.

In order to further extend the indications for treating early gastric cancer with less invasive surgery, *endoscopic resection combined with laparoscopic regional lymph-node dissection* have been implemented [2-4].

PATHOLOGICAL ASSESSMENT AFTER ENDOSCOPIC RESECTION

Endoscopic resection has generally been unpopular in the West, because of the very low incidence of suitable early gastric cancer cases. The diagnostic difficulties related to endoscopy seem to be a factor, but the low incidence of early gastric cancer may also be explained by the different histological criteria applied in the West and Japan; that is to say, most intestinal-type mucosal cancer in Japan is not regarded as a cancer in the West [82]. Whatever the case, such lesions ought to be diagnosed as neoplastic or dysplastic on histology, in line with the Vienna classification [83], and they should be subjected, where appropriate, to endoscopic resection.

The importance of meticulous pathological staging after endoscopic resection cannot be overemphasized. Accurate staging can only be achieved when the specimen is properly oriented by the endoscopist or their assistant immediately after excision in the endoscopy unit prior to the specimen being immersed in formaldehyde. Orientation of the specimen is best performed by fixing its periphery with thin needles inserted into an underlying plate of rubber or wood. The submucosal side of the specimen is placed in contact with the plate (Figure 8r).

After fixation, the specimen is sectioned serially at 2-mm intervals parallel to a line that includes the closest resection margin of the specimen, so that both lateral and vertical margins are assessed.

The report must include histological type along with the degree of differentiation, the depth of tumor invasion (T), size, location, and macroscopic appearance. The presence of ulceration and lymphatic and/or venous involvement, and the status of the resection margins should be reported in detail to determine the curability [62].

PATIENT'S CARE AND COMPLICATIONS OF ENDOSCOPIC RESECTION

Vital signs such as blood pressure, oxygen saturation, and electrocardiograms must be checked during endoscopic procedures [60]. After the procedure standard doses of proton-pump inhibitors twice a day are prescribed for 8 weeks, and patients are typically fasted for 24 hours after the procedure [53], followed by clear liquid on the second day. With adequate medication pain after resection is typically mild or absent at all [42]. If the patient's symptoms, laboratory findings, and chest and abdominal radiographs were unremarkable the day after ESD, a light meal was permitted, and the patient was then discharged within 1 week. Probably the administration of proton pump inhibitors might be moderately effective for ulcer healing of post resection defect, but it's no doubt, that it's quite effective for prevention bleeding complications or to treat them [26]. If complications occurred, the schedules were changed according to the individual patient's condition.

The major complications of endoscopic resection for early gastric cancer include bleeding, perforation [Table 5] and much rare - stricture formation (after circumferential resection in cardia or pylorus).

Table 5. Complication rate of endoscopic resection

Techniques	Complication rate	
	Bleeding	Perforation
ERHSE [33]	6.7% (25/373)	2.9%(11/373)
EMR [45]	3.3% (26/790)	3.0% (24/790)
ESD with the tip of an electrosurgical snare (thin type)/a flex knife [99]	1.7%(1/59)	3.4%(2/59)
ESD with sodium hyaluronate and small-caliber tip transparent hood [101]	1% (1/70)	0% (0/70)
ESD with a hook knife [71]	-	1.5%(3/204)
ESD (Inoue H., 2009)	3.2% (12/370)	3.0% (11/370)
ESD [45]	4.0% (20/500)	2.0% (10/500)
ESD [23]	5,1% (14/276)	4,0(11/276)

Table 6. Relationships between delayed bleeding and tumor location, size, and ulcer findings [30]

		Delayed bleeding	P value
Location	Upper third of stomach	1% (1/176)	
	Middle third of stomach	6% (24/431)	0.001
	Lower third of stomach	7% (31/426)	<0.001
Size (mm)	≤20	5% (35/719)	
	21–30	7% (13/176)	0.184
	≥31	8% (11/138)	0.139
Ulcer finding	Positive	5% (13/243)	
	Negative	6% (46/790)	0.781

Bleeding is the most common complication (Figure 10a-c), occurring in up to 8% of patients undergoing standard **endoscopic mucosal resection** and in up to 7% of patients undergoing **endoscopic submucosal dissection** [63, 89] (Tables 5, 6). Most bleeding occurs during the procedure or within 24 hours. Immediate bleeding appears more common with resections of tumors located in the upper third of the stomach. During endoscopic submucosal dissection, immediate minor bleeding is not uncommon, but it can be successfully treated by grasping and coagulation of the bleeding vessels, using hemostatic forceps [19]. Endoclips are often deployed for severe bleeding.

Delayed bleeding, manifested as hematemesis or melena at 0 to 30 days after the procedure, is treated by emergency endoscopy performed after fluid resuscitation, using techniques similar to those described [69]. Delayed bleeding is common after endoscopic submucosal dissection and is closely related to tumor location and size [85].

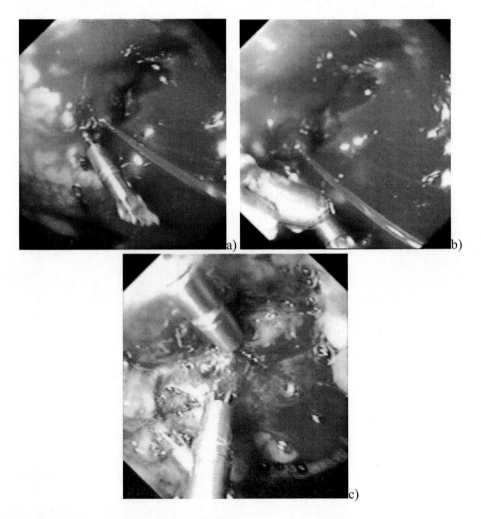

Figure 10a-c. Management of bleeding during ESD.
a) Arterial bleeding from submucosal layer; unsuccessful placement of the first hemostatic clip.
b) The attempt to stop bleeding with the hot biopsy forceps and 80-W soft-mode coagulation.
c) Final hemostasis with endoscopic clips.

Perforation is uncommon during endoscopic mucosal resection, but is seen relatively more commonly during endoscopic submucosal dissection. The risk of perforation during endoscopic submucosal dissection is around 4% (Table 7).

Table 7. Relationships between risk of perforation and tumor location, size, and ulcer findings [30]

		Risk of perforation	P value
Location	Upper third of stomach	7% (13/176)	<0.001
	Middle third of stomach	4% (16/431)	<0.05
	Lower third of stomach	1% (6/426)	
Size (mm)	≤20	3% (18/719)	
	21–30	3% (6/176)	0.184
	≥31	8% (11/138)	0.139
Ulcer finding	Positive	6% (14/243)	<0.05
	Negative	3% (21/790)	

Immediately recognized perforation can be successfully closed with endoclips (Figure 11a-c) and conservatively observed with nasogastric suction and antibiotics, without emergency laparoscopy or laparotomy [57, 98], because the stomach in patients during gastric endoscopic mucosal resection or endoscopic submucosal dissection is thought to be comparatively clean due to antibacterial effect of gastric acid. If pneumoperitoneum (Figure 11b) and even tension pneumothorax and subcutaneous emphysema due to perforation are severe, breathing and cardio-vascular deterioration or neurogenic shock can occur. To prevent/treat abdominal compartment syndrome, decompression of the pneumoperitoneum must be performed under transabdominal ultrasonographic guidance or laparoscopically, as well as drainage tube insertion to thoracic cavity in case of pneumothorax. To reduce the risk of compartment syndrome CO_2 insufflation during the procedure is recommended.

Delayed perforation is thought to occur because of the excessive electrical coagulation of the vessels lying within the submucosal or muscular layers. When these vessels need coagulation, care must be taken not to push the device to the gastric wall and not to coagulate for long intervals.

Surgical intervention is required for large defects and/or development of peritonitis [87].

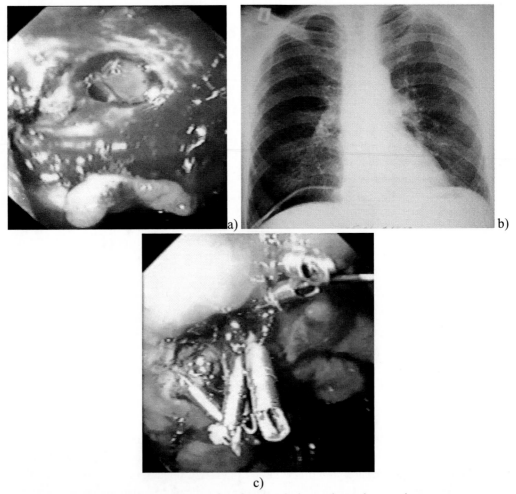

Figure 11a-c. Diagnosis and management of perforation during endoscopic resection.
a) Opening in the gastric wall caused by electrosurgical knife.
b) Pneumoperitoneum due to perforation. The X-ray demonstrated moderate volume of free air in the abdominal cavity.
c) Complete closure of the opening with endoscopic clips.

OUTCOMES OF ENDOSCOPIC RESECTION

The outcomes of endoscopic resection have been studied in details and still being investigated precisely around the world [23, 49]. The successful outcomes of endoscopic mucosal resection observed from major institutions in Japan [64], Korea [45,], Europe and USA have allowed endoscopic mucosal resection to become the standard treatment for early gastric cancer not only in Japan, but step by step – in the other countries [90].

Collected data from Japanese series on the inject, lift, and cut, endoscopic mucosal resection with cap or endoscopic mucosal resection with previous ligation of early gastric cancer indicate that en-bloc resection can be achieved in approximately 75% of cases. The inject, lift, and cut technique resulted in a little higher en bloc resection rate than the inject, suck, and cut technique for tumors ≥11mm and ≤20 mm in size. However, if the tumors exceeded 20mm in size, en bloc resection rates became extremely low in both techniques.

As previously mentioned, standard endoscopic mucosal resection techniques are associated with risks of recurrence, especially when resections are not performed en bloc, or when the resection margins are involved by tumor. The incidence of local recurrences after endoscopic mucosal resection ranged from 2% to 35%, particularly in cases of piecemeal resection or no clear tumor margins [49]. Average local recurrent rates were around 10% in the former, but local recurrent rates of the latter were less than 5% (Table 8).

Table 8. En bloc resection and recurrence rates after endoscopic resection for early gastric cancer [30]

Techniques	En bloc resection rate ≤20mm tumor >20 mm		Local recurrent rate
ERHSE [33]	55,1% (183/332)	19% (7/37)	2.3% (8/349)
EMR [45]	90.2% (607/660)	77.7% (101/130)	3.3% (13/287)
Strip biopsy, EAM [94]			3.5% (15/423)
EMR + Laser Ida et al.			6.7% (11/165)
Strip biopsy, EMR + laser NCCH (1978–1998)			8.5% (53/620)
Strip biopsy Mitsunaga et al.			18.2% (54/296)
Strip biopsy, EMR-C Kawaguchi et al.			36.5% (97/266)
ESD with isolated tip knife [Gotoda]	97% (231/238)	94% (141/150)	-
ESD with the tip of an electrosurgical snare (thin type)/a flex knife [99]	95% (56/59)		-
ESD with sodium hyaluronate and small-caliber tip transparent hood [101]	100% (37/37)	97% (32/33)	-
ESD [23]	97.8% (175/179)	97.0% (65/67)	0,9% (2/212)
ESD [45]	92.1% (267/292)	91.0% (151/166)	0.3% (1/359)
ESD with a hook knife [71]	95%(194/204)		0.5%(1/204)

EAM, Endoscopic aspiration mucosectomy; EMR-C, endoscopic mucosal resection with cap; ERHSE, endoscopic mucosal resection with local injection of hypertonic saline-epinephrine.

The disease-specific survival rates are close to 99-100% within follow-up periods varying between 4 months and 11 years, although not all studies reported long-term outcomes. In comparison the 5-year cancer-specific survival rates after gastrectomy with lymph node dissection of early gastric cancer limited to the mucosa or the submucosa are 99% and 96%, respectively [80].

Endoscopic submucosal dissection is still investigational and demands an extremely high level of skill. In some specialized centers in Japan, the long-term outcomes of patients who have had endoscopic resection using the extended criteria are currently being studied [12, 91]. Follow−up endoscopy for surveillance of recurrence is carried out at 2 or 3 months after ESD in the first year, and annually thereafter. In immature stages of endoscopic submucosal dissection, en bloc resection rates were not as good in comparison with those of the other techniques. After maturity of the techniques of endoscopic submucosal dissection, en bloc resection rates became greater than 90%, regardless of size of the tumor (Table 8). Recent results are really promising and demonstrate very low local recurrence rates of 0 − 0,5%, but still within a relatively limited (in comparison with EMR) follow-up (Figure 12a,b).

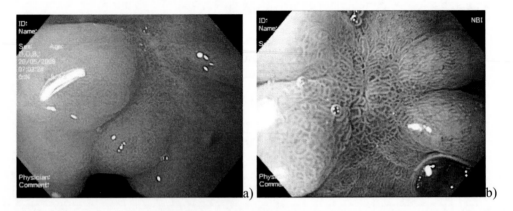

Figure 12 a, b. One year after ESD - no signs of recurrent tumor.
a) Postoperative scar in the conventional white light.
b) Same postoperative scar in the NBI mode.

The incidence of metachronous multiple gastric cancer in patients who have undergone endoscopic resection for the first lesion should be prospectively investigated to determine the interval of sufficient surveillant endoscopy [59, 61].

CONCLUSIONS

Endoscopic resection is a promising and rapidly evolving technique represents an important advance in endoscopic therapy, making it possible curative treatment of selected cases of early gastric cancer. It is well established as a standard therapy in Japan and is increasingly becoming accepted all over the world [1]. Endoscopic mucosal resection is less invasive than surgical resection, and thus morbidity and mortality is lower, however it is technically demanding and are sometimes hazardous. Compared to photodynamic therapy and argon plasma coagulation, endoscopic mucosal resection can more easily remove mucosa and submucosa, without damaging the underlying muscle and permits histologic evaluation of all the resected mucosa. Improved endoscopic tools will allow wider endoscopic mucosal resections to be performed. Endoscopic submucosal dissection, a modification of endoscopic mucosal resection, has been developed to allow the resection of larger lesions in an en-bloc manner; the early results so far have been really encouraging, although the long-term outcome data are still being monitored [74]. However, randomized trials comparing endoscopic mucosal resection with surgery or other ablative endoscopic techniques are lacking, and more data are needed on the long-term results. Although several problems still remain, endoscopic submucosal dissection is one of the best ways for patients suffering from early gastric cancer to preserve their stomach and protect their quality of life [108].

Patients need careful evaluation prior to endoscopic mucosal resection, and only those with superficial lesions and no lymph node involvement should undergo the procedure. So there is a strong need to detect gastric cancer at an earlier stage. The application of endoscopic submucosal dissection requires substantial learning period and should be performed in centers with all options for endoscopic, laparoscopic and open procedures for the adequate clinical care of patients, especially in case of complications.

In the field of endoscopy, technological development and theoretical progress will present us an innovative method for the treatment of early gastric cancer, which may result in better outcomes [96].

ACKNOWLEDGEMENTS

My cordial gratitude to my parents for the opportunity and to my beloved family – Lena, Olya and Dima – for their love, patience and assistance. I would like also to thank my teachers – A.Grinberg, V.Minz, Yu.Gallinger, A.Boodzinsky, M.Classen and P.Cotton for difficult but outstanding lessons and my Japanese colleagues and friends – R.Narisawa, H.Maguchi, T.Oyama, H.Inoue, H.Kashida, I.Oda, N.Yahagi - for inspiration. I also wish to express my gratitude to all my co-workers and friends from our department and particularly to – M.Timofeev, Z.Galkova, E.Ivanova, P.Tchernyakevich and O.Yudin – for their invaluable collaboration and support in preparing this publication.

REFERENCES

[1]   Aabakken L. Endoscopic diagnosis and treatment of gastric tumors. *Endoscopy* 2007; 39: 974-977

[2]   Abe N, Mori T, Izumisato Y, Sasaki H, Ueki H, Masaki T, et al. Successful treatment of an undifferentiated early gastric cancer by combined en bloc EMR and laparoscopic regional lymphadenectomy. *Gastrointest Endosc* 2003;57:972–5.

[3]   Abe N, Mori T, Takeuchi H, Yoshida T, Ohki A, Ueki H, et al. Laparoscopic lymph node dissection after endoscopic submucosal dissection: a novel and minimally invasive approach to treating early-stage gastric cancer. *Am J Surg* 2005;190:496–503.

[4]   Abe N., Toshiyuki Mori, Hirohisa Takeuchi, Hisayo Ueki, Osamu Yanagida, Tadahiko Masaki et al. Successful treatment of early stage gastric cancer by laparoscopy-assisted endoscopic full-thickness resection with lymphadenectomy. *Gastrointest Endosc* 2008;68:1220-4

[5]   Ahmad NA, Kochman ML, Long WB, Furth EE, Ginsberh GG. Effi cacy, safety, and clinical outcomes of endoscopic mucosal resection: a study of 101 cases. *Gastrointest Endosc* 2002;55: 390–6.

[6]   Akahoshi K, Chijiwa Y, Hamada S, Sasaki I, Nawata H, Kabemura T, et al. Pretreatment staging of endoscopically early gastric cancer with a 15 MHz ultrasound catheter probe. *Gastrointest Endosc* 1998;48:470–6.

[7]   Akiyama M, Ota M, Nakajima H, Yamagata K, Munakata A. Endoscopic mucosal resection of gastric neoplasms using a ligating device. *Gastrointest Endosc* 1997;45:182–6.

[8]   Bonenkamp JJ, Songun I, Hermans J, Sasako M, Welvaart K, Plukker JT, et al. Randomised comparison of morbidity after D1 and D2 dissection for gastric cancer in 996 Dutch patients. *Lancet* 1995;345:745–8.

[9]   Chen P-J., Chu H-C., Chang W-K., Hsieh T-Yu., Chao Yo-C. Endoscopic submucosal dissection with internal traction for early gastric cancer (with video) *Gastrointest Endosc* 2008;67:128-32

[10]   Choi IJ, Kim CG, Chang HJ, Kim SG, Kook MC, Bae JM. The learning curve for EMR with circumferential mucosal incision in treating intramucosal gastric cancer. *Gastrointest Endosc* 2005; 62:860–5.

[11]   Chung Il-K., Jun Haeng Lee, MD, Suck-Ho Lee, MD, Sun-Joo Kim, MD, Joo Young Cho, MD Won Young Cho, MD Therapeutic outcomes in 1000 cases of endoscopic submucosal dissection for early gastric neoplasms: Korean ESD Study Group multicenter study. *Gastrointest Endosc* 2009; doi:10.1016/ j.gie.2008.09.027

[12]   Conio M, Ponchon T, Blanchi S, Filibertiet R. Endoscopic mucosal resection. *Am J Gastroenterol* 2006;101:653–63.

[13]   Deyhle P, Largiader F, Jenny S, Fumagalli I. A method for endoscopic electroresection of sessile colonic polyps. *Endoscopy* 1973; 5:38–40.

[14]   Eguchi T, Gotoda T, Oda I, Hamanaka H, Hasuike N, Saito D. Is endoscopic one-piece mucosal resection essential for early gastric cancer? *Dig Endosc* 2003;15:113–6.

[15]   Ell C, May A, Gossner L, Pech O, Gunter E, Mayer G, et al. Endoscopic mucosectomy of early cancer and high-grade dysplasia in Barrett's esophagus. *Gastroenterol* 2000;118:670–7.

[16]   Etoh T, Katai H, Fukagawa T, Sano T, Oda I, Gotoda T, et al. Treatment of early gastric cancer in the elderly patient: results of EMR and gastrectomy at a national referral center in Japan. *Gastrointest Endosc* 2005;62:868–71.

[17]   Farrell JJ, Lauwers GY, Brugge WR. Endoscopic mucosal resection using a cap-fi tted endoscope improves tissue resection and pathology interpretation: an animal study. *Gastric Cancer* 2006;9: 3–8.

[18]   Fujii K, Okajima K, Isozaki H, Hara H, Nomura E, Sako S, et al. A clinicopathological study on the indications of limited surgery for submucosal gastric cancer (in Japanese with English abstract). *Jpn J Gastroenterol Surg* 1998;31:2055–62.

[19]   Fujishiro M, Ono H, Gotoda T, Yamaguchi H, Kondo H, Saito D. Usefulness of Maalox for detection of the precise bleeding points and confi rmation of hemostasis on gastrointestinal hemorrhage. *Endoscopy* 2000;32:196.

[20]   Fujishiro M, Yahagi N, Kashimura K, Matsuura T, Nakamura M, Kakushima N, et al. Tissue damage of different submucosal injection solutions for EMR. *Gastrointest Endosc* 2005;62:933–42.

[21]   Fujishiro M, Yahagi N, Nakamura M, Kakushima N, Kodashima S, Ono S, et al. Successful outcomes of a novel endoscopic treatment for GI tumors: endoscopic submucosal dissection with a mixture of high-molecular-weight hyaluronic acid, glycerin, and sugar. *Gastrointest Endosc* 2006;63:243–9.

[22] Fujishiro M., O. Goto, N. Kakushima, S. Kodashima, Y. Muraki, M. Omata. Endoscopic submucosal dissection of stomach neoplasms after unsuccessful endoscopic resection. *Digestive and Liver Disease* 39 (2007) 566–571.

[23] Goto O et al. M. Fujishiro, S. Kodashima, S. Ono, M. Omata. Outcomes of ESD for early gastric cancer with special reference to validation for curability criteria. *Endoscopy* 2009; 41: 118-122

[24] Goto O., M. Fujishiro , N. Kakushima , S. Kodashima , S. Ono, H. Yamaguchi et al. Endoscopic submucosal dissection as a staging measure may not lead to worse prognosis in early gastric cancer patients with additional gastrectomy. *Digestive and Liver Disease* 40 (2008) 293–297

[25] Gotoda T, Friedland S, Hamanaka H, Soetikno R. A learning curve for advanced endoscopic resection. *Gastrointest Endosc* 2005;62:866–7.

[26] Gotoda T, Kondo H, Ono H, Saito Y, Yamaguchi H, Saito D, et al. A new endoscopic mucosal resection (EMR) procedure using an insulation-tipped diathermic (IT) knife for rectal fl at lesions. *Gastrointest Endosc* 1999;50:560–3.

[27] Gotoda T, Sasako M, Ono H, Katai H, Sano T, Shimoda T. An evaluation of the necessity of gastrectomy with lymph node dissection for patients with submucosal invasive gastric cancer. *Br J Surg* 2001;88:444–9.

[28] Gotoda T, Yanagisawa A, Sasako M, Ono H, Nakanishi Y, Shimoda T, et al. Incidence of lymph node metastasis from early gastric cancer: estimation with a large number of cases at two large centers. *Gastric Cancer* 2000;3:219–25.

[29] Gotoda T. A large endoscopic resection by endoscopic submucosal dissection (ESD) procedure. *Clin Gastroenterol Hepatol* 2005; 3:S71–3.

[30] Gotoda T. Endoscopic resection of early gastric cancer *Gastric Cancer* (2007) 10: 1–11

[31] Gotoda T., Ichiro Oda, MD, Katsunori Tamakawa, PhD, Hirohisa Ueda, PhD, Toshiaki Kobayashi, MD, PhD, Tadao Kakizoe, MD, PhD Prospective clinical trial of magnetic-anchor–guided endoscopic submucosal dissection for large early gastric cancer (with videos). *Gastrointest Endosc* 2009;69:10-5.)

[32] Hiki Y. Endoscopic mucosal resection (EMR) for early gastric cancer. (in Japanese with English abstract). *Jpn J Surg* 1996;97: 273–8.

[33] Hirao M, Masuda K, Ananuma T, Nala H, Noda K, Matsuura K, et al. Endoscopic resection of early gastric cancer and other tumors with local injection of hypertonic saline-epinephrine. *Gastrointest Endosc* 1988;34:264–9.

[34] Hosokawa K, Yoshida S. Recent advances in endoscopic mucosal resection for early gastric cancer (in Japanese with English abstract). *Jpn J Cancer Chemother* 1998;25:483.

[35] Hull MJ, Mino-Kenudson M, Nishioka NS, Ban S, Sepehr A, Puricelli W, et al. Endoscopic mucosal resection: an improved diagnostic procedure for early gastroesophageal epithelial neoplasms. *Am J Surg Pathol* 2006;30:114–8.

[36] Inoue H, Takeshita K, Hori H, Muraoka Y, Yoneshima H, Endo M. Endoscopic mucosal resection with a cap-fitted panendoscope for esophagus, stomach, and colon mucosal lesions. *Gastrointest Endosc* 1993;39:58–62.

[37] Ishikawa S., Akihiko Togashi, Mituhiro Inoue, Shinobu Honda, Fumiaki Nozawa, Eiichirou Toyama et al. Indications for EMR/ESD in cases of early gastric cancer:

relationship between histological type, depth of wall invasion, and lymph node metastasis. *Gastric Cancer* (2007) 10: 35–38

[38] Isshi K, Tajiri H, Fujisaki J, Mochizuki K, Matsuda K, Nakamura Y, et al. The effectiveness of a new multibending scope for endoscopic mucosal resection. *Endoscopy* 2004;36:294–7.

[39] Itoh H, Oohata Y, Nakamura K, Nagata T, Mibu R, Nakayama F. Complete 10-year postgastrectomy follow-up of early gastric cancer. *Am J Surg* 1989;158:14–6.

[40] Japanese Gastric Cancer Association. Gastric cancer treatment guideline (in Japanese). 2nd ed. Kanehara-Shuppan, Tokyo, 2004.

[41] Japanese Gastric Cancer Association. Japanese classification of gastric carcinoma–2nd English edition. *Gastric Cancer* 1998;1: 10–24.

[42] Kaneko E, Hanada H, Kasugai T, Ogoshi K, Niwa K. The survey of gastrointestinal endoscopic complications in Japan (in Japanese). *Gastroenterol Endosc* 2000;42:308–13.

[43] Kantsevoy S., Adler D.G., Conway J.D., Diehl D.L., Farraye F.A., Richard Kwon, et al. Endoscopic mucosal resection and endoscopic submucosal dissection. *Gastrointest Endosc* 2008;68:11-18

[44] Katsube T, Konno S, Hamaguchi K, Shimakawa T, Naritaka Y, Ogawa K, et al. The effi cacy of endoscopic mucosal resection in the diagnosis and treatment of group III gastric lesions. *Anticancer Res* 2005;25:3513–6.

[45] Kim Jae J., Jun Haeng Lee, Hwoon-Yong Jung, Gin Hyug Lee, Joo Yong Cho, Chang Beom Ryu et.al. EMR for early gastric cancer in Korea: a multicenter retrospective study. *Gastrointest Endosc* 2007;66: 693-700

[46] Kitamura T, Tanabe S, Koizumi W, Mitomi H, Saigenji K. Argon plasma coagulation for early gastric cancer: technique and outcome. *Gastrointest Endosc* 2006;63:48–54.

[47] Kobayashi T, Gotoda T, Tamakawa K, Ueda H, Kakizoe T. Magnetic anchor for more effective endoscopic mucosal resection. *Jpn J Clin Oncol* 2004;34:118–23.

[48] Kodashima S., Fujishiro m., Yahagi N., Kakushima n., Masanori Nakamura, Omata M. Endoscopic submucosal dissection for recurrent gastric tumors. *Digestive Endoscopy* (2006) 18, 151–153

[49] Kojima T, Parra-Blanco A, Takahashi H, Fujita R. Outcome of endoscopic mucosal resection for early gastric cancer: review of the Japanese literature. *Gastrointest Endosc* 1998;48:550–4.

[50] Kondo H, Gotoda T, Ono H, Oda I, Kozu T, Fijishiro M, et al. Percutaneous traction-assisted EMR by using an insulationtipped electrosurgical knife for early stage gastric cancer. *Gastrointest Endosc* 2004;59:284–8.

[51] Korenaga D, Haraguchi M, Tsujitani S, Okamura T, Tamada R, Sugimachi K. Clinicopathological features of mucosal carcinoma of the stomach with lymph node metastasis in 11 patients. *Br J Surg* 1986;73:431–3.

[52] Kume K, Yamasaki M, Kubo K, Mitsuoka H, Ota T, Matsuhashi T, et al. EMR of upper GI lesions when using a novel soft, irrigation, prelooped hood. *Gastrointest Endosc* 2004;60:124–8.

[53] Lee SY, Kim JJ, Lee JH, Kim YH, Rhee PL, Paik SW, et al. Healing rate of EMR-induced ulcer in relation to the duration of treatment with omeprazole. *Gastrointest Endosc* 2004;60:213–7.

[54] Ludwig K, Klautke G, Bernhard J, Weiner R. Minimally invasive and local treatment for mucosal early gastric cancer. *Surg Endosc* 2005;19:1362–6.

[55] Maruyama K, Okabayashi K, Kinoshita T. Progress in gastric cancer surgery in Japan and its limits of radicality. *World J Surg* 1987;11:418–25.

[56] Matsuzaki K, Nagao S, Kawaguchi A, Miyazaki J, Yoshida Y, Kitagawa Y, et al. Newly designed soft prelooped cap for endoscopic mucosal resection of gastric lesions. *Gastrointest Endosc* 2003;57:242–6.

[57] Minami S, Gotoda T, Ono H, Oda I, Hamanaka H. Complete endoscopic closure using endoclips for gastric perforation during endoscopic resection for early gastric cancer can avoid emergent surgery. *Gastrointest Endosc* 2006;63:596–601.

[58] Nagano H, Ohyama S, Fukunaga T, Seto Y, Fujisaki J, Yamaguchi T, et al. Indications for gastrectomy after incomplete EMR for early gastric cancer. *Gastric Cancer* 2005;8:149–54.

[59] Nakajima T, Oda I, Gotoda T, Hamanaka H, Eguchi T, Yokoi C, et al. Metachronous gastric cancers after endoscopic resection: how effective is annual endoscopic surveillance? *Gastric Cancer* 2006;9:93–8.

[60] Naruse M., Shuji Inatsuchi. Risk management in endoscopic submucosal dissection in upper gastrointestinal endoscopy *Digestive Endoscopy* (2007) 19 (Suppl. 1), S2–S4

[61] Nasu J, Doi T, Endo H, Nishina T, Hirasaki S, Hyodo I. Characteristics of metachronous multiple early gastric cancers after endoscopic mucosal resection. *Endoscopy* 2005;37:990–3.

[62] Nunobe S, Gotoda T, Oda I, Katai H, Sano T, Shimoda T, et al. Distribution of the deepest penetrating point of minute submucosal gastric cancer. *Jpn J Clin Oncol* 2005;35:587–90.

[63] Oda I, Gotoda T, Hamanaka H, Eguchi T, Saito Y, Matsuda T, et al. Endoscopic submucosal dissection for early gastric cancer: Technical feasibility, operation time and complications from a large series of consecutive cases. *Dig Endosc* 2005;17:54–8.

[64] Oda I., Daizo Saito, Masahiro Tada, Hiroyasu Iishi, Satoshi Tanabe, Tsuneo Oyama et al. A multicenter retrospective study of endoscopic resection for early gastric cancer *Gastric Cancer* (2006) 9: 262–270

[65] Ohashi S, Segawa K, Okamura S, Mitake M, Urano H, Shimodaira M, et al. The utility of endoscopic ultrasonography and endoscopy in the endoscopic mucosal resection of early gastric cancer. *Gut* 1999;45:599–604.

[66] Ohgami M, Otani Y, Kumai K, Kubota T, Kitajima M. Laparoscopic surgery for early gastric cancer (in Japanese with English abstract). *Jpn J Surg* 1996;97:279–85.

[67] Ohta H, Noguchi Y, Takagi K, Nishi M, Kajitani T, Kato Y. Early gastric carcinoma with special reference to macroscopic classification. *Cancer* 1987;60:1099–106.

[68] Oizumi H, Matsuda T, Fukase K, Furukawa A, Mito S, Takahashi K. Endoscopic resection for early gastric cancer: the actual procedure and clinical evaluation (in Japanese with English abstract). *Stomach and Intestine* 1991;26:289–300.

[69] Okano A, Hajiro K, Takakuwa H, Nishio A, Matsushita M. Predictors of bleeding after endoscopic mucosal resection of gastric tumors. *Gastrointest Endosc* 2003;57:687–90.

[70] Ono H, Kondo H, Gotoda T, Shirao K, Yamaguchi H, Saito D, et al. Endoscopic mucosal resection for treatment of early gastric cancer. *Gut* 2001;48:225–9.

[71] Oyama T, Kikuchi Y. Aggressive endoscopic mucosal resection in the upper GI tract — Hook knife EMR method. *Min InvasTher Allied Technol* 2002;11:291–5.

[72] Park S., Hoon Jai Chun, Chul Young Kim, Ju Young Kim, Jin Su Jang, Yong Dae Kwon et al. Electrical Characteristics of Various Submucosal Injection Fluids for Endoscopic Mucosal Resection. *Dig Dis Sci* (2008) 53:1678–1682

[73] Rembacken BJ, Gotoda T, Fujii T, Axon ATR. Endoscopic mucosal resection. *Endoscopy* 2001;33:709–18.

[74] Repici A. Endoscopic submucosal dissection: established, or still needs improving? *Gastrointest Endosc* 2009;69:16-17

[75] Rosch T, Sarbia M, Schmacher B, Deinert K, Frimberger E, Toermer T, et al. Attempted endoscopic en bloc resection of mucosal and submucosal tumors using insulated-tip knives: a pilot series. *Endoscopy* 2004;36:788–801.

[76] Saitoh Y, Obara T, Watari J, Nomura M, Taruishi M, Orii Y, et al. Invasion depth diagnosis of depressed type early colorectal cancers by combined use of videoendoscopy and chromoendoscopy. *Gastrointest Endosc* 1998;48:362–70.

[77] Sano T, Kobori O, Muto T. Lymph node metastasis from early gastric cancer: endoscopic resection of tumour. *Br J Surg* 1992;79: 241–4.

[78] Sano T, Okuyama Y, Kobori O, Shimizu T, Morioka Y. Early gastric cancer; endoscopic diagnosis of depth of invasion. *Dig Dis Sci* 1990;35:1340–35.

[79] Sano T, Sasako M, Kinoshita T, Maruyama K. Recurrence of early gastric cancer. Follow-up of 1475 patients and review of Japanese literature. Cancer 1993;72:3174–8.

[80] Sasako M, Kinoshita T, Maruyama K. Prognosis of early gastric cancer. *Stomach and Intestine (in Japanese; abstract in English)* 1993;28:139–46.

[81] Sasako M. Risk factors for surgical treatment in the Dutch gastric cancer trial. *Br J Surg* 1997;84:1567–71.

[82] Schlemper RJ, Itabashi M, Kato Y, Lewin KJ, Riddell RH, Shimoda T, et al. Differences in diagnostic criteria for gastric carcinoma between Japanese and Western pathologists. *Lancet* 1997;349:1725–9.

[83] Schlemper RJ, Riddell RH, Kato Y, Borchard F, Cooper HS, Dawsey SM, et al. The Vienna classifi cation of gastrointestinal epithelial neoplasia. *Gut* 2000;47:251–5.

[84] Seol Sang-Yong Current techniques and devices for safe and convenient endoscopic submucosal dissection (esd) and korean experience of esd. *Digestive Endoscopy* (2008) 20, 107–114

[85] Shiba M, Higuchi K, Kadouchi K, Montani A, Yamamori K, Okazaki H, et al. Risk factors for bleeding after endoscopic mucosal resection. *World J Gastroenterol* 2005;14:7335–9.

[86] Soetikno R, Gotoda T, Nakanishi Y, Soehendra N. Endoscopic mucosal resection. *Gastrointest Endosc* 2003;57:567–79.

[87] Soetikno R, Kaltenbach T, Yeh R, Gotoda T. Endoscopic mucosal resection for early cancers of the upper gastrointestinal tract. *J Clin Oncol* 2005;23:4490–8.

[88] Tada M, Shimada M, Murakami F, Mizumachi M, Arima K, Yanai H, et al. Development of strip-off biopsy (in Japanese with English abstract). *Gastroenterol Endosc* 1984;26:833–9.

[89] Tada M. *One piece resection and piecemeal resection of early gastric cancer by strip biopsy* (in Japanese with English abstract). Tokyo: Igaku-Shoin; 1998; p. 68–87.

[90] Takekoshi T, Baba Y, Ota H, Kato Y, Yanagisawa A, Takagi K, et al. Endoscopic resection of early gastric carcinoma: results of a retrospective analysis of 308 cases. *Endoscopy* 1994;26:352–8.

[91]   Takenaka R., Yoshiro Kawahara, Hiroyuki Okada, Keisuke Hori, Masafumi Inoue, Seiji Kawano, et al. Risk factors associated with local recurrence of early gastric cancers after endoscopic submucosal dissection. *Gastrointest Endosc* 2008;68:887-94

[92]   Takeuchi Y., Noriya Uedo, Hiroyasu Iishi, Sachiko Yamamoto, Shunsuke Yamamoto, Takuya Yamada, et al. Endoscopic submucosal dissection with insulated-tip knife for large mucosal early gastric cancer: a feasibility study (with videos) *Gastrointest Endosc* 2007;66: 186-193

[93]   Takizawa K., I. Oda, T. Gotoda, C. Yokoi, T. Matsuda, Y. Saito, D. Saito, H. Ono. Routine coagulation of visible vessels may prevent delayed bleeding after endoscopic submucosal dissection - An analysis of risk factors. *Endoscopy* 2008; 40: 179-183

[94]   Tanabe S, Koizumi W, Mitomi H, Nakai H, Murakami S, Nagaba S, et al. Clinical outcome of endoscopic aspiration mucosectomy for early stage gastric cancer. *Gastrointest Endosc* 2002;56: 708–13.

[95]   Tanaka K., Hideki Toyoda, Yasuhiko Hamada, Masatoshi Aoki, Ryo Kosaka, Noda T. et al. Endoscopic submucosal dissection for early gastric cancer using magnifying endoscopy with a combination of narrow band imaging and acetic acid instillation *Digestive Endoscopy* (2008) 20, 150–153

[96]   Tanaka M., Hiroyuki Ono, Noriaki Hasuike, Takizawa K. Endoscopic Submucosal Dissection of Early Gastric Cancer. *Digestion* 2008;77(suppl 1):23–28

[97]   Tsujitani S, Oka S, Saito H, Kondo A, Ikeguchi M, Maeta M, et al. Less invasive surgery for early gasric cancer based on the low probability of lymph node metastasis. *Surgery* 1999;125: 148–54.

[98]   Tsunada S, Ogata S, Ohyama T, Ootani H, Oda K, Kikkawa A, et al. Endoscopic closure of perforations caused by EMR in the stomach by application of metallic clips. *Gastrointest Endosc* 2003;57:948–51.

[99]   Yahagi N, Fujishiro M, Kakushima N, Kobayashi K, Hashimoto T, Oka M, et al. Endoscopic submucosal dissection for early gastric cancer using the tip of an electrosurgical snare (thin type). *Dig Endosc* 2004;16:34–8.

[100]   Yamamoto H, Kawata H, Sunada K, Sasaki A, Nakazawa K, Miyata T, et al. Successful en bloc resection of large superficial tumors in the stomach and colon using sodium hyaluronate and small-caliber-tip transparent hood. *Endoscopy* 2003;35:690–4.

[101]   Yamamoto H, Kawata H, Sunada K, Satoh K, Kaneko Y, Ido K, et al. Success rate of curative endoscopic mucosal resection with circumferential mucosal incision assisted by submucosal injection of sodium hyaluronate. *Gastrointest Endosc* 2002;56:507–13.

[102]   Yamao T, Shirao K, Ono H, Kondo H, Saito D, Yamaguchi H, et al. Risk factors for lymph node metastasis from intramucosal gastric carcinoma. *Cancer* 1996;77:602–6.

[103]   Yamazaki H, Oshima A, Murakami R, Endoh S, Urukata T. A long term follow-up study of patients with gastric cancer detected by mass screening. *Cancer* 1989;63:613–7.

[104]   Yanai H, Matsubara Y, Kawano T, Okamoto T, Hirano A, Nakamura Y, et al. Clinical impact of strip biopsy for early gastric cancer. *Gastrointest Endosc* 2004;60:771–7.

[105]   Yanai H, Noguchi T, Mizumachi S, Tokiyama H, Nakamura H, Tada M, et al. A blind comparison of the effectiveness of endoscopic ultrasonography and endoscopy in staging early gastric cancer. *Gut* 1999;44:361–5.

[106] Yano H, Kimura Y, Iwazawa T, Monden T. Laparoscopic management for local recurrence of early gastric cancer after endoscopic mucosal resection. *Surg Endosc* 2005;19:981–5.

[107] Yasuda K, Shiraishi N, Suematsu T, Yamaguchi K, Adachi Y, Kitano S. Rate of detection of lymph node metastasis is correlated with the depth of submucosal invasion in early stage gastric carcinoma. Cancer 1999;85:2119–23.

[108] Yasuhiro Onozato Y., Satoru Kakizaki,2 Hiroshi Ishihara,1 Haruhisa Iizuka,1 Naondo Sohara,Shinichi Okamura et al. Feasibility of endoscopic submucosal dissection for elderly patients with early gastric cancers and adenomas. *Digestive Endoscopy* (2008) 20, 12–16.

In: Gastric Cancer: Diagnosis, Early Prevention, and Treatment   ISBN 978-1-61668-313-9
Editor: V. D. Pasechnikov, pp. 267-284   © 2010 Nova Science Publishers, Inc.

Chapter VIII

SURGICAL TREATMENT OF EARLY GASTRIC CANCER

Corrado Pedrazzani[1], Armands Sivins[2],
*Daniele Marrelli[1], Franco Roviello[1, *]*

[1]Department of Human Pathology and Oncology, Unit of Surgical Oncology,
University of Siena, Siena, Italy
[2]Riga Eastern University Hospital, Latvia Oncology Center and University of Latvia,
Riga, Latvia

ABSTRACT

Early gastric cancer (EGC) is defined as a tumour that spreads no further than the submucosa layer irrespective for the presence of lymph node metastasis. Management of EGC varies widely between Far East and West countries. Endoscopic resection is ordinarily adopted in Japan and Korea, whilst surgical treatment is still the most adopted option in Europe and United States. Surgical treatment of EGC is herein discussed. Indications regarding the extent of gastric resection as well as the degree of lymph node dissection are reported. Short- and long-term results are analyzed together with mode of recurrence. Quality of life after subtotal and total gastrectomy is described with regards to the type of reconstruction. Finally, new technologies and practices, i.e. laparoscopy, function preserving surgery and sentinel node biopsy, are critically examined.

*   Author responsible for correspondence: Prof. Franco Roviello, Dipartimento di Patologia Umana e Oncologia, Sezione di Chirurgia Oncologica, Policlinico 'Le Scotte', Viale Bracci 2, 53100 Siena, Italy; Telephone: ++39 (0)577 585156; Fax: ++39 (0)577 233337; E-mail: roviello@unisi.it

INTRODUCTION

Early gastric cancer (EGC) is defined as a tumour that spreads no further than the submucosa layer irrespective for the presence of lymph node metastasis. Such extent corresponds to the T1 category according to the TNM classification of the Union International Contre le Cancer (UICC) and American Joint Committee on Cancer (AJCC). As a result, it is typically characterized by a favourable prognosis with a 5-year survival rate exceeding 90-95%. [1-4]

EGC in West and Far East Countries

EGC management underwent with time to a gradual revolution due to the better diagnostic and therapeutic techniques. Although the clinicopathological features of the disease are similar between Far East and West countries, its management varies widely. Surgery is ordinarily adopted by European and North American surgeons, [4-6] whereas less invasive techniques, such as endoscopic mucosal resection (EMR) and endoscopic submucosal dissection (ESD) are frequently employed by Japanese colleagues. [1]

Endoscopic resection (EMR/ESD) is comparable in many respects to conventional surgery, with the advantage of being less invasive and more cost-effective. The extremely low incidence of lymph node involvement in specific subsets of EGC allows to achieve a precise staging and cure by such local treatment. Patients who are identified to have virtually no risks of lymph node metastasis are good candidates for endoscopic resection. [7] Current indications include the resection of small intramucosal EGCs of Lauren intestinal histotype. Rationale for this recommendation is based upon the knowledge that larger-size lesions or lesions with diffuse histology histotype are more likely to extend into the submucosal layer and have lymph node metastasis. In addition, resection of larger lesions has demonstrated to be technically demanding in "non-Japanese" hands. Thus, the accepted indications for EMR/ESD are: (1) elevated cancers equal or less than 2 cm in diameter and (2) small (≤1 cm) depressed lesions without ulceration. These lesions must be well-differentiated cancers confined to the mucosa with no lymphatic or vascular involvement. Some extended criteria have been recently proposed in Japan where ESD is currently under evaluation for tumours equal or less than 3 cm confined to the mucosa or with a minute infiltration of the submucosa (SM1, <500μm from the muscolaris mucosa). [1,7] Noteworthy, endoscopic resections are frequently used as diagnostic and staging tools which allow stratification and refinement of further surgical treatment.

Taking into account these data one should consider that the proportion of EGC in Japan encompasses 50% of all gastric cancer cases and that almost 10,000 cases are diagnosed each year. Differently, in Europe and United States, the number of EGCs is much lower and the learning curve of EMR and ESD is at the beginning and is stepping forward slowly.

The overall accuracy of endoscopy (EGD), multi-detector computed tomography (MDCT) and endoscopic ultrasound (EUS) in diagnosing EGC were reported to be 84–97%, 78–94% and 76–96%. In a recent series by Ahn and colleagues, the predictive values for EGC of EGD, MDCT, and EUS were 87%, 92%, and 94%, respectively. Once again, these studies were from specialized centres mainly from Japan and the last referenced analyzed more than 400 Korean patients operated within one-year period. [8]

In EGC nodal involvement is an infrequent event. In a series on 652 EGC patients by the Italian Research Group for the Study of Gastric Cancer, the percentage of node positive cases was 14%. It was 5% for mucosal and 24% for submucosal tumours. [4] These data match with those reported by other Western centres. [3,9]

In our opinion the management of EGC is very much influenced by the possibility of having the lesion resected by endoscopic treatment. The endoscopic 'en bloc' resection (EMR/ESD) allows the removal of the tumour and an appropriate staging of the lesion. When EMR/ESD is not available, the chance of understaging the depth of tumour invasion and lymph node involvement should be always taken into account. Similarly, 'piece meal' resection as well as other endoscopic techniques, which do not provide a complete pathological specimen, may remove the lesion without providing a complete prognostic estimation and the need for additional therapy.

In conclusion, unless carried out within randomized controlled trials, standard surgical resection still represents the mainstay of therapy for other than intestinal or elevated EGCs and for lesions greater than 2 cm. In centres where lack of endoscopic skills compromise a proper diagnosis and staging, standard surgical resection is strongly recommended.

EXTENT OF GASTRIC RESECTION

Distal Subtotal Gastrectomy

The preferred surgical treatment for tumour of the lower and lower/middle third of the stomach is the distal subtotal gastrectomy (DSG), consisting in the resection of four-fifth of the stomach (Figure 1a).

Two randomized controlled trials showed no difference in long-term results or quality of life after DSG compared to total gastrectomy. [10,11]

Japanese guidelines for the treatment of gastric cancer suggest to perform a modified distal subtotal gastrectomy (MDSG) in mucosal tumour equal or less than 2 cm other than well-differentiated or in submucosal tumour equal or less than 1.5 cm. MDSG consists in the resection of less than two-thirds of the distal stomach (Figure 1b).

This management is based on EMR/ESD results and it is not always feasible in European and United States centres where preoperative diagnostic assessment is less accurate. Cases where clinical downstaging is possible should be treated according to guidelines for T2 and T3 tumours. For tumours with expanding growth a resection margin of at least 3 cm is considered to be safe, whilst a 5 cm margin should be preferred for infiltrative tumours. [7]

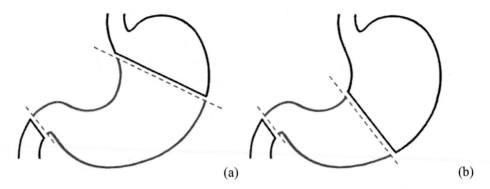

Figure 1. Resection line in distal subtotal gastrectomy (a) and in modified distal subtotal gastrectomy (b) according to the Japanese guidelines for the treatment of gastric cancer.

Total Gastrectomy

Total gastrectomy (TG) represents the standard treatment for upper third tumours and tumours of the middle third in which a safe resection margin is not achievable with DSG. Otherwise, TG is never justified either in consideration of Lauren histotype or the possibility of a second metachronous malignancy of the gastric remnant. An exceptional indication for TG could be the presence of an EGC in a CDH1 (E-cadherin) germline mutation carrier that configures the hereditary cancer syndrome of the Hereditary Diffuse Gastric Cancer (HDGC). In this case, a complete resection of the gastric mucosa at proximal and distal margin is mandatory. [12]

Proximal Gastrectomy

Function-preserving surgery has been performed more frequently with the aim of improving the postoperative quality of life. Proximal gastrectomy (PG) has been proposed by several authors to improve the quality of life by preserving half of the stomach in patients with upper third EGC. No randomized controlled trials have been published to date comparing proximal and total gastrectomy. Up to date conflicting data are presented in observational series about similarities between PG and TG with regards to long-term results and quality of life. In our opinion PG should be carried out in controlled trials in view of the risk of missing an advanced form (T2 o T3), and in absence of evidences that this procedure is able to offer a better quality of life. Furthermore, the small number of procedures carried out in non-specialized centres could lead to an increased morbidity and mortality.

EXTENT OF LYMPH NODE DISSECTION

Basis for Extended Lymphadenectomy, D1-α and D1-β

The extent of lymphadenectomy is a matter of debate in advanced as well as in EGC surgery. Certainly D2 lymphadenectomy leads to a higher number of examined nodes and hence to a better staging. AJCC and UICC recommend a minimum of 15 nodes for adequate staging. Even though D2 lymphadenectomy has been demonstrated to lead to better long-term results in several prospective non-randomized trials, no significant survival gain was observed in randomized trials published to date. [13,14] One of the speculations added to explain the lack of benefit from D2 lymphadenectomy in the MRC [13] and Dutch [14] series was the high number of T1 tumors with a small percentage of N positive cases. In EGC is certainly very difficult to demonstrate a significant survival benefit after extended (D2) lymphadenectomy. Also in a recent series by Roviello and colleagues, no statistical difference in disease free survival was observed in relation to the extent of lymphadenectomy. Nonetheless, the risk of recurrence diminished with the increased number of dissected nodes, particularly when more than 15 nodes were retrieved. This result was similar, in an apparently paradoxical way, when only node negative patients were considered. These data seem to confirm the studies by Baba et al. [15] and Siewert et al. [16] who claimed that D2 lymphadenectomy improves prognosis in patients without lymph node metastases probably because cancer cells are present in regional nodes even in cases classified as N0. [16]

One could argue that the routinarely use of D2 lymphadenectomy in EGC leads to an overtreatment in the majority of cases. Conversely, limited lymphadenectomy could be the cause of residual tumour since one out of 4 T1sm patients have lymph node metastasis and 2-10% have lymph node metastasis in second tier nodes. Certainly, an improper lymph node clearing may affect the prognosis of patients with a very high chance of cure.

In order to limit surgical over-treatment, Japanese guidelines tailors the extent of lymphadenectomy on EMR/ESD results. A D1 lymphadenectomy plus left gastric artery nodes (station no. 7) is proposed in mucosal tumours equal or less than 2 cm other than well-differentiated and in well-differentiated submucosal tumour equal or less than 1.5 cm (D1-α lymphadenectomy) (Figure 2a). A D1 lymphadenectomy plus left gastric artery, anterior hepatic artery (station no. 8a) and celiac trunk (stations no. 9) nodes is preferred for submucosal tumours equal or less than 1.5 cm other than well-differentiated (D1-β lymphadenectomy) (Figure 2b). [7] Once again, in absence of a definite preoperative diagnosis of EGC a D2 or at least a D1-β lymphadenectomy is advisable. In any case a proper division of gastric vessels at their origin from main trunks must be performed (Figure 3).

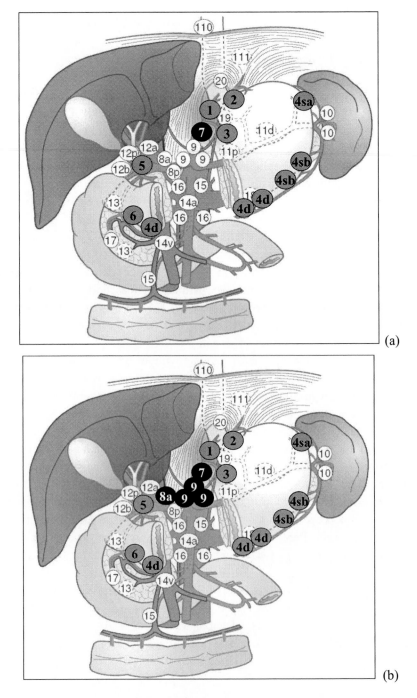

Figure 2. Schematic representation of D1-α (a) and D1-β lymphadenectomy (b) according to the Japanese guidelines for the treatment of gastric cancer.

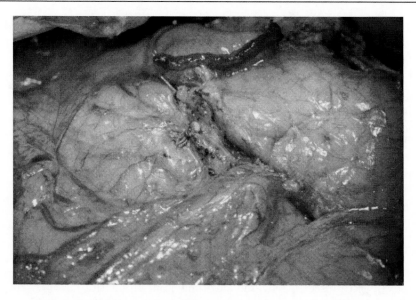

Figure 3. Intraoperative view of the division of right gastroepiploic vessels at their origin with complete dissection of infrapyloric lymph nodes (Station 6).

Short- and Long-term Results after Surgery for EGC

Morbidity and Mortality

In gastric cancer surgery morbidity and mortality vary widely depending on expertise and case volume of the surgeon and centre. Postoperative mortality after extended lymphadenectomy (D2) is reported to be 0.8% or even absent in randomized trials from East Asia, and less than 2% in the Japanese nationwide registry. In Western observational studies, it found to increase to 2–5%, with a peaked of up to 5–13% in European clinical trials. Similarly postoperative morbidity after extended lymphadenectomy is low (17–21%) in East Asian trials, intermediate (21–35%) in European observational studies, and the high in European and United States phase III trials (43– 46%).

The Italian Research Group for the Study of Gastric Cancer reported a postoperative mortality rate of 2%. [4] Similarly, the series from Latvia Oncology Center presented a 3% mortality after gastrectomy for early and advanced gastric cancer. [17]

Survival and Prognostic Factors

Five-year survival rate after surgical resection for EGC varies between 82% and 100%. [1-4] Table 1 reports main clinicopathological characteristics and long-term results after surgical treatment in some Japanese and Western series.

Table 1. Lymph node groups (Level 1 - 3) by location of tumour according to the JGCA classification. D2 lymphadenectomy requires the dissection of lymph nodes of Level 1 and 2 which vary depending on tumour location

Country (year)	No. of cases	% of EGC	Mean age	Postop mortality	% of T1sm	% of N+	Survival	
							5-year	10-year
Japan (2000) [18]	5265	-	-	-	43	9	97	-
Japan (2001) [19]	1051	50	62	0.4	41	9	>90	-
Korea (2003) [20]	1452	33	53	-	50	13	90	>85
U.S.A. (1999) [21]	165	11	67	-	60	31	88	-
Austria (1999) [22]	130	16	66	2.0	46	12	75	62
France (2000) [3]	332	13	64	4.2	52	10	82	-
Portugal (2002) [23]	91	15	60	5.7	50	6.5	85	80
Italy (2006) [4]	665	16	65	1.9	49	14	94	89

In curatively (R0) resected EGC the most important prognostic factor is represented by nodal involvement. Both the number (AJCC/UICC classification) and the site (JGCA classification) of lymph node metastasis demonstrated to accurately predict the prognosis. [3,4,24,25]

Table 2. Main clinicopathological characteristics and long-term results in some large Japanese, Korean and Western surgical series

Lymph node station	Location	Lower third	Middle third	Upper third
1	Rt paracardial	2	1	1
2	Lt paracardial	M	3	1
3	Lesser curvature	1	1	1
4sa	Short gastric	M	3	1
4sb	Lt gastroepiploic	3	1	1
4d	Rt gastroepiploic	1	1	2
5	Suprapyloric	1	1	3
6	Infrapyloric	1	1	3
7	Lt gastric artery	2	2	2
8a	Anterior comm. Hepatic	2	2	2
8p	Posterior comm. hepatic	3	3	3
9	Celiac artery	2	2	2
10	Plenic hilum	M	3	2
11p	Proximal plenic	2	2	2
11d	Distal splenic	M	3	2
12a	Lt hepatoduodenal	2	2	3
12p	Posterior hepatoduodenal	3	3	3
13	Retropancreatic	3	3	M
14v	Superior mesenteric vein	2	3	M
14a	Superior mesenteric artery	M	M	M
15	Middle colic	M	M	M
16a2,b1	Paraaortic	3	3	3

M: Lymph nodes regarded as distant metastasis.

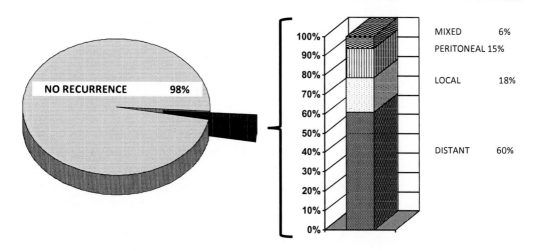

Figure 4. Percentage and mode of recurrence after surgical treatment of EGC. Literature review on 11954 cases and 244 recurrences (2%).

Node negative patients showed 5 and 10-year disease specific survival rates approaching 100%. Conversely, patients with more than 6 positive nodes showed a poor prognosis and an increased risk of cancer recurrence. Lee and colleagues reported 28% recurrence rate for patients with more than 6 positive nodes. In our series, 5-year survival rate was beyond 90% in patients with 1 to 6 positive nodes and it was less than 30% in patients with more than 6 metastatic nodes. [4,25]

Several studies investigated clinico-pathological factors associated with lymph node involvement. Interestingly, the great majority of series were from Far East countries (Japan, Korea, China and Taiwan) while only a few came from Western hemisphere. Amongst the factors analysed, lymphatic invasion (Ly), depth of tumour invasion (mucosa or submucosa), tumour diameter, Lauren histotype and differentiation, Kodama histotype and age were significantly associated to nodal metastasis.

Noteworthy, two large series from Korea recently reported no possibility of lymph node involvement in undifferentiated EGC less than 2-2.5 cm in diameter. [26,27]

Time and Mode of Recurrence

Although prognosis and recurrence rate of EGC are quite rare after surgical resection, cancer relapse may occur in certain cases (1.5%-12%) (Figure 4). Recurrence of advanced gastric cancer has been widely investigated and described, conversely mode and timing of EGC recurrence is less known due to the low number of adverse events.

Lee and colleagues described a group of 1452 EGC patients treated with D2 curative gastrectomy and a median follow-up period of 58 months. Four types of recurrence were described: locoregional (locoregional lymph nodes), distant (liver, lung, brain and distant lymph nodes) peritoneal and mixed. Twenty-one patients relapsed. Among these, submucosal invasion was present in 16 cases, lymph node involvement in 14. The majority of patients recurred within 24 months (13 cases), 6 between 24 and 60 months and 2 beyond 5 years. Locoregional recurrence was evident in 4 cases, distant recurrence occurred in 9 cases and peritoneal in 2. Six patients died of mixed recurrence, in 5 of them a systemic recurrence was diagnosed. [20]

TYPE OF RECONSTRUCTION AND QUALITY OF LIFE

Since the first total gastrectomy was performed by Schlatter in 1897, the significant adverse events related to the operation have been identified. The demanding postoperative phase and the nutritional and metabolic changes related to the removal of the stomach frequently lead to a difficult recovery. Postprandial symptoms are common after total gastrectomy, and this operation often leads to weight loss, malabsorption, and impaired dietary intake. Conversely, preserving the gastric remnant undoubtedly allows a better quality of life. Subtotal gastrectomy is now considered the treatment of choice for lower and middle-lower third gastric cancer and the routine use of total gastrectomy has been definitively abandoned by the majority of authors (Figure 5).

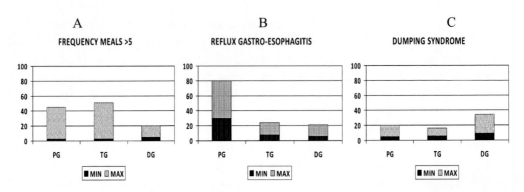

Figure 5. Main symptoms observed after distal subtotal gastrectomy, total gastrectomy and proximal gastrectomy. Minimum and maximum percentages reported by current literature are illustrated.

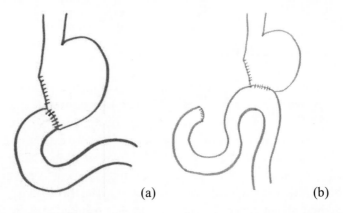

Figure 6. Main reconstruction methods after subtotal gastrectomy. Billroth I (a), Billroth II (b) and Roux-en-Y (c) reconstruction are depicted.

Reconstruction after Subtotal Gastrectomy

Reconstruction methods available after subtotal gastrectomy are Billroth I, Billroth II and Roux-en-Y (Figure 6).

Key issues in the evaluation of post-gastrectomy digestive function are eating capacity, reservoir performance of the gastric remnant, presence of reflux symptoms, and occurrence of dumping syndrome.

With respect to reservoir performance of the gastric remnant and eating capacity, symptoms control is essential to minimize impairment in everyday life after gastrectomy. Loss of body weight (74%–94%), loss of appetite (32%– 40%), and increase in the number of daily meals (63%–67%) are common complaints after gastrectomy. As highlighted by Svedlund and colleagues [28], weight loss continued during the first trimester after surgery, after which it remained stable. Nevertheless, just after one year, loss of appetite is marginal, the great majority of patients consume an almost regular diet, and they eat less than five meals per day. [29]

Regarding reflux symptoms, gastro-duodenal reflux has been recognized as a major cause of symptoms after gastrectomy. Reflux of bile acids and pancreatic juice may damage gastric and esophageal mucosa and may play a key role in the pathogenesis of gastritis, gastric ulcer, reflux esophagitis as well as esophageal and gastric cancer. For this reason Roux-en-Y reconstruction is preferred by some authors. Two recently published studies from Japan seem to demonstrate Roux-en-Y to be superior compared to Billroth I in preventing bile reflux and post-operative symptoms. We recently analyzed functional results in 195 patients who underwent subtotal gastrectomy with Billroth II reconstruction. Reflux symptoms were reported by about 15% of our patients. This figure is comparable to literature results and, as previously noted, reflux symptoms were fairly stable and mostly well tolerated.

The most characteristic and often disabling postprandial syndrome after gastric surgery is dumping syndrome. Gastric emptying is controlled by fundic tone, antro-pyloric mechanisms and duodenal feedback. Gastric surgery alters these mechanisms in several ways. Gastric resection reduces the fundic reservoir, thereby reducing the stomach's receptiveness to a meal. Similarly, vagotomy increases gastric tone, limiting accommodation. In addition, duodenal feedback inhibition of gastric emptying is lost after gastro-jejunostomy. Accelerated gastric emptying of liquids is a typical feature and a critical step in the pathogenesis of dumping syndrome. Also, hormonal secretions that sustain the gastric phase of digestion are adversely affected. All these factors contribute to the pathogensis of dumping syndrome.

Billroth I reconstruction by keeping the duodenal passage has the theoretical advantage of maintaining the autocrine and paracrine signalling and feedback mechanism. But, lack of clinical evidence exists and, at the moment no procedure is clearly superior to the others. The reported incidence of this disorder varies widely, between 15% and 50%.

Reconstruction after Total Gastrectomy

Impairment of eating capability, reservoir performance and dumping syndrome are observed more frequently after total gastrectomy. Besides, contrary to the general opinion that bile reflux may not cover the whole length of the Roux-en-Y loop, bile acids have been recently demonstrated to reach the distal esophagus after total gastrectomy.

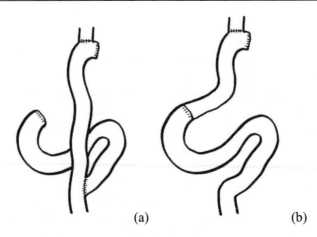

(a)   (b)

Figure 7. Main reconstruction methods after total gastrectomy. Roux-en-Y (a) and Jejunal interposition (b) are depicted.

Several techniques have been described as reconstruction after total gastrectomy with Roux-en-Y and jejunal interposition being the most popular (Figure 7).

Theoretically, the interposition of the jejunum between the esophagus and the duodenum provides advantages to both duodenal passage and endoscopic accessibility of the pancreato-biliary system. Despite that, no definite clinical benefit has been demonstrated and the use of jejunal interposition has not gained popularity among Western surgeons.

More controversies exist on the use of jejunal pouch in Roux-en-Y reconstruction. Some randomized controlled trials showed a better quality of life after jejunal pouch reconstruction. These studies were impaired by the low number of cases which were frequently gastric cancer patients. Therefore, a significant number of patients were lost to follow-up and the results could be biased given that it is well demonstrated that recurrence is the main factor influencing the quality of life. To exclude the influence of cancer recurrence, Kono and colleagues randomized 50 patients receiving total gastrectomy for EGC. In this study, jejunal pouch reconstruction provided better quality of life and less esophageal bile reflux. [30] Recently, Fein and colleagues randomized 138 patients for Roux-en-Y recon struction with or without pouch. An evidence of improvement for the Roux-en-Y with pouch group was evident for disease-free patients especially 2 years after operation. [31] Authors concluded that a pouch is recommended for patients with a good prognosis.

Instead of these data proving a possible benefit in the use of jejunal pouch, simple Roux-en-Y reconstruction is still adopted by the majority of surgeons.

Reconstruction after Proximal Gastrectomy

Proximal gastrectomy has been described as a possibility in EGC of the upper third. Great controversies exist on the appropriateness of this limited procedure and on functional results.

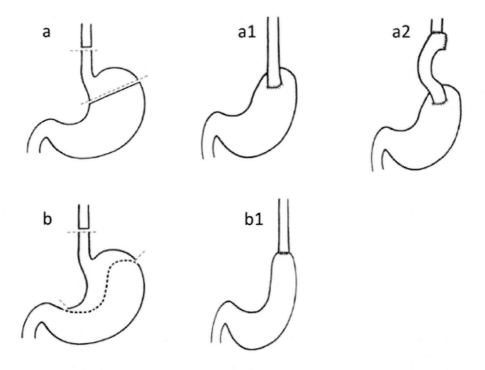

Figure 8. Resection line and main reconstruction methods after proximal gastrectomy (a) with esophago-gastrostomy (a^1) and jejunal interposition (a^2) and after proximal gastrectomy (b) with gastric tube formation (b^1).

Reconstructive options after proximal gastrectomy are esophago-gastrostomy, gastric tube formation or jejunal interposition (Figure 8). The optimal method of reconstruction following proximal gastrectomy is still debated due to the small number of cases and the possibility of severe reflux esophagitis with jejunal interposition that seems to have better results in controlling esophageal reflux. Currently, total gastrectomy remains the standard treatment and the preferred procedure by the majority of surgeons.

MINIMALLY INVASIVE APPROACH TO EGC

Basis for Laparoscopic Gastrectomy

Kitano and colleagues [32] performed the first laparoscopic-assisted gastrectomy for EGC in 1991 and it was first reported in 1994. Advances in surgical technology have made laparoscopic surgery increasingly feasible, and it is rapidly gaining in popularity, although some concerns have been expressed about safety and efficacy.

A recent systematic review by Gemmill and McCulloch [33] analyzed 2546 gastric cancer patients from 23 studies in which laparoscopic surgery was adopted as treatment modality. Two thousand four hundred twenty-seven (2427) patients from 17 studies were from the East (Japan, Korea, China and Taiwan) and 119 patients from 6 studies were from the West. In this setting, minimally invasive gastrectomy demonstrated to be feasible with comparable morbidity and mortality.

The Japanese Laparoscopic Surgery Study Group [34] recently reported the retrospective results on 1294 patients who underwent laparoscopic-assisted gastrectomy (LAG) for EGC in 16 centres. Distal gastrectomy was performed in 1185 patients (91.5%), proximal gastrectomy in 54, and total gastrectomy in 55.

LAG required the dissection of the lesser and greater omentum, ligation and division of the main vessels to mobilize the stomach under pneumoperitoneum, D1-α, D1-β, or D2 lymph node dissection, based on the Guidelines of the JGCA, and resection of the distal two thirds (LADG), proximal third (LAPG), or total stomach (LATG), depending on the location of the tumour. Reconstruction was accomplished by the Billroth-I, esophagogastrostomy, or Roux-en-Y method through a 5- to 7-cm-long minilaparotomy incision. Post-operative complications occurred in 15% of the cases while no post-operative death was reported.

There were 6 cancer recurrences, 1 local recurrence, 1 lymph node recurrence, 2 peritoneal disseminations, 1 liver metastasis, and 1 skin metastasis at the abdominal wall different from the port-site, during the median follow-up period of 36 months (range, 13–113 months). The 5-year disease-free survival rate was 99.8% for node negative patients, 98.7% for N1, and 85.7% for N2.

The authors concluded that LAG is safe for EGC, with an oncologic outcome as good as that of conventional open surgery.

Kim and colleagues [35] reported the results of a prospective randomized trial on 164 patients who underwent LADG or open DG for EGC. The trial was designed to evaluate the quality of life during the early postoperative phase up to 90 days, and the surgical outcome including morbidity and mortality. Statistically significant differences were observed with a more favourable outcome noted in the LADG group with respect to intraoperative blood loss, total amount of analgesics used, postoperative hospital stay, and QOL parameters of global health. Most of the scales on patient functioning including physical, role, emotional, social, and symptom scales such as fatigue, pain, appetite loss, sleep disturbance, dysphasia, gastro-esophageal reflux, dietary restriction, anxiety, and body image were also significantly better in the LADG group compared with the open DG group.

Lapaoscopic surgery is certainly an interesting and enthralling option in the treatment of EGC, anyway some key points should be considered before adopting it in the clinical setting: i) its safety and accuracy must be demonstrated at individual medical institutions; ii) a small number of total gastrectomy have been performed till now; iii) the extent of gastric as well as lymph node dissection must be respected independently from the technique adopted; iv) LAG must be considered an investigational technique and all cases must be included in clinical trials or audited.

Function Preserving Surgery

While some evidences exist about the short-term improvement of QOL after laparoscopic versus open gastrectomy, no definite data have been reported about long-term QOL that seems to be clearly related to organ and function preservation.

Organ preservation have been attempted through laparoscopic and open procedures as intragastric mucosal resection, wedge resection, segmental gastrectomy, pylorus-preserving distal gastrectomy, and proximal gastrectomy. Indications and results of pylorus-preserving distal gastrectomy and proximal gastrectomy have been previously described.

Laparoscopic wedge resection using a lesion lifting method enables complete local resection with full thickness of the stomach wall and organ preservation by a laparoscopic approach. Intragastric mucosal resection also enables a wide range of mucosal resections of lesions located in any part of the stomach except the anterior wall. Although there has been no randomized prospective study to confirm the clinical advantages of these laparoscopic procedures, a survey of the Japan Society for Endoscopic Surgery (JSES) showed limited morbidity and no mortality. Faster recovery and early discharge from hospital were demonstrated by the survey. Laparoscopic wedge resection and intragastric mucosal resection have become well accepted as minimally invasive procedures for mucosal gastric cancer since they began to be performed in the early 1990s. Segmental gastrectomy is an option in cases not suitable for laparoscopic wedge resection and intragastric mucosal resection (mucosal tumour of the lesser curve/anterior wall). Indications to intragastric mucosal resection, wedge resection and segmental gastrectomy resemble those to endoscopic resection.

Sentinel Lymph Node

The first possible site of metastasis along the route of lymphatic drainage from the primary lesion is known as sentinel node (SN). Since the concept of SN was demonstrated in a clinical study involving patients with malignant melanoma, the clinical impact of the SN concept has become a major topic with regard to various solid tumors. Until the late 1990s, the application of the SN concept to gastrointestinal (GI) malignancies met resistance because of the multidirectional and complicated lymphatic flow from the GI tract and the relatively high incidence of anatomical skip metastases. In gastric cancer, this evidence together with some technological and technical difficulties have limited the clinical application of sentinel node navigation till now.

Generally, radio-colloid and the blue-dye-methods are used for detection of SN in gastric cancer as in other gastro-intestinal tumours. The radio-colloid method is a reliable and stable technique for detecting multiple SNs using a gamma probe. Anyway, there are several practical limitations such as the requirement of radiation safety regulations and specific equipment not always available in community hospital. Current available rigid-type laparoscopic gamma probes are fixed by the trocar, thus freedom to search for SN and to avoid the "shine through" effect from the injection site is seriously restricted. Laparoscopic radio-colloid guided SN detection is feasible only in tumours of the lower and middle part of the greater curvature.

The blue-dye-method is also used in gastric cancer but it requires the real-time observation of the lymphatic route that is not possible without prior mobilization of the stomach. Several technical factors may affect the results of blue-dye-method and a learning phase is required. As a results, the combination of both methods is proposed by the majority of authors. Besides other technical limitations, an adjunctive EGD is required for injection of radio-colloid as well as dye tracers.

Retrieval of blue and/or hot lymph nodes is feasible as for usual lymph node dissection. The detection rate reported by a large Japanese series on 348 patients was 96% and the sensitivity to detect metastases 93%. The authors themselves stated that a discrepancy still remains between the validity of the SN concept itself for gastric cancer and clinical feasibility and safety of less invasive surgery based on SN biopsy. Before actual validation of the SN concept by large prospective clinical trials it seems early to apply less invasive approaches without conventional lymph node dissection for cases with a potential risk of lymph node involvement.

SN has to be considered an investigational technique and must be performed exclusively in controlled clinical trials. The next step will be the feasibility of laparoscopic SN biopsy that is actually limited by the above mentioned difficulties.

ACKNOWLEDGEMENTS

Authors thank Lorenzo Garosi who edited figures and tables and Dr. Eleonora Morelli who provided valuable help in collection and analysis of literature data.

REFERENCES

[1]   Gotoda T. Endoscopic resection of early gastric cancer. *Gastric Cancer*. 2007;10(1):1-11.

[2]   Morita S, Katai H, Saka M, Fukagawa T, Sano T, Sasako M. Outcome of pylorus-preserving gastrectomy for early gastric cancer. *Br J Surg*. 2008 Sep;95(9):1131-5.

[3]   Borie F, Millat B, Fingerhut A, Hay JM, Fagniez PL, De Saxce B. Lymphatic involvement in early gastric cancer: prevalence and prognosis in France. *Arch Surg*. 2000 Oct;135(10):1218-23.

[4]   Roviello F, Rossi S, Marrelli D, Pedrazzani C, Corso G, Vindigni C, Morgagni P, Saragoni L, de Manzoni G, Tomezzoli A. Number of lymph node metastases and its prognostic significance in early gastric cancer: a multicenter Italian study. *J Surg Oncol*. 2006 Sep 15;94(4):275-80.

[5]   Macdonald JS, Smalley SR, Benedetti J, Hundahl SA, Estes NC, Stemmermann GN, Haller DG, Ajani JA, Gunderson LL, Jessup JM, Martenson JA. Chemoradiotherapy after surgery compared with surgery alone for adenocarcinoma of the stomach or gastroesophageal junction. *N Engl J Med*. 2001 Sep 6;345(10):725-30.

[6]   Cunningham D, Allum WH, Stenning SP, Thompson JN, Van de Velde CJ, Nicolson M, Scarffe JH, Lofts FJ, Falk SJ, Iveson TJ, Smith DB, Langley RE, Verma M, Weeden S, Chua YJ, MAGIC Trial Participants. Perioperative chemotherapy versus surgery alone for resectable gastroesophageal cancer. *N Engl J Med*. 2006 Jul 6;355(1):11-20.

[7]   Nakajima T. Gastric cancer treatment guidelines in Japan. *Gastric Cancer*. 2002;5(1):1-5.

[8]   Ahn HS, Lee HJ, Yoo MW, Kim SG, Im JP, Kim SH, Kim WH, Lee KU, Yang HK. Diagnostic accuracy of T and N stages with endoscopy, stomach protocol CT, and endoscopic ultrasonography in early gastric cancer. *J Surg Oncol*. 2009 Jan 1;99(1):20-7.

[9]   Everett SM, Axon AT. Early gastric cancer in Europe. *Gut*. 1997 Aug;41(2):142-50.

[10] Bozzetti F, Marubini E, Bonfanti G, Miceli R, Piano C, Gennari L. Subtotal versus total gastrectomy for gastric cancer: five-year survival rates in a multicenter randomized Italian trial. Italian Gastrointestinal Tumor Study Group. *Ann Surg.* 1999 Aug;230(2):170-8.

[11] Gouzi JL, Huguier M, Fagniez PL, Launois B, Flamant Y, Lacaine F, Paquet JC, Hay JM. Total versus subtotal gastrectomy for adenocarcinoma of the gastric antrum. A French prospective controlled study. *Ann Surg.* 1989 Feb;209(2):162-6.

[12] Pedrazzani C, Corso G, Marrelli D, Roviello F. E-cadherin and hereditary diffuse gastric cancer. *Surgery.* 2007 Nov;142(5):645-57.

[13] Cuschieri A, Weeden S, Fielding J, Bancewicz J, Craven J, Joypaul V, Sydes M, Fayeers P. Patient survival after D1 and D2 resections for gastric cancer: long-term results of the MRC randomized surgical trial. Surgical Co-operative Group. *Br J Cancer.* 1999 Mar;79(9-10):1522-30.

[14] Bonenkamp JJ, Hermans M, Sasako M, van de Velde CJH. Extended lymph-node dissection for gastric cancer. *N Engl J Med.* 1999 Mar 25;340(12):908-14.

[15] Baba H, Maehara Y, Takeuchi H, et al. Effect of lymph node dissection on the prognosis in patients with node negative early gastric cancer. *Surgery.* 1995 Apr;117(4):380-5.

[16] Siewert JR, Kestlmeier R, Busch R, et al. Benefits of D2 lymph node dissection for patients with gastric cancer and pN0 and pN1 lymph node metastases. *Br J Surg.* 1996 Aug;83(8):1144-7.

[17] Sivins A, Pedrazzani C, Roviello F, Ancans G, Timofejevs M, Pcholkins A, Krumins V, Boka V, Stengrevics A, Leja M. Surgical treatment of gastric cancer in Latvia: results of centralized experience. *Eur J Surg Oncol.* 2009 May;35(5):481-5. Epub 2008 Dec 30.

[18] Gotoda T, Yanagisawa A, Sasako M, Ono H, Nakanishi Y, Shimoda T, Kato Y. Incidence of lymph node metastasis from early gastric cancer: estimation with a large number of cases at two large centers.*Gastric Cancer.* 2000 Dec;3(4):219-225.

[19] Shimada S, Yagi Y, Shiomori K, Honmyo U, Hayashi N, Matsuo A, Marutsuka T, Ogawa M. Characterization of early gastric cancer and proposal of the optimal therapeutic strategy. *Surgery.* 2001 Jun;129(6):714-9.

[20] Lee HJ, Kim YH, Kim WH, Lee KU, Choe KJ, Kim JP, Yang HK. Clinicopathological analysis for recurrence of early gastric cancer. *Jpn J Clin Oncol.* 2003 May;33(5):209-14.

[21] Hochwald SN, Brennan MF, Klimstra DS, Kim S, Karpeh MS. Is lymphadenectomy necessary for early gastric cancer? *Ann Surg Oncol.* 1999 Oct-Nov;6(7):664-70.

[22] Pertl A, Jagoditsch M, Jatzko GR, Denk H, Stettner HM. Long-term results of early gastric cancer accomplished in a European institution by Japanese-type radical resection. *Gastric Cancer.* 1999 Aug;2(2):115-121.

[23] Nogueira C, Silva AS, Santos JN, Silva AG, Ferreira J, Matos E, Vilaça H.Early gastric cancer: ten years of experience. *World J Surg.* 2002 Mar;26(3):330-4.

[24] Huang B, Zheng X, Wang Z, Wang M, Dong Y, Zhao B, Xu H. Prognostic significance of the number of metastatic lymph nodes: is UICC/TNM node classification perfectly suitable for early gastric cancer? *Ann Surg Oncol.* 2009 Jan;16(1):61-7.

[25]   Folli S, Morgagni P, Roviello F, De Manzoni G, Marrelli D, Saragoni L, Di Leo A, Gaudio M, Nanni O, Carli A, Cordiano C, Dell'Amore D, Vio A; Italian Research Group for Gastric Cancer (IRGGC). Risk factors for lymph node metastases and their prognostic significance in early gastric cancer (EGC) for the Italian Research Group for Gastric Cancer (IRGGC). *Jpn J Clin Oncol.* 2001 Oct;31(10):495-9.

[26]   Ye BD, Kim SG, Lee JY, Kim JS, Yang HK, Kim WH, Jung HC, Lee KU, Song IS. Predictive factors for lymph node metastasis and endoscopic treatment strategies for undifferentiated early gastric cancer. J Gastroenterol Hepatol. 2008 Jan;23(1):46-50.

[27]   Li C, Kim S, Lai JF, Oh SJ, Hyung WJ, Choi WH, Choi SH, Zhu ZG, Noh SH.Risk factors for lymph node metastasis in undifferentiated early gastric cancer. *Ann Surg Oncol.* 2008 Mar;15(3):764-9.

[28]   Svedlund J, Sullivan M, Liedman B, Lundell L. Long term consequences of gastrectomy for patient's quality of life: the impact of reconstructive techniques. *Am J Gastroenterol.* 1999 Feb;94(2):438-45.

[29]   Pedrazzani C, Marrelli D, Rampone B, De Stefano A, Corso G, Fotia G, Pinto E, Roviello F. Postoperative complications and functional results after subtotal gastrectomy with Billroth II reconstruction for primary gastric cancer. *Dig Dis Sci.* 2007 Aug;52(8):1757-63.

[30]   Kono K, Iizuka H, Sekikawa T, Sugai H, Takahashi A, Fujii H, Matsumoto Y. Improved quality of life with jejunal pouch reconstruction after total gastrectomy. *Am J Surg.* 2003 Feb;185(2):150-4.

[31]   Fein M, Fuchs KH, Thalheimer A, Freys SM, Heimbucher J, Thiede A. Long-term benefits of Roux-en-Y pouch reconstruction after total gastrectomy: a randomized trial. *Ann Surg.* 2008 May;247(5):759-65.

[32]   Kitano S, Iso Y, Moriyama M, Sugimachi K. Laparoscopy-assisted Billroth I gastrectomy. *Surg Laparosc Endosc.* 1994 Apr;4(2):146-8.

[33]   Gemmill EH, McCulloch P. Systematic review of minimally invasive resection for gastro-oesophageal cancer. *Br J Surg.* 2007 Dec;94(12):1461-7.

[34]   Kitano S, Shiraishi N, Uyama I, Sugihara K, Tanigawa N; Japanese Laparoscopic Surgery Study Group. A multicenter study on oncologic outcome of laparoscopic gastrectomy for early cancer in Japan. *Ann Surg.* 2007 Jan;245(1):68-72.

[35]   Kim YW, Baik YH, Yun YH, Nam BH, Kim DH, Choi IJ, Bae JM.Improved quality of life outcomes after laparoscopy-assisted distal gastrectomy for early gastric cancer: results of a prospective randomized clinical trial. *Ann Surg.* 2008 Nov;248(5):721-7.

INDEX

A

acetic acid, 250, 265

achlorhydria, 157

acidity, 63

activity level, 48

adenocarcinoma, 2, 3, 14, 15, 16, 22, 23, 25, 29, 33, 34, 38, 42, 58, 61, 64, 69, 70, 73, 88, 90, 91, 95, 98, 104, 105, 106, 107, 108, 111, 116, 126, 129, 130, 131, 133, 135, 138, 139, 140, 142, 144, 146, 147, 148, 163, 168, 174, 178, 213, 215, 217, 220, 227, 236, 238, 239, 282, 283

adenoma, 17, 44, 73, 85, 96, 107, 132, 145, 146, 176, 178, 189, 211, 217, 221, 222, 231

adhesion, 44, 46, 60, 69, 71, 75, 78, 86, 98, 109, 133, 134

adiposity, 48

adjustment, 48, 49, 51

adolescents, 84

adult stem cells, 80

adulthood, 40

adverse event, 275, 276

aetiology, 47

Africa, 3, 4, 8, 9, 67

African Americans, 16

aggregation, 44

aggressiveness, 75

aging population, 1

AIDS, 90

Albania, 7

alcohol abuse, 187

alcohol consumption, 37, 89, 187, 196

alcohol use, 22

allele, 45, 60, 61

alpha-tocopherol, 40, 54

aluminium, 29

amines, 49, 55, 186

anatomy, 152, 221

anemia, 152

aneuploidy, 65, 66

angiogenesis, 56, 75, 76, 109, 110, 112, 184, 193, 217

angulation, 241

annual rate, 14

antibiotic, 164, 176, 182

antibiotic resistance, 182

antibody, 78, 79, 111, 154, 169, 171, 173, 181

anti-cancer, 186

anticoagulant, 156

antigen, 60, 67, 98, 153, 155, 156, 165, 166, 175, 181, 182

anti-inflammatory drugs, 77, 132

antioxidant, x, 25, 26, 39, 40, 52, 53, 58, 62, 69, 91, 143, 185, 194, 195

antrum, 12, 57, 122, 125, 144, 153, 156, 157, 159, 160, 161, 162, 165, 166, 180, 203, 204, 212, 219, 221, 222, 226, 227, 231, 244, 250, 283

anxiety, 280

APC, 46, 65, 66, 72, 73, 103, 104, 105, 117, 133, 146

apoptosis, 56, 61, 62, 66, 69, 77, 78, 95, 98, 107, 112, 116, 172, 186, 191

ARC, 87

arginine, 110

argon, 250, 258

arrest, 56, 59, 78, 186

artery, 271, 274

asbestos, 29, 30, 41, 42, 87

ascorbic acid, 26, 27, 39, 53, 91, 99, 194, 195

Asia, 3, 4, 7, 9, 20, 25, 32, 36, 58, 174, 188

Asian countries, 9, 135

assessment, xi, 55, 121, 124, 125, 132, 135, 136, 137, 143, 155, 156, 157, 159, 169, 174, 177, 178, 180, 181, 184, 201, 211, 228, 230, 237, 269

asymptomatic, ix, 17, 32, 44, 63, 86, 142, 151, 155, 168, 179, 198, 228

atherosclerosis, 165

E

W

X